Health is the Foundation of Success

by

Grandmaster Y. K. Kim

Y. K. Kim Productions, Inc.   Orlando

Health is the Foundation of Success

ISBN 1-879873-01-X

Library of Congress Catalog Number: 95-78794

Notice

This book is NOT intended to give medical advice or prescribe treatment for any particular illness in a specific situation. The book contains common-sense health recommendations that have worked for the author, and MAY also work for other people. Each of us has a unique physiology and lives in a unique environment. Always consult a health care professional when applying general recommendations to a particular situation.

The author has attempted to provide the most accurate and up-to-date information available. However, research in the fields of health, fitness, and nutrition is constantly growing and improving. It is imperative that you consult a health care expert before you make any significant changes in your daily routine, to protect yourself from following outdated or inappropriate advice.

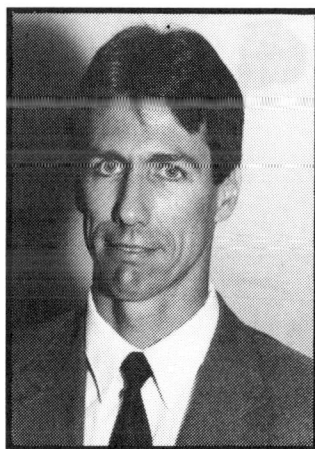

Special Acknowledgment to
Tim McCarthy

Co-Author
Master Tim McCarthy
President of the World Martial
Arts Research Foundation

This book is your beautiful new, strong, and healthy baby. It is the result of your dedication, sacrifice, special talents, and the gift of your great writing skills.

Without you, this book would still be on the shelf. I cannot find any words to adequately show my appreciation for what you have done to complete this book.

It is a great honor and pleasure to associate with you in the field of the martial arts. I am proud to say that you are my best student. You are my teacher. You are my brother. Some day the whole world will recognize your special dedication.

We are now at the middle point of the journey to reaching our dream: building a four year martial arts university, dedicated to providing outstanding leaders for the future of the world. Our strong, unbreakable bond will guide and comfort us on this journey to making a more peaceful world.

Sincerely,
Grandmaster Y. K. Kim

Acknowledgments

Health is the Foundation of Success has only been possible through the true love, respect, and warm support of my family:

First, my life-long mentor and supplier of spiritual energy, the most respected person in my life, my mother.

I am also indebted to my most caring and respectable mother- and father-in-law, Mr. and Mrs. Yun, for caring for my two children during the writing of the book, for encouraging me to complete it, and for reviewing and editing the actual writing.

The most important people in my life: my lover and my best friend, my wife Son Ja, and our hope and mirror, our lovely children Jackie and Min Chul, have encouraged me and supported me as I wrote every night and weekend.

I also would like to extend my special thanks to those who encouraged and supported me throughout the writing, and helped with the editing:

My adopted sister Nickie Sarner, host of the television show Inside Central Florida.

My student and Instructor, retired Colonel, former POW and decorated hero from W.W.II, Instructor Bert Powell.

My student and author of the book Natural Guide to Better Health, Petie Clapper.

My medical advisor and medical editor, Dr. Ronald Chernov.

Almost every picture that appears in this book was taken by Instructor Ted Allguire, who dedicated countless hours to insuring the professional quality of all the photography.

I also would like to thank my staff and students, who have been so understanding and supportive of the time it took to produce this book.

No one creates anything alone, least of all me. This book is the product of all the teachers in my life, all the friends I have known, and all the students I have taught. They each have helped me in their own way, and they have guided me to become the person that I am today. I hope I have put all that they have taught me to good use.

CONTENTS

A Letter from the Doctor

Finally, a book on health and the prevention of disease that *everyone* can understand and benefit from.

The concepts presented in Grandmaster Y. K. Kim's <u>Health is the Foundation of Success</u> are time tested, true, accurate, and essential for a good, healthy, and full life. He explains in easy to understand language . . . . only you have the ability to make things come out right for you. Grandmaster Y. K. Kim explains how you and you alone can change your health <u>before</u> the doctor has to use drugs to do it for you. Just think of the savings you will receive by <u>preventing</u> the situations that could lead you to financial devastation. Think of how much more productive you can be at everything you do when you feel good and strong and healthy.

In my thirty years experience as a surgeon, clinician, healer, and friend to my patients, the most provoking ailment of all my patients has been STRESS. It is my observation that stress is the underlying cause of the majority of life's maladies as we know them today. Grandmaster Y. K. Kim's thoughts on stress make a very clear picture in order for everyone to better understand and correct our behaviors regarding this devastating illness. No one individual has better put into words my own feelings regarding stress than Grandmaster Y. K. Kim.

I highly recommend everyone that can read, read this book. The savings could be greater than you think . . . it could save your life!

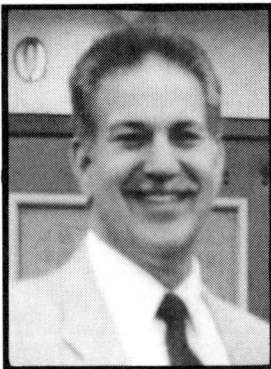

Dr. Ronald L. Chernov

Why I Wrote
Health is the Foundation of Success

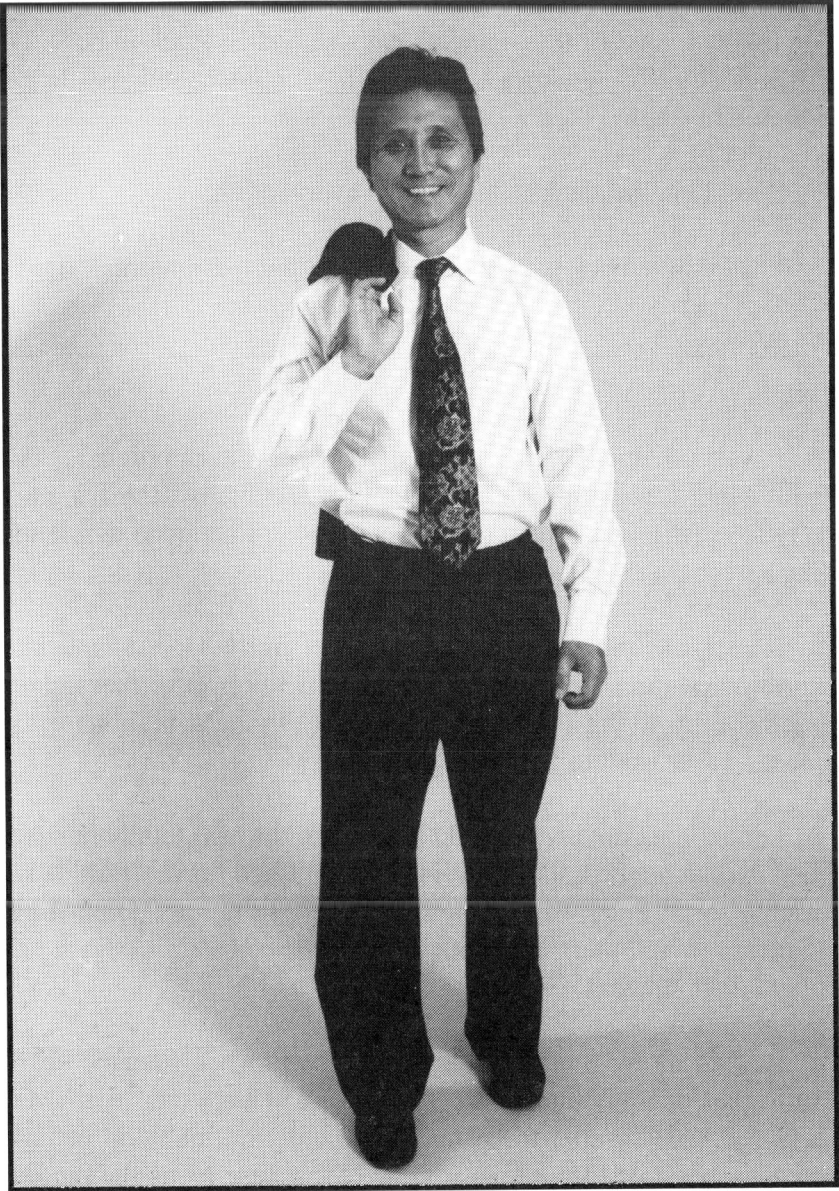

Health is the most important thing in my life.

I truly believe that health is the foundation of success in life.

No matter who you are: rich or poor, educated or uneducated, famous or unknown, young or old, male or female, black, white, or yellow, NO ONE -- not you or me -- wants to get sick and be stuck in bed. No one likes that feeling of weakness; no one likes to look and feel terrible. I know I didn't want to.

Sure, I had headaches, but doesn't everybody?

I had a little back pain once in a while, but that's normal, right?

Wrong.

I was ashamed of myself and extremely disappointed. All the while I thought I was building myself up, I was actually destroying myself. My very foundation was shattered and everything I believed in fell apart. I felt like a hypocrite and a charlatan.

Here I was the top martial arts master in the U. S. -- maybe even the world -- teaching thousands of people how to improve themselves, yet I was physically living in pain, and mentally living a nightmare. I was ashamed. I never want to live like that again.

I don't think anybody should have to go through totally unnecessary pain and mental anguish like that. I did, but I asked for it. (I didn't know I was asking for it, but I was.) That's why I'm writing this book: I believe that there are some other people out there -- maybe you? -- who are asking for it but don't realize it.

If I can show you what you are doing wrong, just maybe I can save you from that pain and anguish. If you don't believe me, fine. Maybe I can help you recover after the pain comes, and you finally do believe me. I know there are lots of dummies out there, because I was the biggest one of all. You can buy a new car; you can buy a new house; but you can NOT buy a new body. You only get one, so you had better take care of it.

I used to think I was healthy and strong because I could smash concrete eight feet in the air with my feet in the blink of an eye. My exhibitions would bring thousands of people to their feet, cheering. I practiced hard physically and mentally every day to become a Tae Kwon Do Master. I felt strong and healthy, and long hours of practice did not bother me at all.

After a long day of hard training, I would be starving. I ate anything that didn't move: fats, sugars, caffeine, junk food, even some good food. I would always eat too much, especially late at night, but I had no digestive problems and wasn't getting fat, so I didn't worry. (Maybe all the fat was going to my head). On top of that, I used to smoke.

Can you imagine anyone being that dumb: working out all day long to build a strong body and a sound mind, then eating garbage food and smoking? That's about as smart as taking a shower and then rinsing off with mud. But I did it. I was slowly destroying my beautiful body, but I was doing it in places that I couldn't see: my heart, lungs, liver, kidneys, spleen, and stomach. I figured as long as I looked healthy, I must be healthy.

To make things worse, I was teaching others to follow me. I had some of my students ask me how to improve their diet. I told them, "Work out hard and eat whatever you like." After all, that's what I did, and I was healthy, wasn't I?

Actually, my advice wasn't too bad. I was pretty healthy, because I was young, and my bad habits hadn't had time to catch up with me, yet. I was not smart enough to know that if you have good health, you must take care of it or you will lose it. Before long, those habits started to catch up with me.

It all started innocently enough with a stomach ache. No problem: just take a little medicine. That's the American Way, right? If you have a pain, take something to kill the pain. Don't worry your pretty little head about what caused the pain. As long as the pain goes away, everything is O.K. (Does this sound familiar to you?)

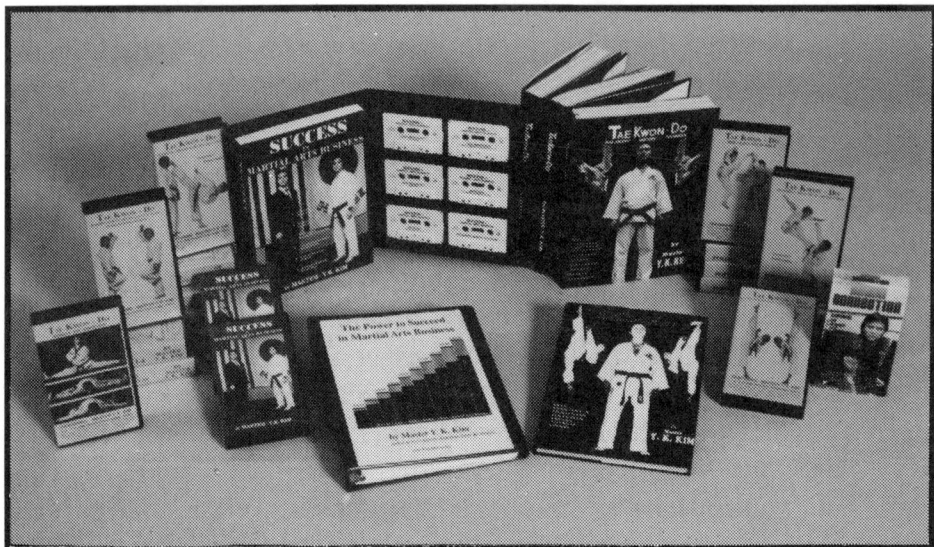

Martial Arts Books and Videos written and produced by Grandmaster Y. K. Kim

So the stomach aches came and went, and soon became diarrhea or constipation. I wasn't very smart. My body was sending me signals, and I was ignoring them. I developed a close relationship with milk of magnesia. This was not the smartest time of my life.

One major complication that I had is that I love what I am doing. My work is my life. Working twenty-five hours a day, eight days a week was not enough for me. I wanted ten more bodies just so I could do more work (I was also beginning to want another body that didn't have so many problems.) People told me I was a work-a-holic, and I thanked them for the compliment.

I felt a lot of pressure from the worries and responsibilities, but I kept working day and night. Sometimes I got headaches.· (Don't you?) No problem: just pop a few aspirin and keep working. I had no idea that pills and potions had side effects. I was only interested in one effect: stop the pain so I can do some work. I didn't even try to release the tension.

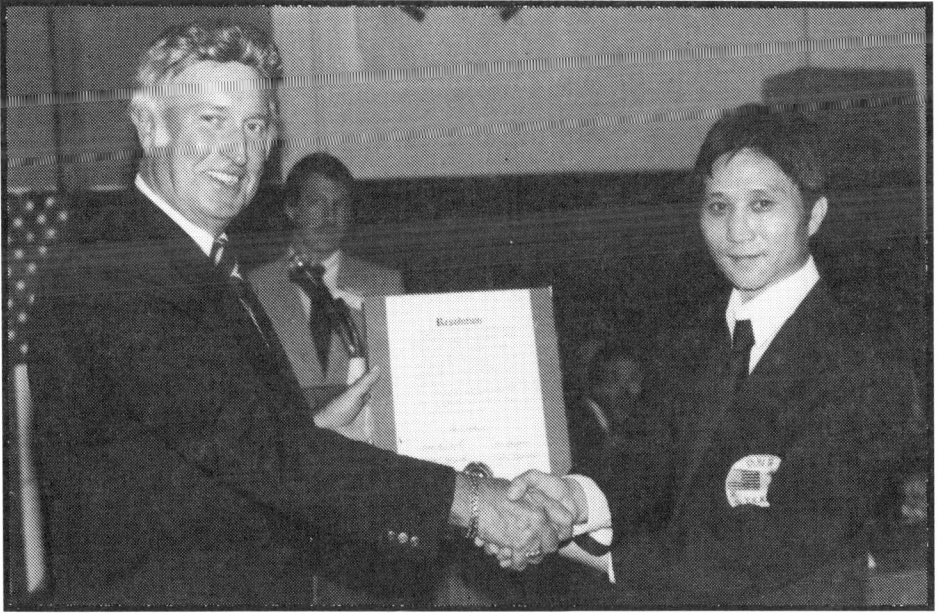

December 1, 1984: "Y. K. Kim Day" proclaimed in Central Florida

I did pretty good for myself. I lived the American dream in the classic rags to riches style. I came to this country with only the uniform in my hand and a head full of dreams. By the time the headaches started I had already built one of the largest martial arts schools in the U. S., expanded to develop a powerful international martial arts organization, written a world-wide best-selling book, produced and starred in my own major action film, was honored with public service awards, and had "Y. K. Kim Day" proclaimed in Central Florida for all I had done for the community.

I had already achieved many professional martial artist's life dreams, and I wasn't even forty. I was making more than enough money for my needs, and had a bright future. My choice of career not only let me stay healthy (or so I thought), but allowed me to teach others how to become healthy and confident. My fitness center was open twenty-four hours a day, seven days a week, for the benefit of my members.

I continued to work as hard as I possibly could. I taught that the body is just a tool of the spirit, and my spirit was very strong. If my body felt tired, my spirit could give me the energy I needed to keep going. I was very happy to teach Tae Kwon Do every day so that my students

5

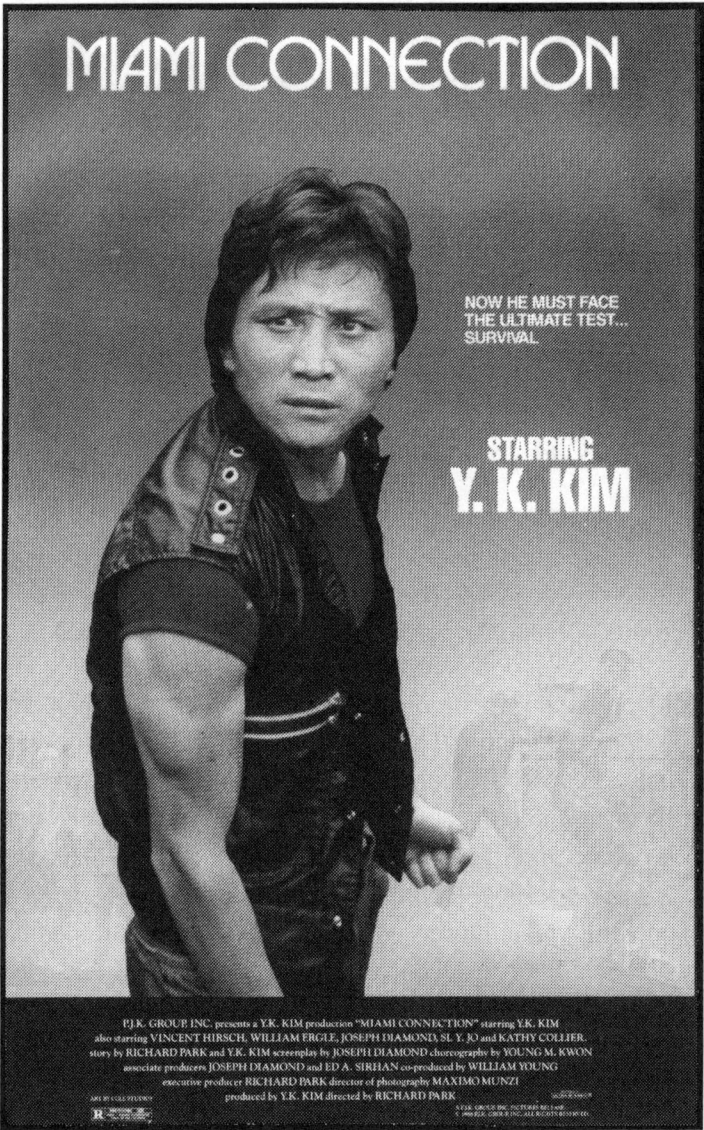

Poster from "Miami Connection" starring writer and producer Master Y. K. Kim

could improve themselves physically, mentally, and spiritually. I solved many students' health problems. Aside from teaching, though, I was managing and operating my school and organization. I was constantly marketing and promoting to gain new students.

Then one day my neck began to feel awkward. I could not turn it to the left or right, and I was in constant pain. I think a lot of people have had this once in a while. I didn't really like the idea of taking pain killers, but I needed to continue my work. My students were more important than a few pills, so I sacrificed. I bought one of those smelly creams that make your muscles warm, rubbed it on my neck, and was able to work. I probably just slept in the wrong position. Isn't that what you tell yourself when it happens to you? After a couple of days, everything was O.K., so I continued my routine.

When the pain came back, I went to a chiropractor. He did some manipulations, and I felt great. In less than twenty minutes, though, the pain came back. This was getting serious. I felt a little ashamed as a Tae Kwon Do Master to be in such pain. I had to hide my pain from my students. I did not understand what was happening, because I was healthy and strong . . . . . . or so I thought.

I used some more muscle cream and went back to work with renewed determination. I had a strong spirit. I had overcome problems before, so I was confident I could overcome this. It was just a matter of not letting little things stop me. I had no idea what stress was, or how to release it safely. So it just built up.

About a month later the pain came back again, only this time it was deeper. Not only my neck but now my middle back was stiff, and the pain was more intense. I rubbed in my smelly muscle cream and made up my mind that I would have to really work hard to overcome my problems. So I did.

Now, ever since I was young I've had back problems. I had an accident, and since then my back has always required a lot of attention. I also discovered at a young age that the more exercise I got, the stronger my back became and the better it felt. So it was a simple relationship: when my back felt weak, I would exercise. If it felt very weak, I would exercise a lot. So what did I do about this intense weakness in my back? Do some intense exercise. This time it felt different, though. It was very hard to move, let alone exercise.

7

One night my neck and back locked up tight, and I literally couldn't move. I was home alone, but fortunately the telephone was right beside me. I called one of my trusted students and also called a colleague (a Master from a neighboring town). They came over to my house and took me to the emergency room. The doctor took X-rays and told me there was nothing wrong. I felt better mentally, knowing there was nothing wrong. On the other hand, there is nothing more frustrating than someone telling you there is nothing wrong when you can feel some very real pain. He gave me some pain killers and muscle relaxers, told me to rest, and suggested I wear a lower back support belt. If you can imagine the humiliation of a Tae Kwon Do master wearing a support belt, you can begin to understand how I felt. Pain is a strong motivator, though, so I wore the belt. It was the only way I could continue to work.

I know now how stupid I was. Ninety per cent of what I was doing was right, but that ten per cent was really bothering me. I just wasn't paying attention to the messages I was getting. The doctor even told me in plain English to relax, but I didn't hear that part. I focused on the symptoms of my problems without trying to find the cause. I always had goals to motivate me, and I was very successful in achieving those goals. I had accomplished everything through hard work, so I firmly believed that the harder I worked, the more successful I would become. I knew I had a strong spirit, and my spirit was what had allowed me to succeed where others had failed. Personal pain became just another obstacle to overcome (as it had always been in my Tae Kwon Do training). So I ignored the pain, focused on my goals, and pushed myself even harder. I didn't realize what my body was trying to tell me. I didn't realize that working the way I was working could destroy me, or that there was another way to reach my goals without destroying myself.

One day my whole back, from my neck down to my tail bone, stiffened up like a rock. I couldn't move -- not even one inch. On top of that I felt like someone was stabbing me with an ice pick. This time I couldn't go to the hospital . . . . an ambulance had to come to pick me up. It was difficult to even take an X-ray, but they did. Can you guess what they found? Nothing. They gave me a shot of pain killers, pills, ice bags, heating pads, and sent me home. I was stuck on my back for a few days, but my mind was still able to work. I thought and planned and organized, took my pills, rubbed my ointments, used the hot and cold packs, and in a couple of days I was back on my feet and back to work. I thought I was being strong.

I had this happen several times over the next couple of years: my back would lock up and paralyze me, I would go to the hospital in excruciating pain, they would find nothing wrong, and send me home. The last time it happened it was so bad that I couldn't even move enough to go to the bathroom. Like a baby, I would have to be cleaned and changed by my loving wife. I was ashamed, but I had been through this before, and in a couple of days I would be fine. I took my pain killers and muscle relaxers, rubbed in the ointments, used hot and cold packs, but to no avail. A week later I was worse instead of better.

I was disappointed in my life. I began to question everything. I wasn't afraid to die, but I was ashamed to live like this (besides, it was very painful). I thought that maybe I damaged my nerves and would be paralyzed forever. My life was ruined: I was a Tae Kwon Do master who couldn't kick. That's like a baseball pitcher who loses his throwing arm.

After two weeks nothing had changed. Since I had left my native land of Korea I had been too busy to even visit my beloved mother. My best friend and life partner was reduced to cleaning my diapers. My darling daughter would never know a father she could be proud of. All my Tae Kwon Do training, all my physical abilities, all my spirit, had left me worse than a newborn baby -- at least the baby could move. I couldn't even lie still without pain! What good was all the money I had earned, all the awards I had won, my books, my movie? What good was any of that, now?

It was at this point that I realized what the most important thing in my life was: my health. Without health I not only could not reach my dreams, and could not use what I had already accomplished, but I was now a burden on my loved ones. My dreams and ambitions were dead. Rigor mortis had pre-maturely claimed my body. I was unable to face my loyal students.

Up until this point I did not know what stress meant. Besides, I was too busy to worry about it. I sure found out, though. I was strong physically, but I did not realize that the real foundation of health depends

9

upon how attitude, breathing, diet, and exercise work as a team to affect my (and your) health.

Physically, mentally, spiritually, I had reached the bottom. There was no place to turn (and even if there were, it hurt too much to turn). If I had been spiritually weak, I might never have recovered. On the other hand, if I had been mentally weak, I never would have been able to push myself to that point of TOTAL exhaustion.

I had to re-organize. I had to learn to care about myself. The doctor no longer had to tell me to relax -- my body wouldn't let me do anything else. I thought about everything, and re-evaluated many of my basic beliefs:

Was I doing the right kind of exercise?

Must I eat everything on my plate?

Is non-stop hard work, to the point of self-destruction, the only way to succeed?

Are aspirin and other pills the best way to cure pain?

I asked some questions I never had time to ask before. I made up my mind that I would find the answers, so this would never happen to me again.

After about the fourth week my despair turned to anger. I had given myself time enough to recover. I was a man, not a baby. I was a Tae Kwon Do master: that truly means I am a master of my body, my mind, and my spirit. It was time to think positively about the future and turn those thoughts into reality. By sheer force of will and the energy generated by four weeks of shame, frustration, and anger, I was able to get up out of bed, pain and all, and start my life over. I was very lucky to have this chance and not be paralyzed forever, but without positive thinking I never would have made this chance. I was determined to make some changes.

Since that day I've done a lot of research. I had never paid attention to other exercise and health experts, because I thought my program was the best. How narrow minded I was! I began to meet with and listen to professionals and experts from different areas of health: exercise specialists and physiologists, aerobics experts, nutritionists, breathing experts, medical doctors, and acupuncturists. I read as many books as possible, and watched tapes. This time I listened to my body. Through taking care of my health, I was able to re-condition my body. I changed the things I put in my body. I changed the way I breathed. I changed the way I exercised. I changed the way I worked. Before long I was able to achieve the same amazing martial arts techniques I could when I was twenty.

The answer I found was so simple that it amazed me: health is harmony with nature. All my life I had been trying to conquer what I thought were my weaknesses. I was working on the symptoms instead of the causes. In fact, all I had to do was cooperate with my nature, and I would have saved myself a lot of pain and anguish. Harmony involves the four supports of proper mental attitude, proper breathing, proper diet, and proper exercise. The four together build a strong foundation. I was foolish enough to believe I could build my house with one support: exercise. The exercise was good, but it was not enough. Just like a house, I needed support from all four corners. If even one support is missing, the house will eventually fall.

For a long time I could not jump. I found it difficult to kick, but I kept my positive attitude, continued Power Breathing, ate a proper diet, and did my Power Exercises. Finally, I got my power back. I could feel that I was in the best condition of my life. After a long journey in the tunnel, I could finally see the sunshine.

Just recently, I put on a spectacular Tae Kwon Do exhibition for a crowd of 15,000 for the first time in over five years. I still work hard, but now I work a lot smarter. I listen to my body when it tells me there's a problem. I found out through experience that prevention is much better than cure. I still have a lot of stress in my life, but I have learned to deal with it much better. I take care of the four corners of the foundation of my health every day, because I know that if I don't, my old ghosts will come back to haunt me.

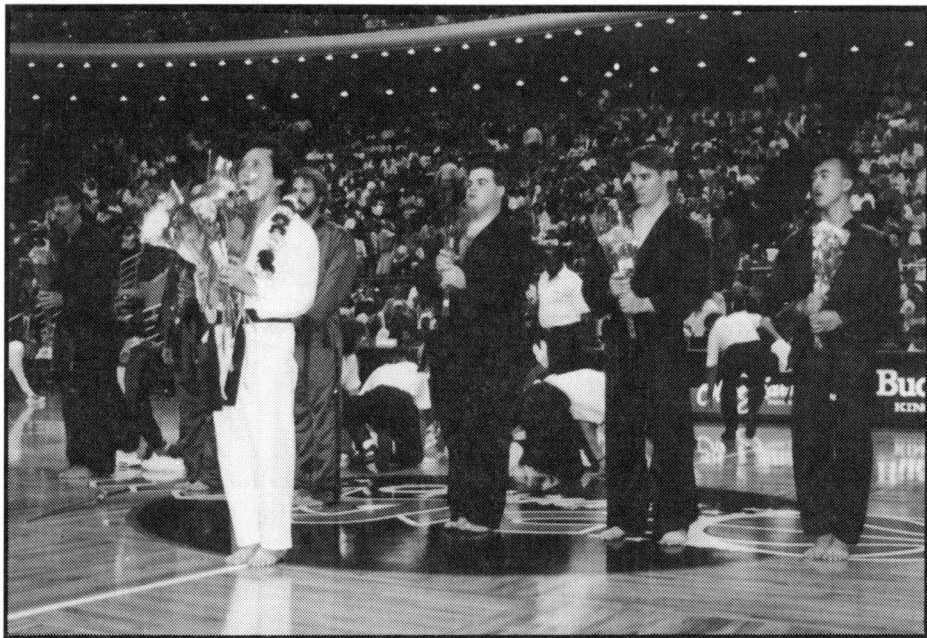
1992 Exhibition at Orlando Arena starring Master Y. K. Kim

I am a teacher: that's what I love to do and that's what I'm good at. When I learned these hard lessons, I felt compelled to teach others what I had learned. I believed there were other people out there who had the same symptoms and same problems. Then I watched President Bush collapse on T.V. in Japan. He had pushed himself too far. I saw President Clinton lose his voice in the middle of his campaign. He had pushed himself too far. I realized that if these two men, two of the greatest citizens of the greatest country in the world, were suffering from the same problem I had, there must be many, many more. This will be the biggest disease of the 21st Century.

In his state of the union address in 1992, President Bush said that Americans spent $750 billion dollars for health care in 1991. He predicted that figure to rise to $800 billion for 1992, and by the year 2005 it would be $2.2 TRILLION. That's more than the defense budget and more than the national debt. Do you realize how much money we could save as a nation if we could eliminate self-inflicted health problems? If we didn't need pain killers? If we could keep ourselves healthy enough not to miss work?

Another great president of this country, John F. Kennedy, once said, "Ask not what your country can do for you, but rather, what you can do for your country." I owe so much to this country, I wish I could pay back even a small part of what I have received. This is the land of opportunity, but if you are not healthy, you cannot take advantage of it. This book is my humble attempt to do something for my country. If people like you can become healthier, you will be happier and more prosperous. Read this book and profit from my experience. Health is the foundation of success.

Do you get headaches?

Does your back hurt?

Are you taking pain killers to take away the symptom rather than trying to find the cause of the problem?

If so, you are now where I was then. You are part of the $800 billion problem. Don't wait until it gets worse. Take steps now to save yourself a lot of pain and suffering. Your health is your most important asset.

Prevention is better than cure.

If you believe that the most important thing in your life is your health, perhaps you can join me in building a stronger, healthier, and happier America.

I hope you read this book at least 10 times.
I hope you practice it forever.
I hope you use it every moment.
I hope you teach as many people as possible.

Together, with a health as our foundation, we can all build successful lives, and a healthy world for our children.

THE FOUNDATION OF HEALTH:
Balancing the Four Corners

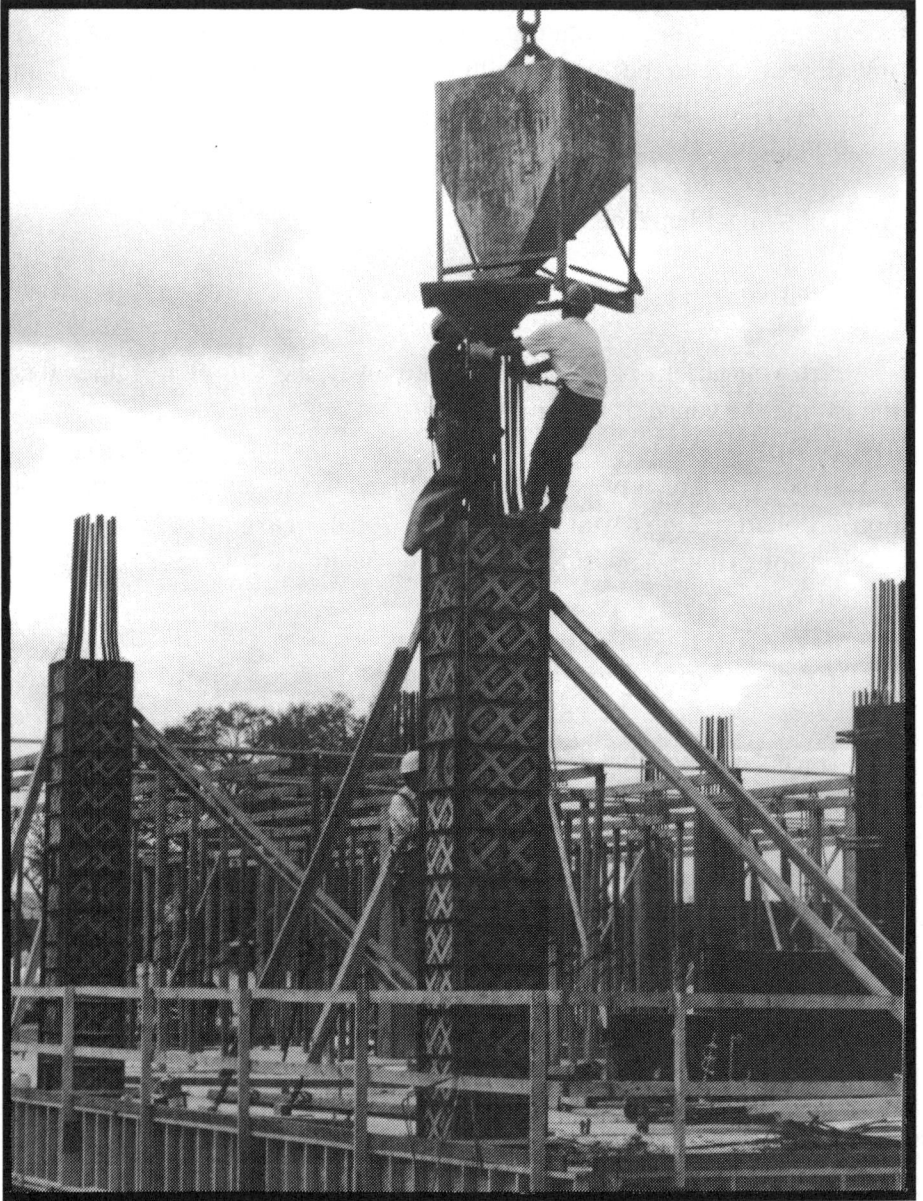

The foundation of health is nature. Nature is harmony. For example, animals inhale oxygen and exhale carbon dioxide; plants take in carbon dioxide and release oxygen. Neither one could survive for very long without the other.

In order to have good health, you have to achieve harmony with nature by balancing the four corners of the foundation of health:

1. Healthy Mental Attitude

2. Power Breathing

3. Natural, Nutritional Food

4. Power Exercises

Let's look at how these four corners work together to support your health and why they need to be balanced. Take the following Health Quiz:

1. You eat only healthy foods, but you cannot digest them because your internal organs, especially your stomach, are bad or weak.
Can you say you are healthy in this case? ___yes ___no

2. You have strong and healthy internal organs now, but you eat junk food all the time and drink a lot of alcohol.
Do you believe you will maintain your health? ___yes ___no

3. You have strong and healthy organs and you eat only natural, nutritional foods, but you are always angry, depressed, nasty, negative, or worried.
Do you think others will say you are healthy? ___yes ___no

4. You have a healthy mental attitude, strong and healthy internal organs, and you eat natural, nutritional food, but you never exercise to release stress or other toxins from your body.
Can you maintain strong health this way? ___yes ___no

The correct answer to all the above questions is "NO." Each and every one of the four corners must be strong to support complete health. These four corners are like the four corners of the foundation of a house. If any one of the corners is weak, the house, no matter how well built, will not stand. Likewise, your health depends on each of the four corner supports. If any one of the corners is weak, your health, no matter how it seems on the outside, will fail.

Let's look at each of the aspects of total health:

1. Healthy Mental Attitude.

A healthy mental attitude is the result of a sound mind that practices positive thinking. Positive thinking requires the self-discipline to clear away the negative and only concentrate on the positive. Self-discipline leads to self-improvement. When you open your mind to positive direction, and discipline yourself to maintain positive thoughts, you will develop a healthy mental attitude. A healthy mental attitude is your most powerful asset. It can change your whole world. By simply changing your mind, you can change your present, and change your future.

We are all familiar with the stories of the self-fulfilling prophesy: an elementary school classroom is randomly divided in half, and the children who are told they are smart believe it, and do the things smart children do; the children who are told they are dumb also believe it, and act like dumb children. The same thing is true of adults: if you believe you are smart or strong or healthy, you will do the things that smart, strong, or healthy people do. People with a healthy attitude are not afraid to exercise and enjoy life, which, in turn, keeps them healthy. They stay healthy because they want to stay healthy.

Likewise, people who believe they are dumb, weak, or sickly, will act dumb, weak, or sickly. No matter how naturally healthy their bodies are, if they do not have a healthy attitude, they will become sick. Someone who believes he is sickly becomes a hypochondriac, giving himself symptoms of every disease he reads or hears about. If he is worried about his job, his spouse, the ozone layer, and everything else, he will worry himself sick with ulcers and other stress-related diseases. If he has a bad temper and is always angry at other people, he will have high blood pressure and other anger-related diseases.

16

Positive brings positive, and negative brings negative. A closed mind will destroy itself; an open mind can build a healthy mental attitude. Self-discipline and meditation will clear your mind of negative thoughts and closed mindedness, and release stress. They will open your mind to positive possibilities, so you can develop and maintain a healthy mental attitude.

2. Power Breathing

Power Breathing is an internal organ exercise. It is deep breathing, which allows you to bring more oxygen into your body with each breath. It also allows you to get rid of more carbon dioxide and noxious gasses by cleaning out your lungs. When there is more oxygen available to your system, all your organs work more efficiently, as does your immune system. The downward movement of your diaphragm also exercises and massages your internal organs, improving your blood circulation, balancing the flow of hormones, and regulating the nervous system. Power Breathing is the resource of health.

If you do not get enough oxygen and blood circulation throughout your system, you will suffer from circulation-related problems like headaches. You will not digest your food properly, and, therefore, will not feed your body effectively. Your organs and immune system will not be working at top efficiency, and you will be more susceptible to infection and disease.

Power Breathing will build up stronger and healthier internal organs. Health is not only skin deep. The appearance of health is often confused with the appearance of beauty. Someone who looks good on the surface is not always healthy on the inside. Real health comes from the inside out: strong organs are the foundation of good health.

3. Natural Nutritional Food

You are what you eat. If you eat natural, nutritional food, you will be naturally healthy. Nature provides you with the perfect foods, in the perfect packages that supply all the nutrients you need for health. As long as you eat natural, nutritional foods in reasonable amounts, you will have all the supplies necessary for excellent health.

17

If you eat junk, you will be junk. It's the "garbage in, garbage out" rule. When you eat processed foods that have some of the natural ingredients removed, these ingredients are usually necessary for proper digestion. We end up eating foods that make us over-fat and under-nourished at the same time.

To go against nature is to go against ourselves, for we are part of nature. When we eat natural foods we keep in harmony with nature, and we can maintain a strong and healthy body and mind.

4. Power Exercises

Power Exercises were designed to give you back your personal power. Your body was designed to move. When you exercise, your muscles grow larger, you burn excess fat, and you utilize oxygen more efficiently. You also move waste products out of your system through increased circulation and sweat. Power Exercises were specifically designed to loosen up and strengthen all your joints, from your toes to your fingers. They will also clean out and relax all your muscles, from your face to your feet. By incorporating Power Breathing, they will strengthen your internal organs to improve your internal health.

Aerobic Self-Defense is a more intense exercise that also gives you the freedom from fear and the peace of mind that comes with the confidence of knowing that you can defend yourself. Whatever form of exercise you do, be sure that it is a proper exercise for each joint, muscle, and internal organ. Power Exercises were designed to be the proper and perfect exercises for the human body.

When you do not exercise, your muscles shrink, you begin storing fat, and your oxygen utilization decreases. Let me give you an example that will help you understand what can happen: if you were to wear the same clothes for a week or more, wouldn't they begin to smell? You need to clean all the dirt and smell out of the clothes, so that they can be fresh again. The same is true of your body. You cannot change bodies like you can change clothes, so you must clean the junk and smell out of the body. How? You can wash the skin in the shower, but that does nothing for your insides. You have to stretch and squeeze the muscles and organs of the internal body to clean them out, just like you would wring out clothes to clean them better than just wetting them. Power Exercises act like a laundry for your body. They will release stress and tension, clean out your muscles and joints, and make them stronger. They are a great way to refresh your body and mind.

You have to balance all four corners of your foundation to maintain your health. Just like a table with four legs, you need strength and support in each corner. If one corner is weak, the table will be out of balance, and everything will slide off. If any one corner is missing or weak in your health program, your body will get out of balance and unhealthy. Unlike a table or a house, though, your body cannot be replaced. You can always buy a new house or a new table; you can never buy a new body. You must take care of it before it breaks; otherwise, it will be too late.

There is a big difference between the East, where I come from (Korea) and the West where I live now (U.S.A.). In the West we concentrate on the physical and the tangible. In the U.S.A. we have thousands of diet books and thousands more of exercise books. Bodybuilding has become a multi-million dollar industry. Yet for a country that has the best doctors and best advice on exercise and nutrition, one out of every five Americans has cancer, and one out of two people has the possibility of developing cancer. We are the sickness super-power of the world.

In the East we are more concerned with the spiritual and intangible. There are lots of books on breathing in Korea, Japan, and China. How many do you know of in the U.S.A.? That is because the effects of breathing are not so easily tangible or measurable. Eastern bodybuilding is internal organ building, not muscle building.

Yet I am not trying to say the East is better than the West. In Korea it has been a tradition to show affection and respect through food. When we really care about someone, we try to feed them as well as we can, encouraging them to eat more and more (this might be left over from the times when food was scarce.) All this over-eating has led to a national health problem. I just recently read in a Korean newspaper that Koreans suffer from stomach problems ten times more than Americans, and that five times more people die of stomach problems.

In the East we have a philosophy: the philosophy that opposites are not only necessary, but complementary. The opposites of male and female, positive and negative, good and evil, Um and Yang (Yin and Yang) make the world go round. Both are necessary for wholeness. In a like manner, the spirituality of the East and the technology of the West must be combined to achieve complete knowledge. When we create a global philosophy, we will have a much more complete view of health. I believe the four corners of the foundation of health is just such a philosophy.

Until I realized that there were four separate and equally important corners to the foundation of health, I was very frustrated about many things that were happening around me. I could not figure out why all of my students would practice Tae Kwon Do so hard, yet some would lose weight and others would not improve at all.

One of my best students, who was big and strong and handsome, worked very hard to become an Instructor. He appeared to be a model of health. Yet one day he had a blood clot, and his one arm swelled up twice its normal size. He went to the hospital, and they told him he would die if he were not careful.

Another of my students had a similar occurrence. He worked out very hard, and also became an Instructor, yet he had varicose veins. He had to have an operation to get rid of the veins.

A third student, who trained with his wife and daughter, was suffering from heart problems. He had the strength and perseverance to become a black belt and Instructor, yet his heart was not healthy.

I could not understand how these students had such bad health when they exercised regularly. Then we had a school party one night, with a buffet dinner. I noticed that all three of these students piled up their plates with fatty meats. I realized then that exercise was not the only factor in good health. These students would practice so hard to clean out their systems, and then right away put more junk back in. Apparently they were shoveling junk in faster than the body could sweat it out. They were not keeping all four corners of their foundation in harmony.

This is one of the main reasons I am writing this book at this moment. I want to teach my beloved Tae Kwon Do students the correct and complete foundation of health. I want to help my own Tae Kwon Do family, and I want to help you, too.

Since I have found harmony with the four corners of the foundation of my own health, I practice them every day, just like eating. I feel younger than ever, healthier than ever, stronger than ever, more confident in myself, more positive, more enthusiastic, and more energetic. I can do anything, and that makes every minute more exciting. I feel like I have doubled my life span and life quality.

You and I have a chance to do something great for our country and the world. By taking a little time to share what we learn with the people around us, we can build a healthier society one person at a time. The healthier people are, the longer they will live, the happier they will be, and the more smiles they will give to us. Isn't that how it's supposed to be?

PREVENTION AND HEALTH

Prevention is better than cure.

Even if I gain the whole world, it means nothing without health.

1. If I were to lose all my money, I would lose something valuable, but it can be replaced.

2. If I were to lose the honor of my name, I would lose a lot, because it is hard to gain back.

3. If I were to lose my health, I would lose everything, including my life. It cannot be replaced, and it would be too late to gain it back.

The most important thing in my life is my HEALTH.

Strong health is the best prevention for any disease. A positive prevention program will build healthier individuals, a healthier society, a healthier America, and A Healthy World.

An ounce of prevention is worth a pound of cure.

Unfortunately, most of us do not know how to prevent. We only know how to cure. So we have to buy cures by the pound, when we could have saved time, money, and energy with a little prevention. Let me give you a simple example. You are driving your car and the OIL light comes on. (This means that there is no oil lubricating your engine.) If you do not turn the engine off immediately, you will destroy the engine. For the price of one or two quarts of oil (less than $3.00), you can save $600 to $2000 to rebuild the motor.

Your body does not have red lights that say "OIL", but it does flash signs to you all the time. If you understood these warnings and would listen to them (follow your own body's directions), you could save yourself a lot of time, money, and pain.

How People Get Sick

Part of maintaining good health is understanding how people get sick. If you understand the causes, you can better avoid them and do the things that create good health.

Very generally, people get sick from 3 causes:

1. Clogged mind.

A clogged mind cannot think, see, or act right. It has blinders on, and does not seek to learn the truth. It is not functioning freely and smoothly; it is slow and unimaginative.

A clogged mind does not realize that it is asking for sickness by acting the way it does.

2. Clogged blood vessels.

When there are clogs in the blood stream, the blood does not flow freely and smoothly. It cannot deliver oxygen and other nutrients to the cells, and it cannot remove the toxins. The blood is over 90% water, and water that does not flow becomes stagnant.

Other things that contribute to clogged blood vessels are negative attitude, shallow breathing, junk food, and lack of exercise. When the blood does not flow freely through a specific area for any reason, that area develops problems.

3. Accident.

Automobile accidents, personal injuries, and infections from other people are rarely sought out. They usually arrive unannounced and without our consciously asking for them. That is why I call them all accidents. However, many "accidents" actually happen because we asked for them. You don't have to travel far on any highway to find someone who drives dangerously. That person, whether he realizes it or not, is asking for an accident. Many personal injuries and infections (like AIDS) occur most often when we voluntarily put ourselves in a high risk situation.

Even when we suffer an "accident", if we have a positive mind and good blood circulation, we can usually recover.

Of the three causes of sickness, two and a half are under our own control. If we keep an active, open mind, good circulation, and do not put ourselves in high-risk situations, we will avoid most sickness, injury, and disease. Only pure accidents that happen to us outside our control will harm us, and healthy circulation of body and mind will help us recover.

Modern Sickness

Medical science has gone a long way to protect us against the diseases and plagues of the past. Vaccinations and antibiotics make many of the infectious and germ-related diseases almost obsolete. Most of the modern sicknesses we still suffer from are more difficult to cure because they are self-inflicted, which means we are destroying ourselves. As we approach the 21st Century, our fast-paced, high-tech lifestyle is creating new diseases every year.

Let's examine together some of the causes of modern sickness, so we can learn how to prevent them, and live a healthier life:

The world we have created is unbalanced: we demand too much of ourselves mentally, and not enough of ourselves physically. We try to make everything easy and convenient: we have washing machines, dishwashers, microwave ovens, heaters and air conditioners, cars, and telephones. In our button-pushing culture, we only need one strong finger to survive. Everything else is done for us. Our bodies go to waste (and in many cases, to waist).

These conveniences make life less physically demanding, but also less healthy. Our bodies are designed to move and work. When we do not move them, and actually imprison them at a desk for many hours a day, they cannot function as they were designed to. Our bodies begin to deteriorate.

Our minds, on the other hand, are working at warp speed. We act and react to all kinds of situations we interpret as threats. Our bodies are designed to deal with a threat physically: we fight or flee. The mental threats we face cause the same physical reactions in our bodies (like the release of adrenaline), but we do not fight or flee to properly dispose of the hormones and energy. This puts our bodies chemically out of balance. We begin to get headaches, stomach aches, nervous twitches, strange pains, rashes, high blood pressure, anxiety, depression, lack of energy, anger, confusion, and an endless list of other symptoms. We are destroying ourselves.

We need to restore our balance. We need to move our bodies to keep the blood from getting clogged. We need to relax our minds to keep them from getting clogged. We need to stop asking for an "accident" to happen.

When you balance the four corners of the foundation of health, you will keep good circulation in your body and mind, and you will always be strong and healthy. In your daily life you need to keep clean, positive habits. If you follow the nine steps to health, you will maintain those clean, positive habits and stay healthy.

You then need to share what you have with those around you by helping them to become more healthy and positive. Helping others is helping yourself.

How to Prevent Injury

I've heard many times that people hurt their backs, strain and pull muscles, twist their ankles or knees, and get a host of other injuries from playing ball, running, aerobics, martial arts, and even swimming. These activities are supposed to be fun and good for them, not harmful.

Even professional athletes in the N.F.L., N.B.A., and the American and National Baseball Leagues suffer from too many unnecessary (and very expensive) injuries. The body is not designed to go from rest to quick motion instantaneously. It needs time to warm up and accustom the muscles and joints to quick movements. If you want to participate in a strenuous activity, you need to warm up your body and mind. Power Exercises were designed as a warm-up for more demanding physical activity.

If you are going to engage in a sport or other physical endeavor:

1. Do the Standing Power Exercises (Chapter 8) to warm up your whole body.

2. Do the Standing Power Exercises and then Concentration Meditation (pp. 166-169) to prepare for a performance.

3. Do Standing Power Exercises, followed by Power Meditation (pp. 178-188), followed by Concentration Meditation in preparation for a special performance or a big game.

You don't want to just warm up your body. Any warm-up routine will do that. Sport-specific routines can even warm up your mind to the sport. Power Exercises and meditation will not only prevent injury, but also give you energy, put you in a positive frame of mind, and increase your confidence, so that you can develop the winning habit. You will cooperate better with your teammates and individually perform at your absolute best, whether on a junior, amateur, or professional level.

How to Prevent Modern Sicknesses by Releasing Stress

Stress is the biggest cause of modern sicknesses in the U.S.A. today. I hear almost every day about health and emotional problems resulting from stress. Many of the people who suffer from these problems do not know why they have them, or, if they know why, do not know how to prevent or relieve the stress. As a result, there are too many victims who are suffering pain and are bed-ridden. I certainly know what I'm talking about, because I was a perfect example of someone who fell victim to exactly that problem. I believe stress is the biggest obstacle to building a healthy society in our modern world.

What is stress?

Stress is pressure or tension that you feel from making yourself work longer or harder than is comfortable.

Stress is not always negative, though. You cannot achieve any worthwhile goal without working for it. In order to expand, or grow, you must put yourself under some stress. The amount of stress you feel, and the way you deal with it, will be the deciding factor in how it affects your health.

Our high-tech world is very competitive: person to person, company to company, nation to nation. Whether we like it or not we have to live with stress. Otherwise, we will be the losers in this competitive world.

Some people try to escape from stress through drugs, alcohol, and other vices. These ways do not help at all. Not only is the problem still there when you sober up, but you have increased your problems by abusing your body. This is a quick way to become a loser.

Other people try to quit because they cannot handle stress. Quitting does not take away all your stress; it just changes the nature of your stress. When you quit, you have to deal with the emotional stress of viewing yourself as a quitter or a failure. In addition, you have lost whatever it is you quit -- like your job. Now you must face the stress of finding a new job, and paying your bills until you find that new job. Often times quitting creates more stress than it solves.

We cannot blame anybody but ourselves for this situation. We must take responsibility for our own health. Making a change does not always mean you quit, though. For example, when you change for the better, you are not giving up -- you are improving. Likewise, when you retire, you have not quit anything.

Fortunately, you do not have to worry at all. I will show you how to handle your stress and have a healthier and more successful life:

1. Find the cause of your stress.

2. Eliminate, change, or improve the cause as much as possible.

3. Release the hormones and energy built up from the stress.

4. Do preventative maintenance to keep stress from building up again.

1. Find the causes of your stress.

The main causes of stress are:

Relationship Pressure

Financial Pressure

Job Pressure

Relationship pressure comes from cooperative living. Whenever two or more people get together, they must sacrifice some of their own freedom for the sake of the group. This is true among lovers, families, friends, and even whole societies. If everyone has complete freedom, there is only anarchy, and no relationship. When people sacrifice their own personal freedoms for the sake of the group, they get many benefits that they would not get when they are alone. The pressure comes about when one person feels that he is giving more than he is getting. Whether or not he really is giving more than he is getting is not nearly as important as how he feels about it.

Many relationship problems, especially marital problems, are rooted in financial trouble. Financial pressure does not come from the amount of money you make. It comes from the relationship between the amount you make and the amount you spend. If you only make $10,000 a year, you will not have any financial pressure if you spend only $9,000 a year. On the other hand, if you make $100,000 a year but you spend $110,000 a year, you will have a lot of pressure. Whether you are dealing with business or personal finances, the solution is to adjust your expenditures to be less than your income. You can increase the income, or reduce the expenses, or do both. If you do not, you will soon be bankrupt.

Job pressure usually comes from forcing yourself to do something you don't want to do. You might be working long hours, but if you love what you are doing, twelve hours a day is not too much. On the other hand, if you hate what you are doing, one hour a day is too much. Try to find a career or a job that you enjoy. If you hate your work, you must change your attitude, change your job, or change both.

Even when you love your work, if it is not varied, your body will rebel:

A. Your head will begin to feel heavy and warm.

B. Your body will become uncomfortable.

C. Your eyes will feel tired.

D. You will get a headache.

29

If you do not take a break, but continue to work, you will lay the foundation for all kinds of sicknesses. Your neck and back will stiffen, and you will begin to get stomach aches, high blood pressure, short temper, and depression. I know where this path leads, and, believe me, you don't want to go there.

2. Eliminate, change, or improve the cause as much as possible.

First of all, no one can make you do anything without your consent (except maybe die). Your boss cannot depress you; you have to allow him to depress you. Your husband cannot make you angry; you have to allow him to make you angry. When you realize this, you can understand that the only pressure is self-imposed pressure. You feel stress when you cannot live up to your own expectations. Other people can influence you to change your expectations (even manipulate you) only if you allow them to do so.

Relationship pressure, financial pressure, and job pressure are all the results of responsibilities you have assumed. They usually center around specific people like your boss, your wife, or your parents, and the pressure you impose on yourself to meet their expectations. Perhaps at the root of the problem is a fear that you will either lose those people or lose their respect. Losing that person or that person's respect will damage your self-worth, and you are back to meeting your own expectations.

Realizing where stress comes from can show you the way to reduce it: change your expectations. You cannot be all things to all people. Not everyone is cut out to be rich. Not everyone is cut out to be a leader. Some have to be smart, some have to be strong. Some have to be fast, some have to be creative. Find out your own strong and weak points, and understand them. Do not expect yourself to be something you are not. Do not get upset when someone else tells you something that you already know about yourself. When you know yourself, you can be confident in your strengths. Confidence is one of the best ways to overcome stress.

You can eliminate or at least reduce most of the causes of stress just by realizing where stress comes from. When you take on certain responsibilities, like children, there are some non-negotiable needs -- like food and shelter. Exactly what kind of food and shelter is negotiable, however, and the amount of financial pressure you put on yourself is completely under your control

If you find yourself getting sick over goals you have set, simply adjust your goals so that they won't make you sick. I'm not saying don't set goals. I'm not saying don't work hard and sacrifice to achieve those goals. I'm just saying don't worry yourself sick. The most important thing in your life is your health, and you cannot enjoy fame or fortune if you are not healthy.

3. Release the hormones and energy built up from the stress.

A. Meditate. Clear your mind of negative thoughts and emotions, and begin to think positively.

B. Exercise. Incorporate an exercise program into your schedule to recharge your energy. I recommend that you do something every day. I strongly recommend that you do Morning Energy Exercises when you first wake up and Night Relaxation Exercises just before you go to bed. You should also do some fairly strenuous Power Exercises sometime during the day -- it doesn't really matter whether it is in the morning, afternoon, or evening. You might also need to do short, specific stress-relieving exercises during the day at the office or whenever you begin to feel stress. It is better to take a short break to release the tension before it builds up, than it is to take a few sick days to recover from a serious problem.

C. Laugh. Laugh as long and as loud as possible. Watch some comedy on television, or establish a "joke of the day" routine with someone at work or at home.

D. Play. Engage in a hobby or some form of "play" in which your mind is active, but not under pressure. This will recharge your energy.

E. Talk. Say your problems out loud to release them. Express your frustrations to someone you trust. They may offer good advice or even solutions, but the important thing is that they listen while you unburden yourself.

If you have violent emotions, it is better not to release them directly on any person, especially someone who cares about you and doesn't deserve the violence. In this case, you should find a secluded spot to yell and scream to release the pent-up tension. If you cannot find a secluded spot to yell without bothering someone else, yell in your car. It is a lot better to look a little funny in the eyes of strangers than it is to say something cruel to someone that you care about.

F. <u>Daydream</u>. When your body is confined to a limited space for long hours, take short trips in your mind. Fantasize. You can remember good times from the past, or dream about good times in the future. After a few moments, when your mind is relaxed, return to work.

G. <u>Practice Tae Kwon Do</u>. Tae Kwon Do is the best overall health program for your body, mind, and spirit. It incorporates proper self-discipline, which creates self-confidence. It will make you physically fit, mentally sound, and give you a positive, successful attitude.

4. Do preventative maintenance to keep stress from building up again.

After you have adjusted your attitude and released your stress, you can continue to deal with your necessary stress through meditation, Power Breathing, good nutrition, and Power Exercises. Meditation will clean your mind of negative thoughts and quiet your body. Power Breathing will help clean your body by increasing circulation and massaging the internal organs. Good nutrition will take away the unnecessary physical stress of digesting junky foods and help restore your body to chemical balance. Power Exercises will massage specific muscles, stretching and contracting them to relax them and allow better circulation. Balance the four corners of the foundation of your health, and develop positive habits through the nine steps to health. Not only will you release stress and tension, you will be healthier, stronger, and more confident in yourself.

This is the beginning of a plan to reduce hundreds of billions of dollars we spend on health care every year. This is money that we could use to balance the federal budget and build a healthier America and A Healthy World.

DEVELOP POSITIVE HABITS:
The Nine Steps to Health

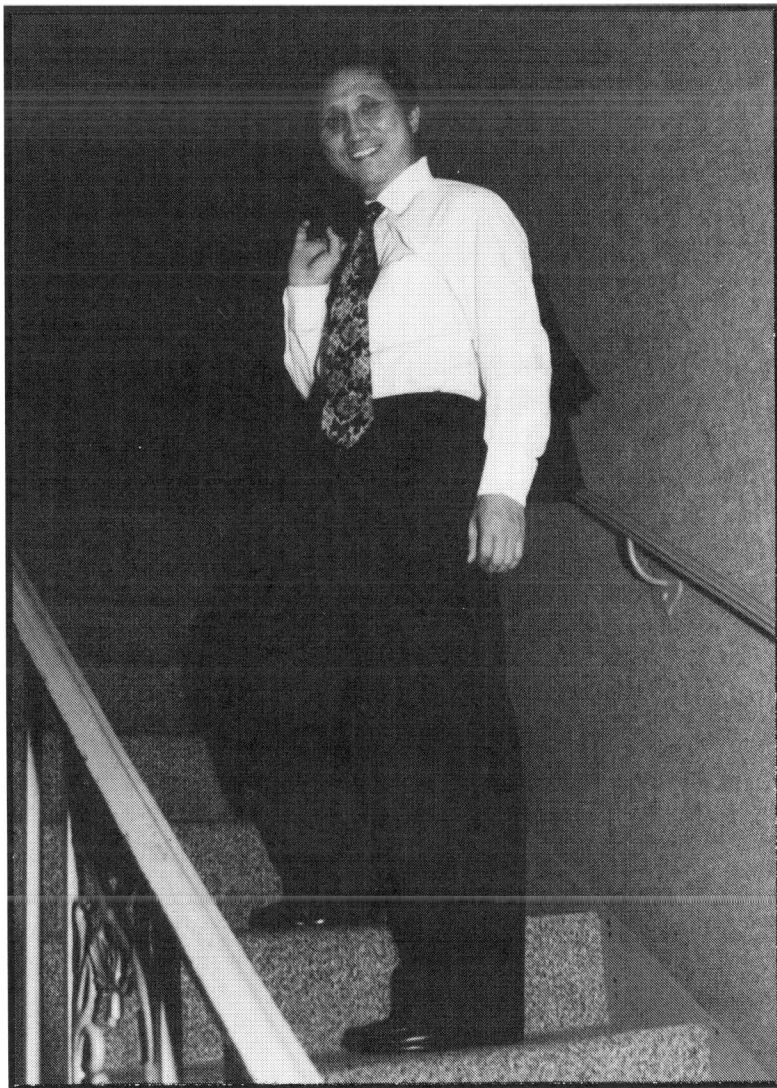

"The Nine Steps to Health will help you become healthier, stronger, more confident, and more energetic throughout your life."   *-- Master Y. K. Kim*

Destroying your health or making it strong is entirely up to you and your daily health habits. You do not need to spend any money or extra time; all it takes is a positive, healthy attitude.

The following nine steps will guide you on your path to health and happiness:

1. Do not be Lazy.

Laziness is health's enemy, success's enemy, and your enemy, because laziness creates negativity. When you are lazy, you do not want to change your life or stick to any plan to reach a goal. If you allow yourself to be lazy, you will never maintain good health because you will not follow these nine steps.

Instead: Be diligent. Develop new positive habits by setting clear personal goals. Do physical activities like walking, cleaning the house, swimming, and cutting the grass. Do mental activities like reading or planning the future. Diligence is health's best friend.

2. Do not lose your temper.

Bad temper, depression, and nasty or negative attitudes destroy you physically, mentally, and emotionally. Anger releases acids that destroy your body, hormones that affect your mind, and emotional vibrations that damage your spirit. This lack of control can be the worst thing for your health.

Instead: Control yourself and your temper. Try to be positive and smile. Make a point to have a good, long, hardy laugh at least three times a day. Throw away all anger, depression, and nasty or negative attitudes through a powerful exercise program that develops self-discipline and self-control like Tae Kwon Do.

34

3. **Do not eat too much; especially do not eat junk food**.

Eating too much will make you lazy and fat, it is often a sign of selfishness. When you eat too much, a lot of blood rushes to your digestive tract, taking blood away from your muscles and brain. You don't want to move, or even think. If you do not use all that food, it will be stored as fat.

On a mental level, selfishness is the same as eating too much: you want everything for yourself, leaving nothing for others. Mental gluttony leads to mental fat, and unhappiness.

Do not drink too much. If you consume alcohol (a poison) in large quantities, you will slowly destroy your liver and other organs.

Junk food creates sickness: garbage in, garbage out. If you use junky building blocks, you will get a junky building. If you eat junk food, your system can only build a junky body.

Instead: Eat natural, nutritional food in reasonable amounts. It will make you strong and healthy. Only take your fair share, whether it's food, money, or any other matter of life.

4. **Do not smoke or do any form of drugs**.

There is enough medical evidence and publicity today to make it obvious to everyone that smoking destroys your health, and drugs destroy your whole life. If possible, try to avoid even prescription drugs and over the counter pills, because they have side effects that are not good for your internal organs.

Instead: Throw away your cigarettes and drugs and do some form of exercise every day, like Tae Kwon Do training, to get natural excitement and euphoria. You will also get the mental discipline and training that will enable you to quit cigarettes, drugs, or any other addicting habit. Power Breathing exercises will also help you clean addicting substances out of your body.

5. Do not carry extra weight.

Being physically fat increases the risk of heart attack and other diseases. It also makes every day more uncomfortable because you have more difficulty moving or doing anything that involves physical activity. Being fat also makes you look bad and feel insecure.

Being mentally fat means you are lazy, negative, or ignorant. From these attitudes you will develop wrong ideas and bad habits.

Instead: Lose weight physically and mentally, and get in shape by Power Exercises and a natural, nutritional diet. You will feel good, look good, be more energetic, more positive, more confident in yourself, and that will give you hope of a brighter future.

6. Do not breathe short, shallow breaths.

Shallow breathing creates a short temper. Shallow breathing does not allow you to inhale enough oxygen for optimum health, and does not allow you to exhale all of the toxins from your lungs.

Instead: Do Power Breathing. It will make you more even-tempered, improve your circulation and waste disposal, and exercise your internal organs. You will feel healthier all the time.

7. Do not allow yourself to feel lonely.

Being alone does not create problems, but feeling lonely invites negative thinking that expresses itself in laziness, bad eating habits, and a search for easy solutions that can lead to drug and alcohol abuse.

Instead: Become active: do positive work by setting clear goals both professionally and personally. You will have the energy and motivation you need to work in a positive direction to achieve them. This is the foundation of self-improvement; you will feel more excited and confident about yourself today and for the rest of your life. You will not have time to feel lonely.

8. **Do not associate with negative people or places**.

Negative people feed your frustration and make you sick. Dishonest people are the most negative of all. Negative places drain your energy and depress you. Negative brings negative. If you live in dirt and filth, you will carry that dirt and filth with you throughout the day. If your home stinks, you will stink.

Instead: Associate with positive people and places. If you are a product of your environment, remove as many of the negative influences as you can from that environment. Choose your friends carefully among those who value truth. Keep your surroundings clean and positive. Positive brings positive, and truth brings truth; together they will bring happiness.

9. **Do not hold on to stress and tension**.

Stress creates all kind of modern sicknesses: ulcers and digestive problems, high blood pressure and heart problems, neuroses and psychological problems, and even cancer. It will destroy your health and create serious emotional trouble in your life.

Instead: Release your stress and tension with a positive exercise program like Power Exercises or Tae Kwon Do Training. You will relax your muscles and release pent-up emotions. You will have more energy today and throughout your life to achieve your goals, and be healthier and happier

I hope you read this part at least ten times until it becomes part of you. Then come back and read it again whenever you need to remind yourself how to maintain excellent health.

Develop the positive habits of the nine steps to health and share them with your family and friends. Remember: when you teach others, you teach yourself, as well.

Develop Positive Habits: The 9 Steps to Health

1. Do not be lazy.
   Be diligent.

2. Do not loose your temper.
   Control yourself and your temper.

3. Do not eat too much; especially do not eat junk food.
   Eat natural, nutritional food in reasonable amounts.

4. Do not smoke or do any form of drugs.
   Throw away your cigarettes and drugs and do some form of exercise every day.

5. Do not carry extra weight.
   Lose weight physically and mentally, and get in shape by Power Exercises, and a natural, nutritional diet.

6. Do not breathe short, shallow breaths.
   Do Power Breathing.

7. Do not allow yourself to feel lonely.
   Become active: do positive work by setting clear goals both professionally and personally.

8. Do not associate with negative people or places.
   Associate with positive people and places.

9. Do not hold on to stress and tension.
   Release your stress and tension with a positive exercise program like Power Exercises or Tae Kwon Do training.
                                        -- Grandmaster Y. K. Kim

POWER BREATHING

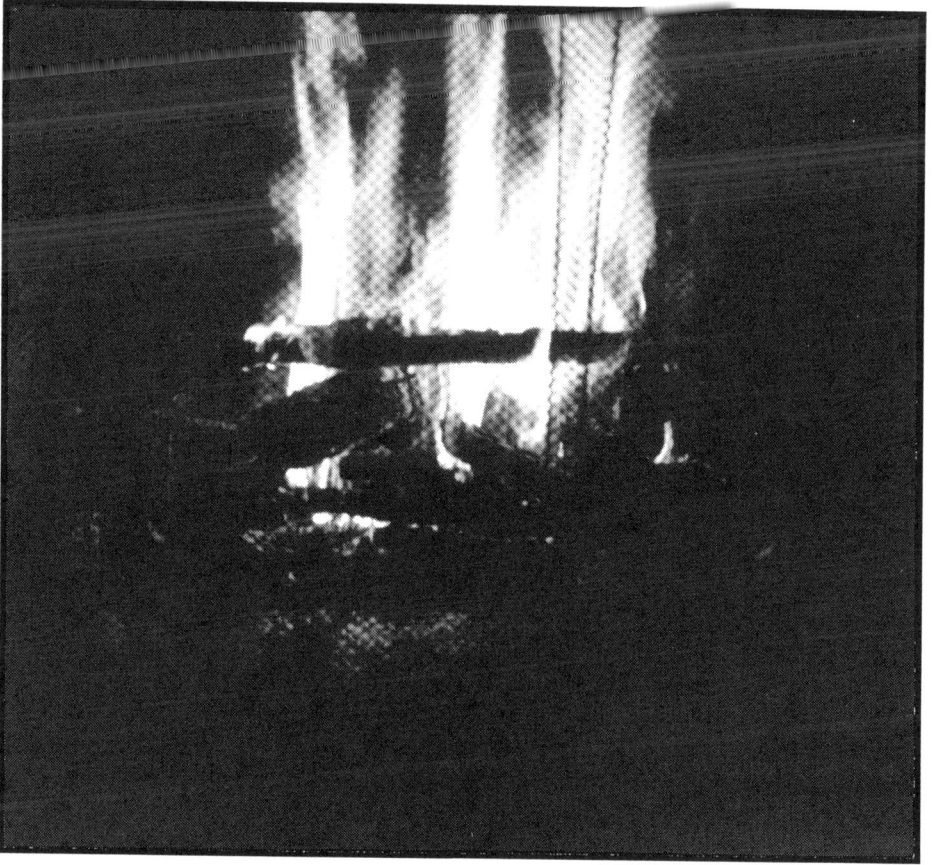

Without air, a fire will die.
With more air, you get more fire.

Without oxygen, you will die.
With more oxygen, you will enliven your body.

Power Breathing is a resource of internal power.

Power Breathing is an internal body exercise.

Power breathing is a resource of natural health that will make you healthier than you have ever been in your life. It will increase the oxygen supply to your body, increase your blood circulation, strengthen your internal organs, improve your digestion system, build up your immune system, balance your hormones, quiet your nervous system, calm your mind, and increase your energy level.

Power Breathing is the best resource of personal power (*ki*).

The Importance of Breathing

People cannot survive without food and oxygen, but there is a big difference. Almost anyone can survive two or three days without food; some can go ten days, twenty days, or longer. No one can survive ten minutes without oxygen.

Breathing is a more immediate need than eating, drinking, sleeping, . . . it is more vitally important than any other activity. Being alive means you are still breathing; when you stop breathing, you are dead. Breath is the difference between life or death. Does it not make sense, then, that the way you breathe will affect the quality of your life?

Power Breathing and Health

In order to have a happy life, people need a healthy body and mind. In order to have a healthy body and mind, people need to balance the four corners of the foundation of health. These four corners are:

1. A Healthy Mental Attitude,
2. Power Breathing,
3. Natural, Nutritional Food,
4. Power Exercise.

Each of the four corners is vitally important, and must be maintained every day. If you ignore any one (or more) of the corner supports, your health will become unbalanced. Just like a building, your health needs a strong foundation. If any one of the corners is weak, the building will eventually fall.

As I explained earlier, harmony is the plan of nature. Animals breathe in oxygen and breathe out carbon dioxide. Plants don't really breathe like animals do, but they take in carbon dioxide and expel oxygen. This great natural balance insures a healthy future for all of us. If we try to go against nature, we will destroy ourselves. If we can live in harmony with nature, we can have a healthy and happy life.

Power Breathing is the natural way to breathe. It is a great gift from nature to people of all walks of life. Unfortunately, many people are ignorant or uneducated about Power Breathing. In our superficial modern society, we judge things by appearance only. We tend to think that someone with large, visible muscles is healthy. Therefore, it seems only logical that building muscle makes you healthy. I'm sorry to say that this just isn't true. Real health begins on the inside, not the outside. What good is it if you can bench press a Cadillac, but you always suffer from headaches or get out of breath before five or ten minutes of jogging or other aerobic exercise? All exercises are not created equal.

If you want to be healthy, start from the inside and work your way out. Make your internal organs healthy, so they can make the rest of you healthy.

Making Your Internal Organs Strong

Organs are made of soft muscle, not striated muscles like your arms or legs. They cannot be exercised by consciously moving them. Instead, you exercise them by moving striated muscles around them, so that they are stimulated and adjusted.

One of the simplest ways to exercise the major organs is to breathe deeply into the lower abdomen, as in Power Breathing. The downward movement of the diaphragm not only exercises these soft muscles of the abdominal organs, but massages them as well. The increased amount of oxygen and blood circulation available from the deep breathing also helps to make these organs more healthy.

Benefits of Power Breathing

1. Power Breathing is a resource of health because it can increase the concentration of oxygen in your body. How? The "normal" breath in an average adult is approximately 300 - 500 c.c.'s (about a pint). Through deep Power Breathing you can triple or even quadruple the amount of air you bring into your lungs with each breath. Doesn't it make sense that if you bring in more oxygen with each breath, you will put more oxygen into your bloodstream? The more oxygen in your bloodstream, the more oxygen available for all your muscles and organs, including the brain, so the better they will work.

Many people suffer from headaches, which are most often due to poor circulation. By increasing the oxygen supply in the blood, and the blood supply to the head, most headaches can be eliminated. Chronic diseases like asthma and high and low blood pressure can be greatly controlled through the improved circulation of oxygen in the bloodstream from Power Breathing.

2. Power Breathing is one of the four corner foundations of health, because it will strengthen your internal organs (liver, heart, spleen, lungs, kidneys, pancreas, gall bladder, stomach, small and large intestines) and improve digestion.

Power Breathing strengthens the different organs according to their different needs. The organs of the torso can be divided into two groups: the upper body organs and the lower body organs, as divided by the diaphragm. The lower body organs enjoy strength, weight, and warmth, while the upper body organs enjoy being light and cool. Again, compare the body to a building: the lower part is strong and heavy, the higher part is light. If the top is heavier than the bottom, the building will collapse.

During Power Breathing, the diaphragm moves downward and compresses the lower body organs, massaging them and making them strong. At the same time, the diaphragm opens the lungs making them airy, light, and cool, and reducing pressure on the heart. Thus, the different organs are strengthened according to their needs.

Secondly, Power Breathing improves digestion. We bring in nutrients to our bodies in only two ways: through lungs or through the stomach. There are no other natural sources of ingestion (I do not consider needles, suppositories, etc., to be natural). If your body needs something, you must either breathe it, or eat (drink) it. Doesn't it make sense that if you want to get the most out of what you eat and drink, your digestive tract must be at top efficiency?

The increased oxygen in the blood will help each organ work more efficiently, as long as that blood can get in to and out of the organs freely. The downward movement of the diaphragm during Power Breathing will compress the digestive organs, moving them and their contents around, and forcing the blood out of the organs. The upward movement of the diaphragm will move the organs and their contents around again, and cause them to fill up with clean, fresh blood. This constant movement of the organs insures even distribution of foods and digestive juices. It also serves to pump stale blood out and fresh blood in.

Indigestion, which is a problem in itself, can be greatly relieved or eliminated by Power Breathing. There are a multitude of other health problems that occur as a result of indigestion, because the body does not get its proper nutrition. These, too, can be relieved or eliminated by Power Breathing.

Digestion related problems like diarrhea and constipation can be corrected by the balancing effect of Power Breathing. Digestion related diseases like diabetes can be greatly controlled by proper (and improper) breathing.

3. Power Breathing will prevent many diseases from starting, and heal many diseases before they get too advanced through improving the immune system. How? The body has a natural defense system to ward off attacks by outside germs and viruses. This immune system can be healthy or unhealthy, like any other part of the body. If your immune system is weak, you are like a country with a weak army: ready to be conquered by the bad guys. There is an old saying that "an army travels on its stomach", which means that the soldiers need nutrition to fight. The same is true of your immune system. If you can improve the nutrition supplied to your immune system, it will be stronger and better able to defend you. Power Breathing increases the amount of oxygen in the blood stream and the efficiency of the digestive system as outlined above. It is only natural, then, that Power Breathing strengthens your immune system along with every other system in the body.

Even when you get sick or injured, Power Breathing will help you heal much faster than "normal", shallow breathing. Diseases like cancer and even AIDS can be warded off by an improved immune system.

4. Power Breathing can improve your nervous system and restore your hormone balance. Think a moment: what is the difference between a nervous person and a calm person? A nervous person is constantly moving, very quickly darting and jabbing from here to there, usually without focus, confusing himself and those around him. A calm person wastes no movement; he is focused, and everything seems to flow smoothly like water. Shallow breathing is quick and short -- the breath of a nervous person. Power Breathing is deep and regular.

Our bodies follow the patterns we design. If we want to be nervous, easily agitated, and on an emotional roller coaster, we should breath quick, shallow breaths. If we want to be calm, even tempered, and peaceful, we should practice Power Breathing.

Life in the 20th and 21st centuries makes us nervous: nervous about our job or business, nervous about sickness, nervous about relationships, nervous about being nervous! This kind of lifestyle is nerve-wracking, and takes it's toll. We become generally uncomfortable, apprehensive, or even painfully terrified. If we cannot fight back, we will have lots of problems. Fear and apprehension cause a release of adrenaline, which stimulates the body for quick reaction to danger. If the danger is not physical, there is no appropriate physical quick reaction to use up the energy, so the body races without going anywhere. We create a hormone imbalance. When we repeatedly feel this apprehension, we repeatedly stimulate the flow of adrenaline, and deplete the adrenal glands. This depletion creates further imbalance. We end up creating weakness and sickness in our otherwise healthy bodies.

Fortunately, we can fight back against nervous living with Power Breathing. When most people face a frightening situation, the adrenaline starts to flow, they breathe short, shallow breaths, and their heart rate increases dramatically. In the first place, Power Breathing can calm you to the point that you are not easily frightened, and stop the adrenaline before it starts. Secondly, even if you become frightened, you can reverse the situation quickly. By consciously taking slow, deep breaths, you slow down your heart rate, calm your mind, and remove the stimulation for the flow of adrenaline. By also increasing the amount of oxygen in the bloodstream and improving the circulation through the diaphragm movement, you will become physically strong and mentally calm once again. Your body will return to its proper rhythms, and your hormones can maintain their natural, healthy balance. Once your body is balanced and calm, diseases and symptoms of nervous tension (like rashes and headaches) will disappear.

5. Power Breathing will increase your energy level, which will improve your strength and stamina. When you increase the amount of oxygen available to the muscles, they can work harder and longer. If, at the same time, you increase the other nutrients necessary for activity, the muscles not only work better, they can recover and grow more quickly. You will have more energy throughout the day, and feel better and more confident in your physical abilities. It will also increase your sexual energy, which you may use in a personal relationship, or re-direct to any passionate or creative act.

6. Power Breathing will give you peace of mind through improved health and a positive mental attitude. The brain, like any other organ, cannot work at peak efficiency without the proper nutrients. When you practice Power Breathing, your brain gets an increased supply of fresh blood, full of oxygen and well-digested nutrients as described above. In addition, the deeper breaths necessarily reduce the number of breaths per minute, slowing down your breathing rhythm. Slower breathing rhythm means a slower -- and, therefore, more relaxed -- body rhythm. When you consciously breathe in Power Breathing, you direct your attention to the action of breathing and away from other distractions. This simple concentration will help you relax your mind. The combination of physical slowing of body rhythms and mental concentration will relax your mind and give it peace. When you are more relaxed and peaceful, you will have a more positive mental attitude.

Stress related problems (headaches, back aches, stomach aches, ulcers, high blood pressure, nervous tension, constipation, and hormone imbalance) can be reduced or eliminated by Power Breathing. As these problems disappear, your attitude will naturally become more and more positive.

7. Power Breathing will improve the quality of your life. In the first place, you will be healthier, with fewer headaches, indigestion problems, colds, etc., to slow you down. You will have more energy to get more done every day. Second, your mind will be sharper and more alert to possibilities. You will be less stressed and more focused on the tasks at hand. Because you feel better, you will look better, and have a more positive attitude. You will have more energy to share with others, both for pursuit of happiness and for productive work. You will be able to enjoy what you are doing and advance and improve.

If you are a student, you will be able to get better grades. If you are an employee, you will have more confidence to bring into your relationship with your co-workers. You will be valuable to your boss and popular amongst your co-workers. If you are an employer, you will have more energy and fresh ideas to make your company grow. Power Breathing is good for your company, good for your individual performance, and good for your personal life.

8. Power Breathing will also help your professional life. Of course, it depends on your profession as to exactly how Power Breathing will help, but it will help almost everyone

A. Anyone who has to use his voice in his job -- a public speaker like a politician, evangelist, motivational speaker, talk show host, announcer, reporter, and especially a singer -- needs Power Breathing to improve his voice. Not only a public speaker, but a professional like a salesman, a teacher, a receptionist, a martial arts instructor, and anyone else who depends on his voice professionally or even personally, needs to practice Power Breathing.   When you practice deep, diaphragmatic, Power Breathing, your voice will be deeper and more powerful. You will create a better, more respect-inspiring image, as well as reduce the stress on your vocal chords. When you speak from your abdomen, you should never "lose your voice" due to extensive speaking like President Clinton did during the 1992 election.

B. Anyone who has to use his body in his job -- a construction worker, an athlete (amateur or professional), a martial arts or other fitness instructor, a garbage collector, a waitress -- needs Power Breathing to keep his body in top condition. Power Breathing not only makes the body stronger and more efficient due to improved circulation and oxygen intake, it makes the body more injury resistant. By calming the body and mind, Power Breathing also allows people to concentrate on their physical performance and clear away excess mental baggage that might interfere or even cause injury. Power Breathing will help you achieve better physical performance and quicker improvement.

Different Ways to Breathe

First of all, you must understand that unconscious breathing is very different from conscious breathing. Unconscious breathing is automatic, and, as I said earlier, the average person only breathes about 300 to 500 c.c.'s of air. Conscious breathing is intentional, and can utilize the full lung capacity, usually from 1000 to 1500 c.c.'s. If you are good with numbers, you can see that most people only use about one-third of their lung capacity in unconscious breathing.

It's not that they only fill up their lungs one-third of the way. It is more accurate that they fill up their lungs two-thirds of the way or more, but never exhale all the way. That leaves roughly the bottom one-third of the lung that never gets cleaned out. That's a lot of stale air. Even if one of these people would consciously take a full breath and fill the lungs up completely, chances are good he would not breathe all the way out and not clean out the stale "dregs". It is not a difficult thing to do, it just is not a developed habit, so it is only done with a conscious effort.

Second, you must realize that there are several kinds of breathing:

1. Chest Breathing
2. Abdominal Breathing
3. Chest and Abdominal Breathing
4. Power Breathing

Chest Breathing is the most common form of breathing among modern adults, and it is the worst of the four. Chest Breathing is necessarily shallow breathing and does not allow enough gas exchange. It does not allow you to clean the stale gasses out of your lungs; it does not allow enough oxygen into the body; it creates short temper; it decreases blood circulation; it decreases the function of all the internal organs; it decreases the effectiveness of the immune system; and it decreases your lifestyle. It is only good for the germs and viruses that want to infect you.

Abdominal Breathing is the natural resting breath for human beings. If you have ever watched a baby breathe, it breathes with its lower abdomen. You can watch the stomach fill and empty like a little balloon. Most modern adults have lost this natural way of breathing and replaced it with shallow, Chest Breathing. I believe the reason is that our high-technology world has made life too easy for us. Everything is automatic: dishwashers, clothes washers, automobiles, elevators, even t.v.'s have remote control switchers. We don't have to move to do anything! When we don't move, we don't need as much oxygen, so our breathing gets lazy. Unfortunately, our bodies need the deep breathing to remain healthy, just as they need the exercise to remain healthy. We need to consciously reverse this trend and return to Abdominal Breathing.

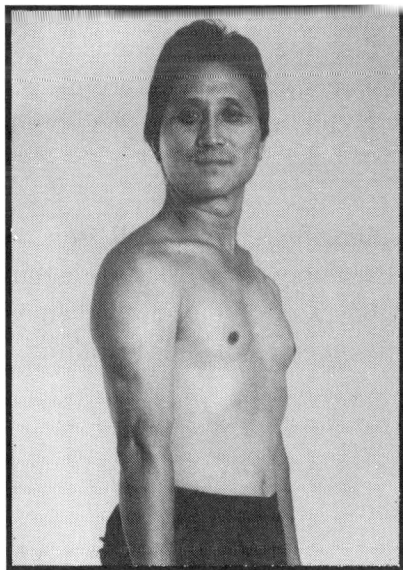

Normal

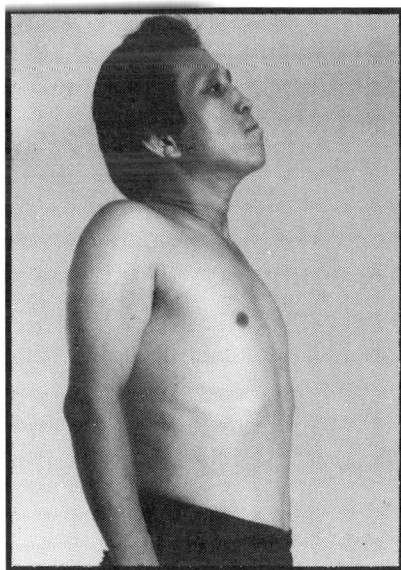

Chest inhale

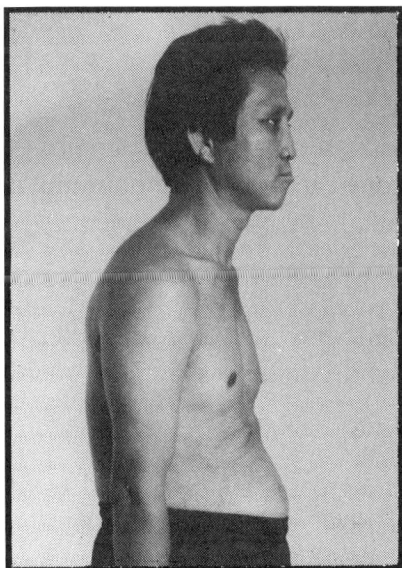

Abdominal inhale

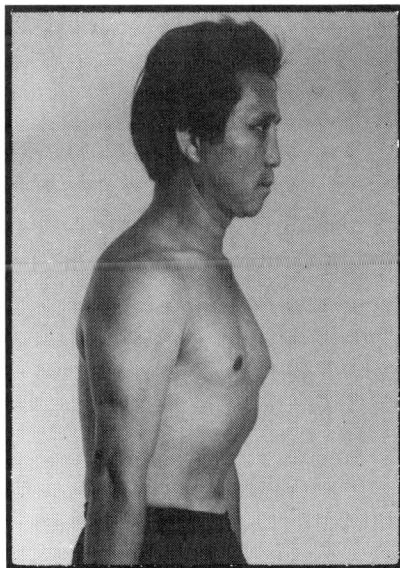

Abdominal exhale

Chest and Abdominal Breathing is a full, deep breath. In Abdominal Breathing we do not always fill up the chest. We use the bottom of the lungs, but we do not use the full top of the lungs. In Chest and Abdominal Breathing, we incorporate both breathing methods to get a full, deep breath. It is the kind of breath we use when we are exerting ourselves physically. It is a very healthy breathing, but not one you can use all of the time.

Power Breathing is the best breathing because it will give you personal power. It utilizes Abdominal Breathing plus Chest Breathing, plus more. By tightening the right combination of muscles when you breathe, you can increase the power and effectiveness of your breathing.

How to Begin Power Breathing

There are two different ways to practice Power breathing:

1. Stationary Power Breathing, and

2. Dynamic Power Breathing.

Stationary breathing is breathing without moving from one place or position to another. It is obvious that no one can breathe without moving at all, but stationary breathing does not entail any extra movement -- just the movements necessary to breathe.

Dynamic breathing is breathing while moving. For example, you could perform dynamic Power Breathing while walking, practicing martial arts, or otherwise exercising.

Both kinds of Power Breathing are a great resource of health, with different strong points and special benefits. I have combined them together into one simple, practical, and beneficial way to learn about breathing. In order that you might understand the different levels and complexities of breathing, I have divided Power Breathing into three different levels, with three levels within each level:

1. Basic Power Breathing 1, 2, and 3.

2. Intermediate Power Breathing 1, 2, and 3.

3. Advanced Power Breathing 1, 2, and 3.

When Power Breathing, you can practice lying down, seated on the floor or in a chair, or standing. You could also practice in any of these positions in different places (i.e., seated in a car, standing in an elevator, standing while walking down the street, etc.) No matter what position, the best and most beneficial breath is

1. Deeper
2. Longer
3. Gentler
4. Quieter
5. Smoother.

Second, you must understand the flow of energy within your body. Eastern medicine is not based only on chemical reactions that can be reproduced in laboratories, as is Western medicine. Eastern medicine is based on energy flow. The energy flows along channels (sometimes called meridians), and gathers around centers (sometimes called *chakras*). Most authorities identify many energy centers (usually seven), but I find that depth unnecessary for the average person. I will only concentrate on the three main energy centers, which, for simplicity, I will call the low, middle, and high energy centers.

The lower energy center (*ha dan jun*) is located one hand's width below and behind your navel. It is your foundation and the center for your physical strength and stamina. The middle energy center (*joong dan jun*) is located about one fist's depth behind your *solar plexus*. It is the emotional center. The high energy center (*sang dan jun*) is located just behind the middle point between your eyebrows, and is sometimes called the third eye. It is the spiritual center.

Ki Energy Centers
Physical Center

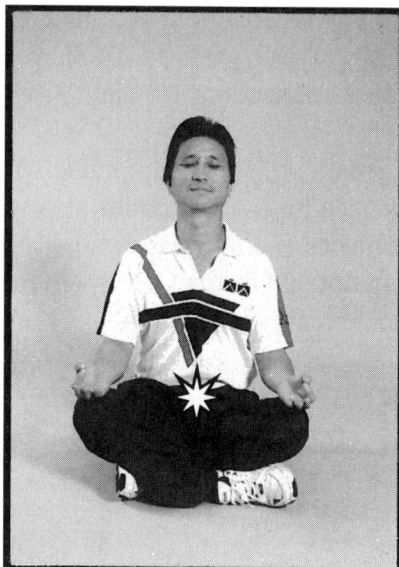

Lower Energy Center
(ha dan jun)

Emotional Center

Spiritual Center

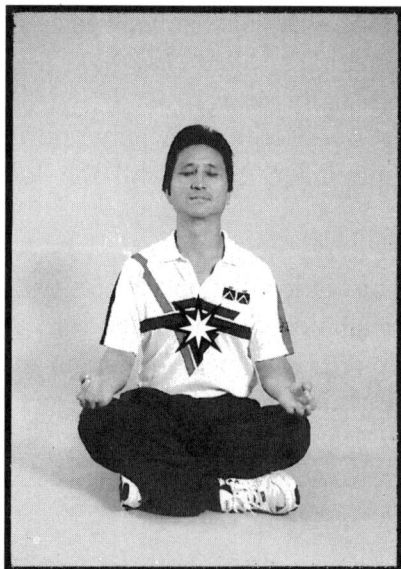

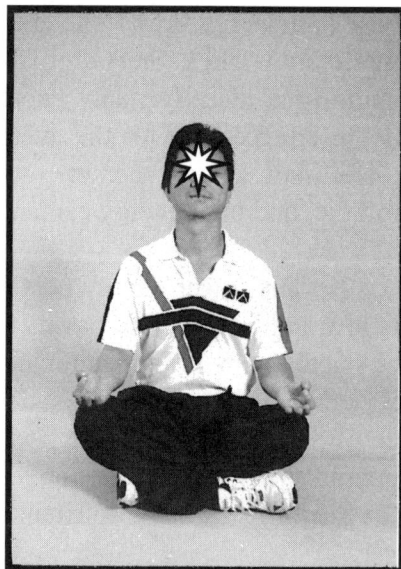

Middle Energy Center
(joong dan jun)

High Energy Center
(sang dan jun)

Basic breathing #1

Basic breathing #1 is retraining to return to abdominal breathing. In order to get the feeling of breathing by extending and contracting the lower abdomen, we will use our hands as a training device to move the lower abdomen.

Preparation:

From a standing position:

1. Assume ready stance (feet shoulder width apart).

2. Loosen up your whole body and mind, including your muscles, joints, and mental tension. (This step is even more important than learning how to breathe.)

3. Straighten your whole body, so that you are equal and balanced from left to right, front to back, and top to bottom. Your center of balance should be your lower energy center, but be careful not to tense any part of your body.

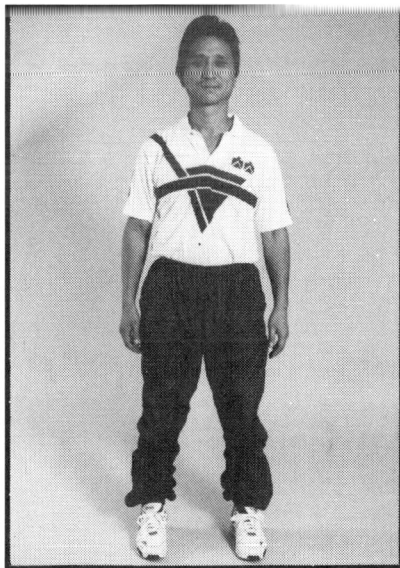

1, 2

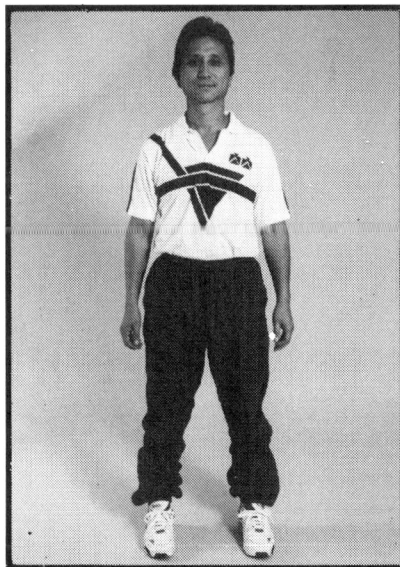

3

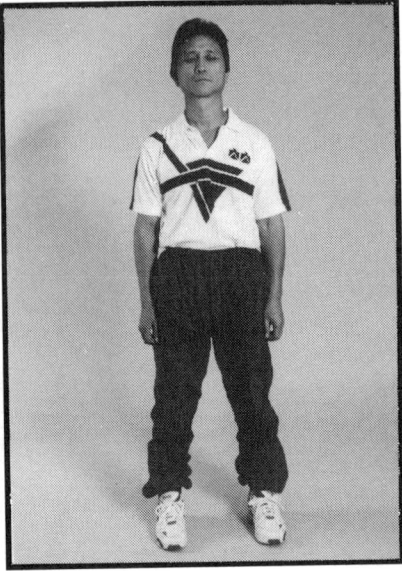

4

4. Slightly close your eyes so that you can barely see. Because your attention will be naturally drawn to things that you see, try not to see anything, so that your mind can go blank without going to sleep.

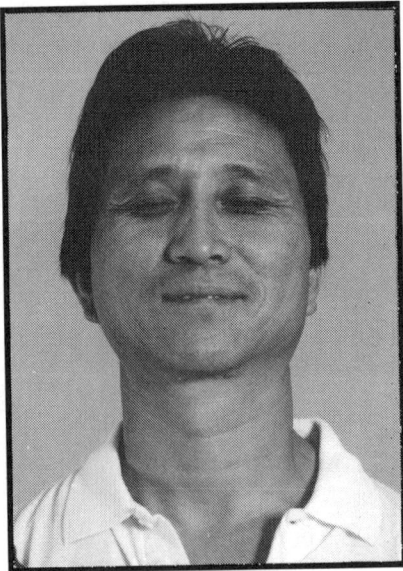

5

5. Maintain a pleasant smile. It will loosen up your face muscles and give you peace of mind.

How to do it:

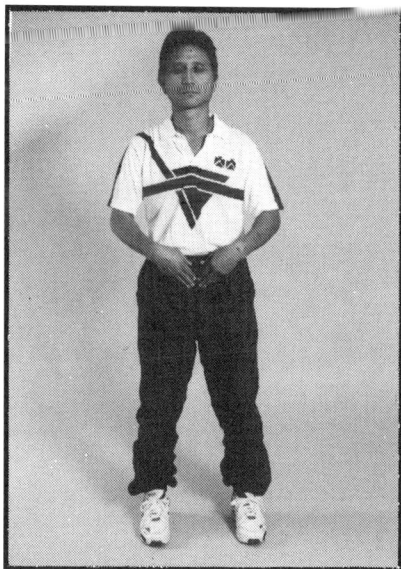

A. Place both your hands on your lower abdomen.

A

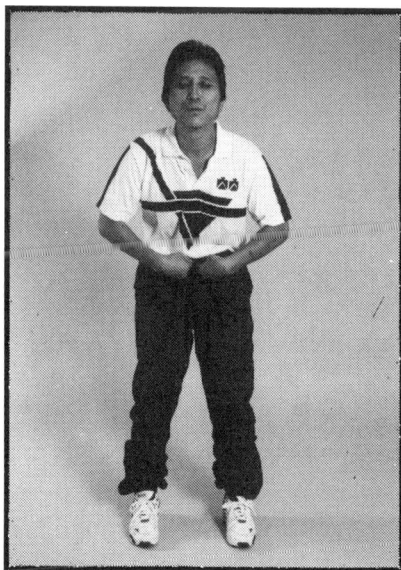

B. Slightly open your mouth and exhale while you use your hands to push in your stomach and bend forward a little bit.

B

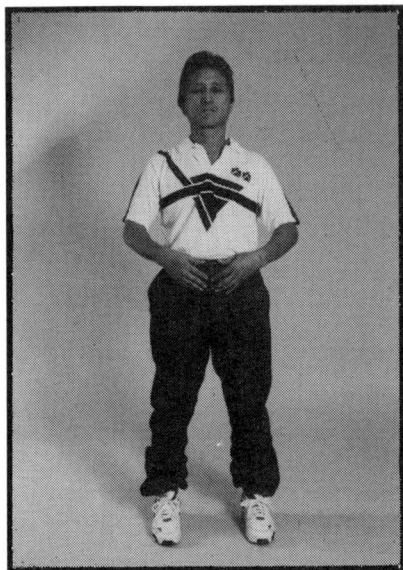

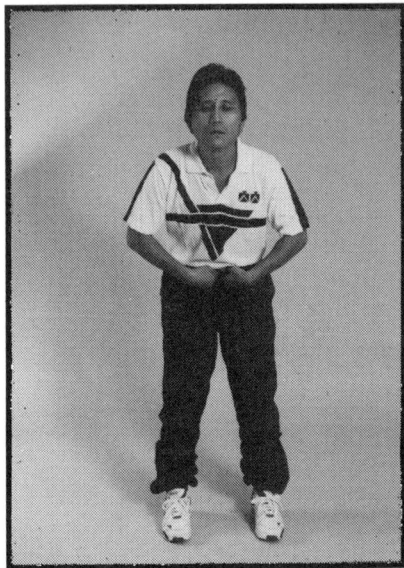

C, D, E   F

C. Intentionally push out your lower abdomen as you straighten your body.

D. Inhale through the nose for three seconds.

E. Hold your breath for three seconds while keeping your abdomen extended.

F. Slightly open your mouth and exhale for three seconds while you push in with your hands and bend forward a little bit.

G. Repeat C through F between five and ten times.

Benefits:

This breathing exercise will:

* increase the supply of oxygen to the body by opening your alveoli (air sacs in your lungs) to allow more oxygen to come in and more carbon dioxide to go out.

* increase the blood circulation throughout the body by squeezing the abdominal organs, which will help pump the blood through the system, making the heart's job easier.

* calm the mind due to the increased oxygen and fresh blood supply to the brain, and the increased carbon dioxide and stale blood moved out.

* strengthen the abdominal muscles through exercise.

* massage the liver and other abdominal organs, due to the downward movement of the diaphragm, which will improve digestion.

* increase energy, strength, and stamina from the natural energy sources of the sun, air, and ground (see page 83).

* release stress and tension.

* build up a strong immune system to prevent you from getting diseases and to help cure diseases that you already have.

When you start, you will probably feel awkward, but continue to practice. When most adults try to do abdominal breathing for the first time, they extend the top of the abdomen, or maybe the middle of the abdomen. Do not get frustrated. It took you many years to forget how to breathe properly, so it may take a little while to remember the correct way. Eventually, you will be able to breathe into the very bottom of your abdomen.

Once you learn the feeling of slow, relaxed breathing (three seconds inhale, three seconds hold, three seconds exhale) you can listen to the rhythm of your own body. Some people can move to a four-four-four rhythm, others may be able to maintain a twelve-twelve-twelve rhythm, or even longer. Do whatever is comfortable for you. You want to breathe as slowly as possible without straining yourself.

When you start as a beginner, attempt to advance slowly. The first time you try basic breathing, you may get dizzy from only the first five to ten breaths. Instead of trying to practice one time for too long, practice for a short time more often. When you feel comfortable with basic breathing #1, slowly build up the number of times you breathe in each practice session until you can do from thirty to one hundred deep breaths in a row. Advancement is completely individual, but an average person can spend about ten to twenty days learning Basic Breathing to the point that Abdominal Breathing comes back as a natural habit, and the hands are no longer needed as a training device.

Practice for five to ten minutes, three times a day: in the morning, during the day, and in the evening. It is not good to practice breathing exercises on a full stomach, so if you are going to coordinate Power Breathing with meal times, do the Power Breathing before you eat, or at least one hour afterward. It is also not good to practice breathing exercises on a totally empty stomach, when you are so hungry that you can't concentrate.

You can practice this breathing anywhere, anytime. Do not worry what other people think, because your health is more important than their narrow mindedness. Do not stop practicing Basic Power Breathing #1 until your natural breathing habit returns the way it was when you were a baby. If you stop practicing Power Breathing it means two things:

1. You have given up on yourself.

2. You are weakening your body and waiting to get sick, so you can be a bother to your family and friends.

58

Be patient and continue practicing Basic Breathing. It will be great for you. After ten to twenty days you will be able to feel some improvements in your body; more energy, a more positive attitude, and more confidence.

If you have a good instructor, it is possible to learn Basic Breathing #1, #2, and #3 at the same time. I recommend that you try to find one who can guide you according to your individual ability. If you cannot find one, follow the plan in the book, but do it slowly. Only advance to Basic Breathing #2 when you have mastered #1 (you can comfortably do at least thirty breaths in a row).

Basic Breathing #2

Basic Breathing #2 is also Abdominal Breathing, but it is a cleansing breath. In basic breathing #1 you learned to push in your stomach to expel all the carbon dioxide and other stale gas. In Basic Breathing #2 you will no longer need to use your hands as a training aid. You will still concentrate on the exhaling process, learning to breathe out all the way so that you can clean out your entire body.

Most people have no problem making a mess. The problem is cleaning the mess properly. Likewise, most untrained people have no problem inhaling all the way, but they seem to have some problem exhaling completely. By emphasizing the exhaling process, you will learn to clean out all the poisons and junk from your system. By emptying your body you will prepare it to receive clean, positive, natural energy (*ki*).

Here is a simple health test to see how completely you can exhale under control:

Cleansing Breath Health Test

Directions: Exhale as long as possible for ten breaths in a row. After the first breath or two, you should stabilize at a consistent level.

If you exhale for:	your breathing development is:
5 seconds	like a baby
10 seconds	on a kindergarten level
15 seconds	on a grammar school level
20 seconds	on a junior high school level
30 seconds	on a high school level
40 seconds	on a college level
50 seconds	on a Master's Degree level
60 seconds	on a Ph.D. level

The Cleansing Breath can help heal heart disease, high blood pressure, liver cancer, diarrhea, nervous weakness, and asthma

Preparation:

The preparations for Basic Breathing #2 are the same as those for Basic Breathing #1. See pages 53 and 54 to review them.

How to do it:

A. Slightly bend your abdomen forward and purse your lips as if blowing out a candle. Exhale completely with the mouth as gently as possible, and naturally shrink your abdomen in as you breathe out for as long as possible.

B. Slightly open your chest and straighten your whole body. Inhale through the nose deeply and intentionally push out your lower abdomen.

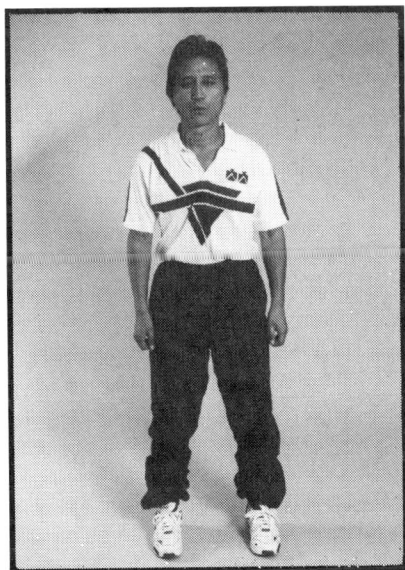

A

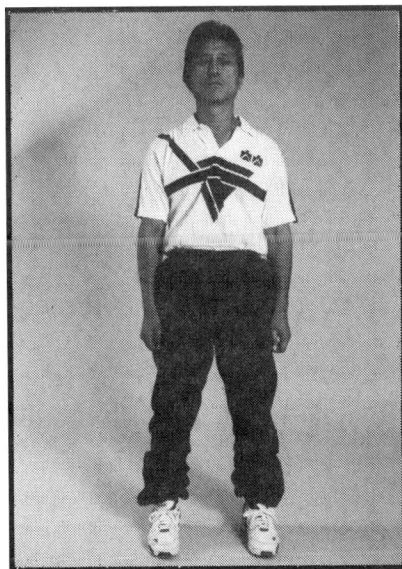

B

61

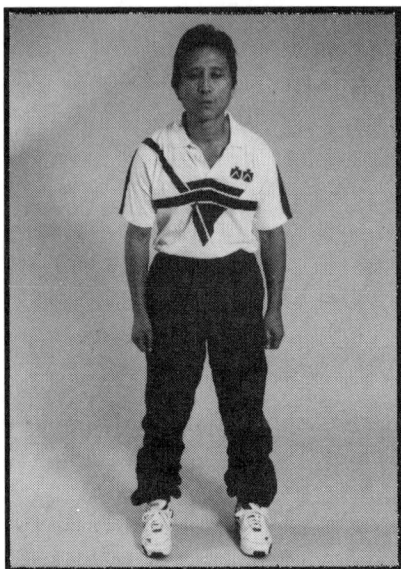

C

C. Do not hold your breath. Exhale immediately through pursed lips for as long as possible, and slowly bend slightly forward as your stomach shrinks. Imagine that you are cleaning out your whole body like a vacuum cleaner, beginning at your toes and working your way up to your head.

D. Repeat B and C between five and ten times.

Benefits:

Basic Breathing #2 has the same benefits as Basic Breathing #1, plus it will:

* clean up your entire internal body.

* help heal many major diseases.

Do not try to do too much at one time. At the beginning, practice for shorter time periods and more often. Slowly build up the number of breaths per session until you can do between thirty and one hundred breaths per session, three times a day. You can practice any where, any time; often travel time is the best: when riding in a plane, bus, or car, or walking.

You may use your nose to exhale, if you wish. Especially during the learning stage, you can control the length of your exhalation much better when you exhale through the mouth. That is why I have recommended mouth breathing as a training aid. Once you have learned the rhythm, though, you can breathe in and out through the nose without diminishing the effect and without drawing attention to yourself when practicing in a public place.

If, at any time, you feel dizzy or uncomfortable in your chest, stop and rest. Change your posture to a more comfortable position, and begin again.

Remember: you are trying to learn to exhale deeper and longer. Imprint this deep exhalation on your unconscious mind through repetition. You will soon have healthy breathing unconsciously.

Basic Breathing is the foundation. When you master Basic Breathing #2, it will be much easier to learn Basic Breathing #3, Intermediate Breathing, Advanced Breathing, and any further Power Breathing.

After ten to twenty days (maybe sooner) you will begin to feel cleaner inside. It is a new and fresh feeling, which will make you feel better about yourself. At this point you should be beginning to feel what I mean when I describe the benefits of Power Breathing. I really appreciate your patience in practicing up to this point, and I believe that now that you can begin to feel the benefits, you will be anxious to advance to Basic Breathing #3.

Basic Breathing #3

Basic breathing #3 is lower abdominal breathing or baby breathing (so called because it is how a baby naturally breathes.) We all naturally breathed this way when we were babies. If you watch a baby breathe while it sleeps, it extends its lower abdomen naturally when it inhales, and shrinks its lower abdomen when it exhales.

Breathe through the nose. The nose was designed for breathing, so use it (we use the mouth in special cases: for learning, and in those instances when we need increased air flow for exercise or cleansing).

It is important that you inhale and exhale the same amount of time. For example, if you inhale for three seconds, exhale for three seconds. You may be comfortable with five seconds, ten seconds, or more. Remember: you want to breathe as deeply and as slowly as possible without straining.

Breathing controls the autonomic nervous system. The autonomic nervous system has two parts: the sympathetic and the parasympathetic. When you pay attention to your exhalation (emphasize it by exhaling longer and stronger), you will stimulate your parasympathetic nervous system. When you pay attention to your inhalation (emphasize it by inhaling longer and stronger), you will stimulate your sympathetic nervous system.

The parasympathetic nervous system releases the flow of involuntary fluids like adrenaline and digestive juices, and dilates the blood vessels. The sympathetic nervous system stops the flow of involuntary fluids like adrenaline and digestive juices, and contracts the blood vessels. The two systems are complementary, and must work in harmony with each other. If either one is out of balance, the body will get chemically out of balance. This is why it is important to breathe in and out for the same length of time.

To put this information into perspective, let's look at an example: when you see or smell good food, especially when you are hungry, your brain automatically starts the flow of digestive juices by stimulating the parasympathetic nervous system. If you do not eat, your brain is supposed to stimulate the sympathetic nervous system to stop the flow. If your brain is tired or stressed out, it may not send the message to stop. At that point the sympathetic nervous center, which is located at the *solar plexus*, is supposed to take over on its own, realize that there is no food to digest, and stop the flow of juices. If the sympathetic nervous center is not able to function properly, due to improper circulation of blood or *ki*, again due to stress, the flow of juices does not get turned off. You end up with a stomach full of high powered acids with nothing to digest, and you begin to get stomach trouble.

Preparation:

The preparations for Basic Breathing #3 are the same as those for Basic Breathing #1. See pages 53 and 54 to review them.

How to do it:

In Basic Breathing #3, do not intentionally push out the lower abdomen when either inhaling or exhaling. Try to let your lower abdomen expand and contract naturally.

A. Exhale through the nose smoothly and count from one to seven.

B. Inhale through the nose smoothly and count from one to seven.

C. Exhale through the nose quietly and count from one to seven.

D. Inhale through the nose quietly and count from one to seven.

E. Exhale through the nose gently and count from one to seven.

F. Inhale through the nose gently and count from one to seven.

G. Exhale through the nose for a long time and count from one to ten.

H. Inhale through the nose for a long time and count from one to ten.

I. Exhale through the nose very deeply and count from one to ten.

J. Inhale through the nose very deeply and count from one to ten.

K. Repeat A through J from five to six times, breathing deeper, longer, gentler, quieter, smoother, until you can breathe to a count of at least ten for both the inhale and exhale.

Benefits:

You will receive all of the benefits of Basic Breathing #2, plus #3 will:

* balance the entire nervous system, and especially control the autonomic nervous system.

* help you achieve unconscious healthy breathing.

* give you good body balance: your lower abdomen will become full and strong while your chest will become flexible and light.

* balance your nervous system and calm your mind.

* balance your mind as your body and mind work together.

The proper speed to breathe at the beginning is to inhale for ten seconds and exhale for ten seconds, for a total of twenty seconds, or three breaths a minute. Slowly increase the length of each breath until you are inhaling and exhaling for fifteen seconds each, twenty seconds each, twenty-five seconds each, or thirty seconds each, at which point your will be breathing only one full breath per minute.

Practice at least three times a day for ten to twenty minutes. You can practice any where any time because, under normal circumstances, no one will know what you are doing. Continue to practice until you come back to the point where you breathe like a baby.

After ten to twenty days you will be able to feel how much you have improved: your digestion and other body functions will have improved so that you will have a much better appetite, you will be calm and secure, and you will have a great feeling about yourself.

I sincerely admire the effort you have made to practice Power Breathing this far. When you have mastered Basic Breathing, it is like you have graduated from elementary school, and are ready to move up to high school. Next you will learn intermediate breathing, which is very interesting and very tough. If you continue to practice as you have so far, you will continue to feel healthier and better about yourself. I know you will make it all the way.

Summary of Basic Breathing

#1. Hands on lower abdomen to learn to breathe deeper: push all the air out through the mouth, inhale through the nose, hold breath, and repeat.

#2. No hands; don't hold the breath. Inhale through the nose and exhale through the mouth for as long as possible to clean junk out of the system.

#3. Inhale through the nose and exhale through the nose for the same length of time to balance the autonomic nervous system, but deeper, longer, gentler, quieter, and smoother.

Intermediate Breathing

In intermediate breathing, you will learn to tighten your lower abdomen. By tightening your lower abdomen, you will learn to make your lower body strong and your upper body light. As I explained earlier, the dividing line between the upper body and lower body is the diaphragm. The organs above the diaphragm enjoy being airy, light and cool. The heart and lungs do not enjoy pressure or heat. The organs below the diaphragm like pressure and heat. The stomach, liver, kidneys, spleen, pancreas, bladder, intestines, etc., need pressure to help the blood flow through them properly, and need heat for protection. Should the upper body become tight and heavy, as in the case of tension localized in the shoulders and neck, the body gets out of balance, and begins to breathe chest breathing. It becomes like a building whose top is heavier than it's foundation: ready for a fall. This is what had happened to me several years ago. To maintain good body balance you need to consciously keep the upper body relaxed and cool, and the lower body strong and warm.

Intermediate breathing takes more attention to perform properly than Basic Breathing. It also can be somewhat dangerous, because the heart and lungs do not like pressure. If you hold your breath while tightening any muscles, it will put pressure on your heart. You can only tighten your lower body muscles while the breath is moving out. If you feel pressure in your chest at any time during intermediate breathing, immediately stop. Move your muscles to find where they are tight, and relax them. Only resume when you feel comfortable.

Positive reactions of better energy circulation:

* Although stationary, you will sweat. You will also be able to warm up (and even make sweat) certain parts of your body at will.

* The flow of saliva will increase in your mouth, improving digestion.

* The stomach will make noise and you will burp and "break wind" as gasses are released.

69

* Your appetite will increase because your digestion is improving.

* Your skin and hair will look rich, shiny, and colorful because of increased circulation and improved digestion.

* You will fall asleep easily and sleep deeper because breathing exercises give you a peaceful and calm mind.

* You will have sharper vision and hearing, and increased sensitivity in touch, taste, and smell.

* You will have increased sexual energy.

Some negative reactions may also occur. They are absolutely normal, so do not worry. Usually, the negative reactions come out before the positive reactions:

* Your whole body will feel tired after breathing exercises because you did not have enough exercise, or the exercise was the wrong kind. Don't worry, just loosen up your whole body before you do breathing exercises.

* You may feel dizzy. Do not worry; do not be impatient. Do not try to do too much at one time. Take your time and build up slowly to a more advanced level.

* If you feel pressure in your chest or a loud heart beat, relax. Loosen up your body, and breathe quietly and gently.

* If your lower back hurts, relax your muscles or change position to change your posture. Maybe even massage the tight muscles to loosen them up.

Generally, negative reactions happen because you did not loosen up your muscles and/or you tried to do too much too soon. Remember, when it comes to breathing exercises, SLOW AND STEADY is the rule. Follow it.

Intermediate Breathing #1

Intermediate breathing was designed to increase autonomic nervous system functions, especially the sympathetic nervous center (the *solar ploxus*), which is sometimes called the second brain. The sympathetic nervous center, or the middle energy center, is located on the bottom side of the diaphragm.

People who are unhealthy, especially overweight people, have a very tight middle energy center (*solar plexus.*) In intermediate breathing #1 we will try to relax and loosen up this area, so that it may function better. We want to keep the lower abdomen tight, while relaxing the middle energy center.

Preparation:

When Power Breathing, you can practice lying down, seated on the floor or in a chair, or standing. You could also practice in any of these positions in different places (i.e., seated in a car, standing in an elevator, standing while walking down the street, etc.,) See pages 53-54 for illustrations of the following descriptions:

1. Assume ready stance (feet shoulder width apart).

2. Loosen up your whole body and mind, including your muscles, joints, and mental tension. (This step is even more important than learning how to breathe.)

3. Straighten your whole body, so that you are equal and balanced from left to right, front to back, and top to bottom. Your center of balance should be your lower energy center, but be careful not to tense any part of your body.

4. Slightly close your eyes so that you can barely see. Because your attention will be naturally drawn to things that you see, try not to see anything, so that your mind can go blank without going to sleep.

5. Maintain a pleasant smile. It will loosen up your face muscles and give you peace of mind.

71

How to do it:

A. Place both hands on the solar plexus so that your fingers are right under the sternum and ribs. Inhale through the nose as deeply as possible.

B. Exhale through a barely opened mouth as you bend slightly forward and slowly massage the solar plexus area with your fingers to help it loosen up and relax.

C. Straighten your back bone without tightening your muscles, relax your whole body, and inhale through the nose as deeply as possible.

D. Exhale through a barely opened mouth as you bend slightly forward and massage the solar plexus area with your fingers to help it loosen up and relax. As you continue to exhale, move your hands to your lower abdomen and feel the muscles of the lower abdomen tighten just a little.

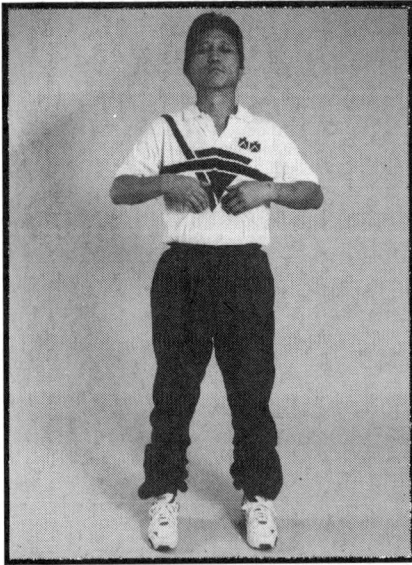

A

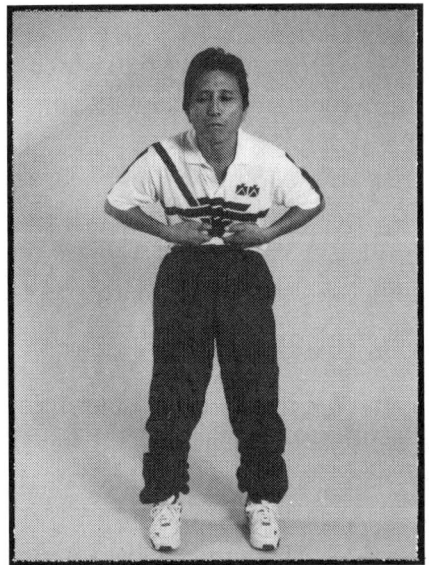

B

E. Straighten your back bone without tightening your muscles, relax your whole body, and inhale through the nose as deeply· as possible.

F. Exhale through a barely opened mouth as you bend slightly forward and massage the solar plexus area to help it loosen up and relax. As you continue to exhale, move your hands to your lower abdomen and feel the muscles of the lower abdomen tighten just a little. Also close your rectum.

G. Straighten your back bone without tightening your muscles, relax your whole body, and inhale through the nose as deeply as possible.

H. Exhale through the mouth as you bend slightly forward and massage the solar plexus area to help it loosen up and relax. As you continue to exhale, move your hands to your lower abdomen and feel the muscles of the lower abdomen tighten just a little. Close your rectum and very lightly tighten the muscles of your legs, too.

I. Repeat G and H approximately six times, increasing the intensity of the leg tightening each time.

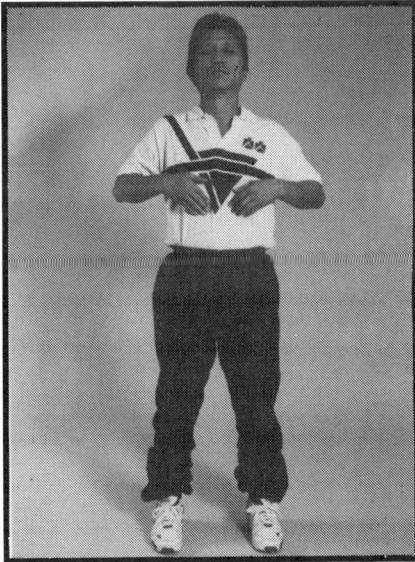

C, E, G

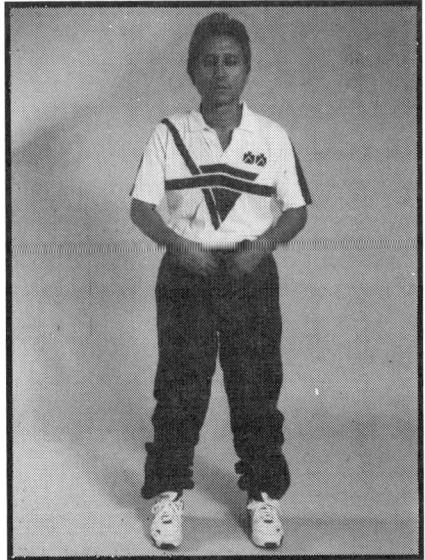

D, F, H

73

Benefits:

Intermediate breathing will give you the same benefits as Basic Breathing #3, plus it will:

* increase the functions of the sympathetic nervous center (*solar plexus*.)

* make your lower body strong and heavy and your upper body flexible and light for good balance, as well as make your body stronger and increase your circulation.

The purpose of the massage is to relax and loosen up the *solar plexus*, or sympathetic nervous center. When you drop your hands to the lower abdomen, you are trying to feel the tightness of the lower abdomen muscles. By using your hands, you should be able to feel the solar plexus area become loose while the lower abdomen becomes tight. By closing the rectum you direct the flow of energy from your lower energy center up your back. When you tighten your legs beginning with the feet, you squeeze the stale blood out of the feet, up the legs, and up to the heart and lungs, where it can be renewed and refreshed.

Try not to do too much at one time. The first time it will probably feel very awkward, but don't worry. Just go slowly and practice often. Soon it will be much easier. The important thing is not to give up. This is the best resource for strong health. When you give up, you not only give up on your own health, you give up on the people who care about you.

Do not hold your breath when you tighten your abdomen, rectum, or legs. When you first tighten your muscles, breathe very gently so as not to strain your chest and heart. As you become more accustomed to it, you may breathe with more power. Also, when you first tighten your muscles, just barely put a little tension through them; do not make them very tight. As you get accustomed to the feeling over time, you can gradually add more tension.

If you feel pressure in your chest, dizziness, pain in your back, or any other form of discomfort, stop immediately. Relax for a while, and only resume when the discomfort is gone.

Every six breaths stop Intermediate Breathing and take two or three relaxed breaths. Do not worry yourself trying to time your inhalation or exhalation, just breathe as deeply and as long as possible.

In Intermediate Breathing you will get a reaction right away to let you know if you are doing it right or not. It is very important to stop immediately if you feel discomfort. You can try to correct yourself after a short rest. If you do not feel discomfort, you are very lucky and should continue to practice. It will take some time to feel really comfortable with it.

In ten to twenty days you should feel a difference. In thirty to forty days you should be able to tell other people of the improvements you feel. After one hundred days it will be your habit. Slowly the time will come when Power Breathing becomes part of your daily life: you eat every day and you practice Power Breathing every day.

If you need any special guidance, try to find an expert in your town to teach you.

Remember: Intermediate Breathing is a little bit tough to do, but it is worth it for you. Only when you feel you have mastered Intermediate breathing #1 should you move on to #2.

Intermediate Breathing #2

Intermediate breathing #2 is complete cleansing breathing. As I mentioned earlier, many people know how to make a mess . . . it seems to come naturally. Few people know how to clean-up their mess properly. Intermediate Breathing #2 will clean out your whole internal body of carbon dioxide and other stale gasses. It is a very deep breathing, beginning down in the feet and working its way up.

In order to get so deep to clean so effectively, you must imagine or visualize what you are trying to do. Intermediate Breathing #2 involves visualization as an integral part of the breathing and cleansing process.

Preparation:

Prepare the same way you would for Intermediate Breathing #1 (see page 71).

How to do it:

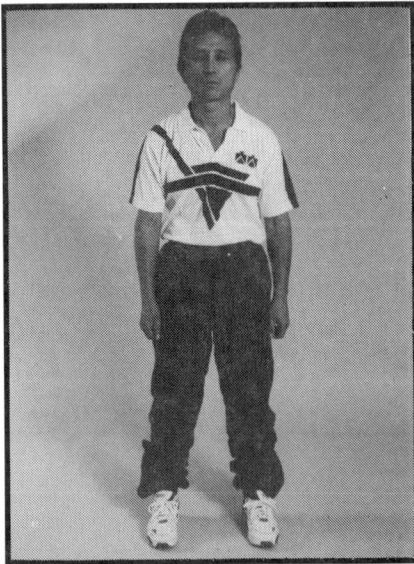

B

A. Relax and inhale through the nose as deeply as possible.

B. Exhale through a barely opened mouth as you bend slightly forward and lightly tighten your lower abdomen. You must visualize that you are cleaning out your entire body, from the foot up to the top of the head.

C. Repeat A and B until you feel comfortable with this style of breathing.

D. Straighten your back bone without tightening your muscles, relax your whole body, and inhale through the nose as deeply as possible.

E. Exhale through a barely opened mouth as you bend slightly forward and lightly tighten your lower abdomen and close your rectum. Again, visualize that you are cleaning out your entire body, from the foot up to the top of the head.

F. Repeat D and E until you feel comfortable with this style of breathing.

G. Straighten your back bone without tightening your muscles, relax your whole body, and inhale through the nose as deeply as possible.

H. Exhale through the mouth as you bend slightly forward and lightly tighten your lower abdomen and close your rectum. Also very lightly tighten the muscles of your legs, too. Continue to visualize that you are cleaning out your entire body, from the foot up to the top of the head.

I. Repeat G and H approximately six times, increasing the intensity of the leg tightening each time.

J. Return to normal, relaxed breathing for a minute or two.

K. Repeat A through J.

Benefits:

Intermediate Breathing #2 will give you all the benefits of Intermediate Breathing #1, plus it will:

* completely clean out all the junk from your body, from your feet to your head, and put in fresh energy.

* help you feel lighter and more closely connected with nature.

* give extra support to the healing of many modern sicknesses.

* completely release internal stress and tension.

Practice only steps A, B, and C until you are very comfortable with this new feeling. When you have become accustomed to tightening your lower abdomen and visualizing the cleansing process, add steps D, E, and F until you become comfortable with them. Eventually, you will be able to practice only G, H, and I as Intermediate Breathing #2.

Do not try to do too much at one time. Breathe out as long as possible: ten seconds, twenty seconds, sixty seconds, or longer, and inhale as deeply as possible. Practice three times a day for ten to twenty minutes. Within ten to twenty days you should feel a difference. After twenty to forty days you will feel like you can fly. After one hundred days it will be second nature to you.

Do not hold your breath while you tighten your abdomen, rectum, or legs. When you first tighten your muscles, breathe very gently so as not to strain your chest and heart. As you become more accustomed to it, you may breathe with more power. Also, when you first tighten your muscles, just barely put a little tension through them; do not make them very tight. As you get accustomed to the feeling over time, you can gradually add more tension.

If you feel pressure in your chest, dizziness, pain in your back, or any other form of discomfort, stop immediately. Relax for a while, and only resume when the discomfort is gone.

If you need any special guidance, try to find an expert in your town to teach you.

Intermediate Breathing #3

Intermediate Breathing #3 is the same as #2, except that you will be breathing through the nose, increasing the length of each breath, increasing the number of breathing sets, and inhaling and exhaling for the same amount of time. Remember to breathe deeper, longer, gentler, quieter, and smoother.

As I said earlier, we only breathe through the mouth for special purposes, like learning. Once we have learned, we can breathe through the nose as our bodies were designed to do.

Preparation:

Prepare the same way you would for Intermediate Breathing #1 (see page 71).

How to do it:

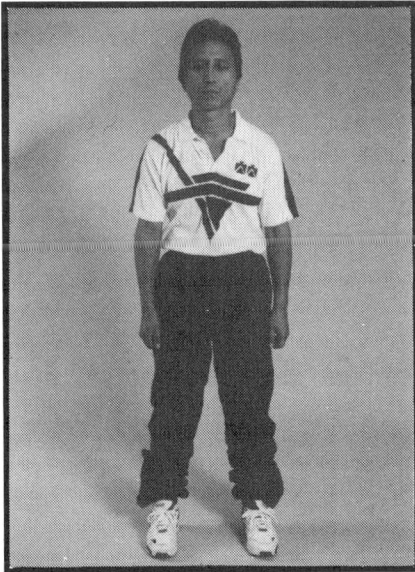

B

A. Relax and inhale through the nose as deeply as possible for at least ten seconds.

B. Exhale through a barely opened mouth for at least ten seconds as you bend slightly forward and lightly tighten your lower abdomen. You must visualize that you are cleaning out your entire body, from the foot up to the top of the head.

C. Repeat A and B until you feel comfortable with this style of breathing.

D. Straighten your back bone without tightening your muscles, relax your whole body, and inhale through the nose as deeply as possible for at least ten seconds.

E. Exhale through a barely opened mouth for at least ten seconds as you bend slightly forward and lightly tighten your lower abdomen and close your rectum. Again, visualize that you are cleaning out your entire body, from the foot up to the top of the head.

F. Repeat D and E until you feel comfortable with this style of breathing.

G. Straighten your back bone without tightening your muscles, relax your whole body, and inhale through the nose as deeply as possible.

H. Exhale through the mouth as you bend slightly forward and lightly tighten your lower abdomen and close your rectum. Also very lightly tighten the muscles of your legs, too, beginning at the foot and moving up to the hips. Continue to visualize that you are cleaning out your entire body, from the foot up to the top of the head.

I. Repeat G and H approximately six times, increasing the intensity of the leg tightening each time.

J. return to normal, relaxed breathing for a minute or two.

K. Repeat A through J.

Benefits:

You will get the same benefits as Intermediate Breathing #2, plus it will:

* completely increase the autonomic nervous system functions and calm the entire nervous system.

* completely relax your entire internal body from the bottom of your feet to the top of your head.

* strongly imprint Power Breathing on your unconscious mind for healthy breathing habits.

* further prevent many unnecessary sicknesses.

Practice only steps A, B, and C until you are very comfortable with this new feeling. When you have become accustomed to lengthening your breaths, add steps D, E, and F until you become comfortable with them. Eventually, you will be able to practice only G, H, and I as Intermediate Breathing #3.

Do not try to do too much at one time. As you practice, you may be able to inhale and exhale for fifteen or twenty seconds at a time. Slowly build up to twenty-five, thirty, sixty seconds or longer. Just be sure the inhalation is the same length as the exhalation and that you do not push yourself too far. Practice three times a day for ten to twenty minutes.

Do not hold your breath while you tighten any muscles; it strains the heart. For better relaxation you may tighten muscles as you inhale. Please see Relaxation Meditation (pp. 173-177) for more details.

If you want more knowledge and greater comfort in Power Breathing, go back to Basic Breathing to learn and practice it all over again. I have done this many times, and I continue to review and practice my basics in order to advance.

Practice Basic and Intermediate Power Breathing when you are exercising. Combining the two increases the benefits of both.

Once again, I really admire the patience and effort you have shown to reach this level. I want to ask you once more to share what you have learned and gained with your family, friends, co-workers, classmates, and neighbors. This resource of health is a great gift from nature.

Do not attempt to move on to Advanced Breathing until you have mastered Intermediate #3.

Summary of Intermediate Breathing:

Intermediate #1 - massage the *solar plexus*, and very lightly tighten the lower abdomen, close the rectum, and tighten the legs.

Intermediate #2: - visualize that you are cleaning out the entire body while you exhale through mouth for as long as possible and very lightly tighten the lower abdomen, close the rectum, and tighten the legs. Exhale for a longer period of time than you inhale.

Intermediate #3 - visualize that you are cleaning out the entire body while you exhale through nose and very lightly tighten the lower abdomen, close the rectum, and tighten the legs. Inhale and exhale for the same length of time.

Advanced Breathing

Advanced Breathing is *ki* or energy breathing. *Ki* breathing is mental breathing, in which you mentally visualize and direct your energy, or *ki*, to a specific location. You can draw *ki*, or energy, from the earth (*chi ki*), air (*dae ki*), and sun or sky (*chun ki*), and store it in your lower energy center.

In the West, we are materialistic, and we believe in only what we can see or touch. When we think of energy, we think of electricity, or of visible sources of energy like gasoline for cars and food for people. In the East, we are more spiritual, and believe in many things we cannot see or touch, as long as we can feel them. For example, heat is a very real form of energy that can be measured, but it is not a physical "thing" that can be seen or touched. It can be easily felt, though. Let's take this one step farther -- think about your favorite dessert: you can probably feel your mouth begin to water; or, as I suggested before, think of a sexual fantasy: you can probably feel the flow of energy in your sexual organs. When you get energy or an actual physical reaction from nowhere but your mind, you are experiencing *ki*.

When ministers and other holy men heal people with the touch of a hand, they are using *ki*. They say the power comes from God. I do not disagree with them; my purpose is not to discover the ultimate source of the power, but to help you understand it so that you can utilize it to make and keep yourself healthy. This healing energy is the same energy that passes from a mother to quiet a frightened child. Children love to be touched because they receive a minute but very real transfer of energy from their parents. This same energy is *ki*. When it is gathered up and intensified, and then directed to a specific area, *ki* can heal many more complicated diseases.

Every living thing on this earth has *ki*. When it loses its *ki*, it will die. A live body and a dead body are chemically the same. The difference is not a measurable amount of any chemical that has been added or taken away. The difference is the process of life or the flow of energy (which can be measured in heart beats or brain waves).

When your flow of *ki* is strong, you have health and confidence. When you are sad or sick, your flow of *ki* is weak. We get *ki* from three different sources:

1. We are born with it.

2. We get it from food.

3. We get it from the air.

Food is not *ki*, but food contains *ki*. Even if the plant or animal has died, it contains a certain amount of *ki* that keeps it fresh. When it is rotten, it has lost almost all of its *ki*. Likewise, oxygen is not *ki*, but oxygen contains *ki*. When a living creature breathes oxygen or eats food, it can extract energy from them.

It is time that we combine the Eastern and Western cultures to make a global culture that takes the best of both worlds. In this way we can truly make a healthier, stronger, and happier life.

Advanced Breathing #1

Advanced Breathing #1 develops your ability to receive *ki*, or energy, from the air (*dae ki)* and store it in your lower energy center (*ha dan jun*). In order to learn to do this, you must clearly visualize that you are receiving strong *ki* from the air and cleaning out all the weak *ki* from your body.

Preparation:

When Power breathing, you can practice lying down, seated on the floor or in a chair, or standing. You could also practice in any of these positions in different places (i.e., seated in a car, standing in an elevator, standing while walking down the street, etc.,)

Wear loose and comfortable clothing. Take off your hat and glasses, if you are wearing them. Try to arrange a time and a place where you won't be interrupted.

1. Sit in a comfortable position. Join the tips of the thumb and index finger of each hand together in a circle. Place the back of the palm of each hand on its respective knee.

2. Loosen up your whole body and mind, including your muscles, joints, and mental tension. (This step is even more important than learning how to breathe).

3. Straighten your body, so that you are equal and balanced from left to right, front to back, and top to bottom. Your center of balance should be your lower energy center, but be careful not to tense any part of your body.

4. Slightly close your eyes so that you can barely see. Because your attention will be naturally drawn to things that you see, try not to see anything, so that your mind can go blank without going to sleep.

5. Maintain a pleasant smile. It will loosen up your face muscles and give you peace of mind.

For Advanced breathing, I recommend the seated position. You may sit however you are comfortable, as long as the back remains straight. You may sit in a chair, especially if you have bad knees. If you sit on the floor, cross your legs in what we call *jung ja*. If you are flexible, you can put one leg on top of the other in the half-lotus, or *ban ka bu ja* position. If you are very flexible, you can put both legs on top of each other in the full lotus or *ka bu ja* position.

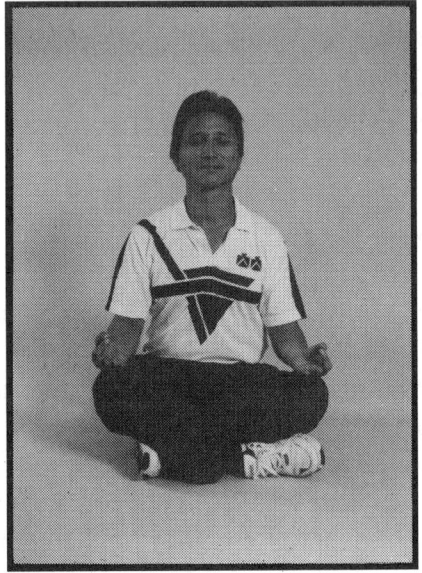

jung ja

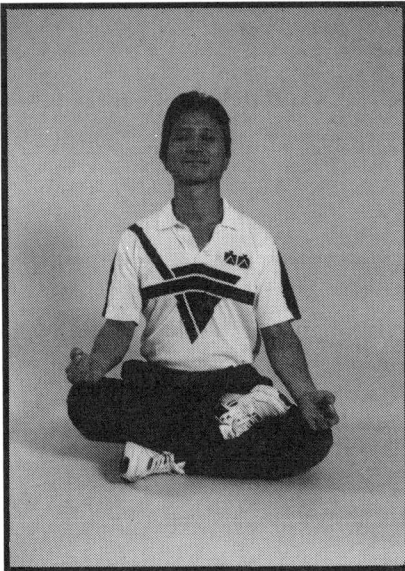

ban ka bu ja

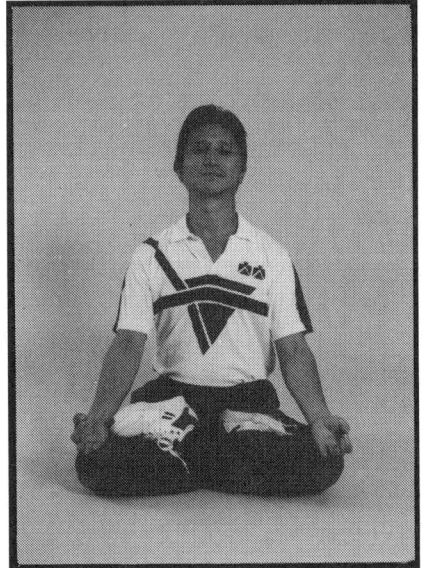

ka bu ja

How to do it:

A. Exhale through the nose, intentionally making a clear mental picture that you are expelling from your body all the weak *ki*, which will take all the junk with it.

B. Inhale through the nose, intentionally making a clear mental picture that you are drawing *dae ki* from the air through the crown of your head and drawing it into your lower energy center.

C. Repeat A and B between ten and twenty times so that you get a clear mental picture of directing and storing the *ki* in your lower energy center. You should get a warm and full feeling in your lower abdomen.

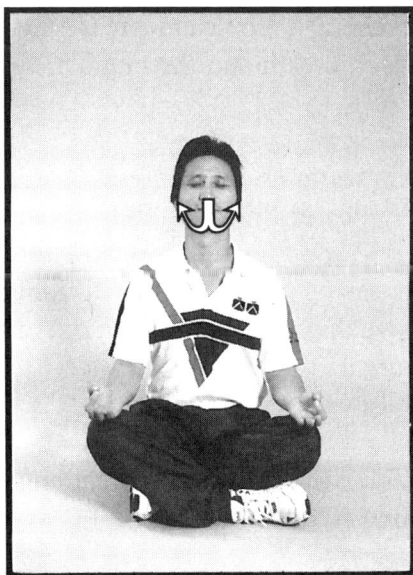

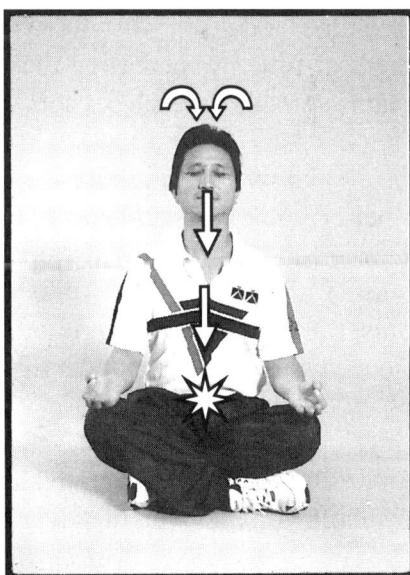

A   B

Benefits:

You will get all the benefits of Intermediate breathing #3, plus Advanced Breathing will:

* increase your physical power.

* increase your mental power.

* improve your immune system even more through the power of *ki*.

The lower energy center (*ha dan jun*) is the center of your physical strength. You do not breathe air directly into your lower energy center; you breathe air into the lungs, which infuses the blood, which goes to the lower abdomen. You can, however, breathe *ki* directly to any part of the body. If you fill up the lower energy center like a storage tank, it will supply *ki* to the rest of the body. When you store a lot of *ki* in your lower energy center, you feel like you are full of strength. It will help balance your lower and upper body.

Practice Advanced Power Breathing #1 for five to ten minutes, three times a day, or whenever you need the energy. You can increase the length of time by increasing the length of each breath and the number of breaths you take in each session.

I know that the first time you read this section it will be pretty hard to believe that you can learn to control *ki* by Power Breathing, but if you practice for a while <u>as if it were true</u>, you will soon be able to feel it for yourself, and then you will believe more easily. Soon you will find yourself trying to explain it to others. I believe that sooner or later modern science will find a way to identify and measure it.

Only when you feel really comfortable with Advanced Breathing #1 should you move on to Advanced Breathing #2.

Advanced Breathing #2

Advanced breathing #2 is an intense visualization of the flow of *ki*. You will draw the energy from several sources and direct it to different places. *Ki* is all around us and readily accessible. We can get energy from the earth (*chi ki*), the air (*dae ki*), and the sun or sky (*chun ki*). Read the meditation section (pp. 178-188) for a more detailed description of the sources of *ki*.

Preparation:

Prepare the same way you would for Advanced Breathing #1 (see page 85).

How to do it:

A. Exhale through the nose, intentionally making a clear mental picture that you are expelling from your body all the weak *ki*, which will take all the junk with it, through your head.

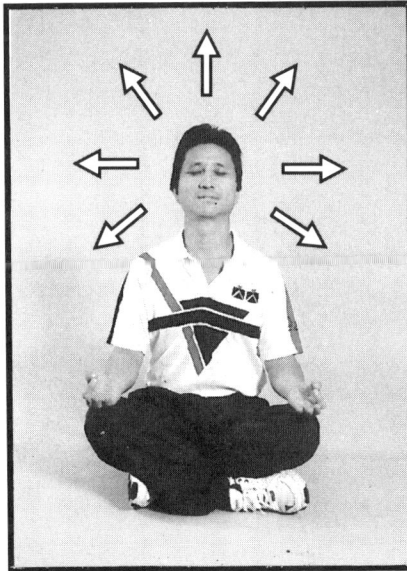

A

B. Inhale through the nose, intentionally making a clear mental picture that you are drawing *ki* from all three sources (the earth, the air, and the sun/sky) into your body through your head, and gathering it in your lower energy center. You should feel full and strong in your lower abdomen.

C. Repeat A and B a few times, intentionally making a clear mental picture that you are gathering the *ki* in the storage tank of your lower energy center until it is full.

D. After a few breaths, exhale through the nose, intentionally making a clear mental picture that you are moving the *ki* from your lower energy center down through your groin, past your rectum, up your spine and neck, and to the top of your head.

E. Inhale through the nose, intentionally making a clear mental picture that you are bringing the *ki* back to your lower energy center from the top of your head down the front of your face, neck, chest, solar plexus and down to the lower energy center.

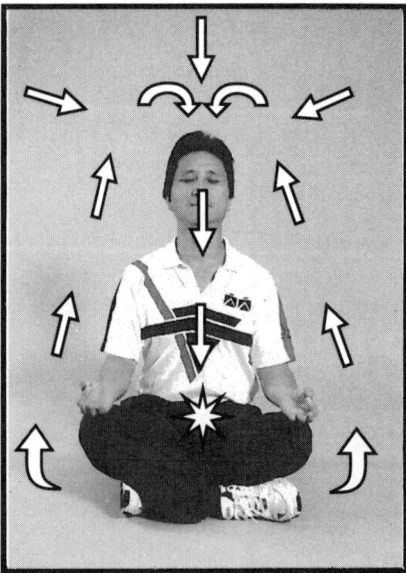

B

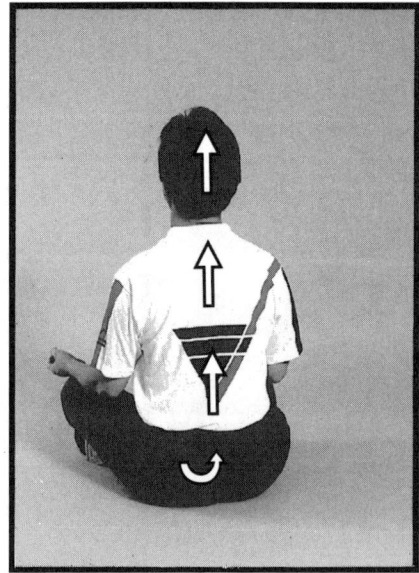

D

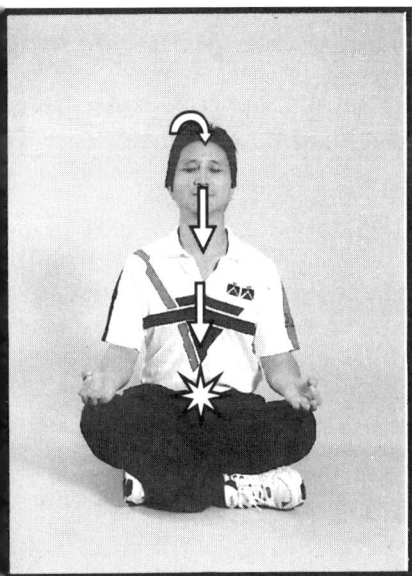

E

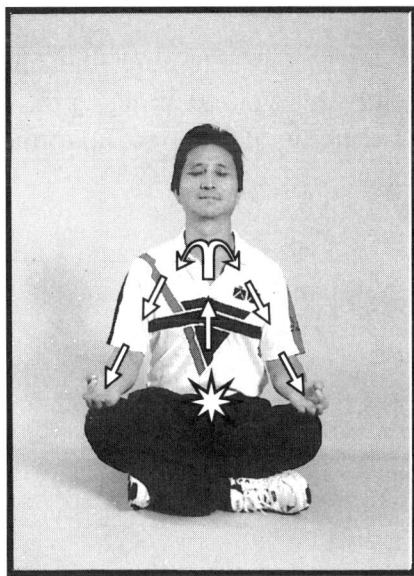

F

F. Exhale through the nose, intentionally making a clear mental picture that you are moving the *ki* up your spine, out to your shoulders, and down each arm to each of your ten fingers.

G. Inhale through the nose, intentionally making a clear mental picture that you are bringing the *ki* back to your lower energy center from the tips of your fingers up through your shoulders, down the front of your chest, solar plexus, and down into the lower energy center.

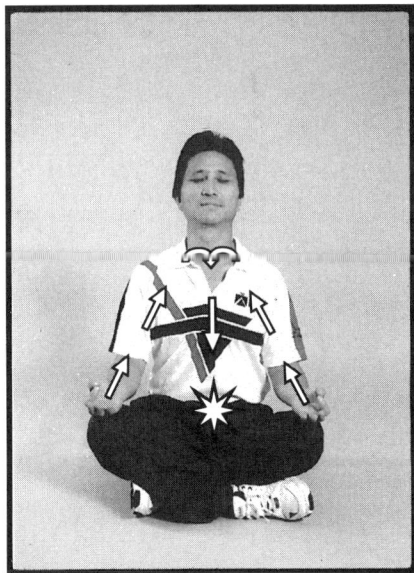

G

H. Exhale through the nose, intentionally making a clear mental picture that you are moving the *ki* from the lower energy center down each leg through the knees to the bottom of the feet, from toes to heels.

I. Inhale through the nose, intentionally making a clear mental picture that you are bringing the *ki* back to your lower energy center from the bottoms of your feet up through your knees and into the lower energy center.

J. Repeat A through I three to five times, for about ten to twenty minutes only two times a day: in the morning and whenever necessary.

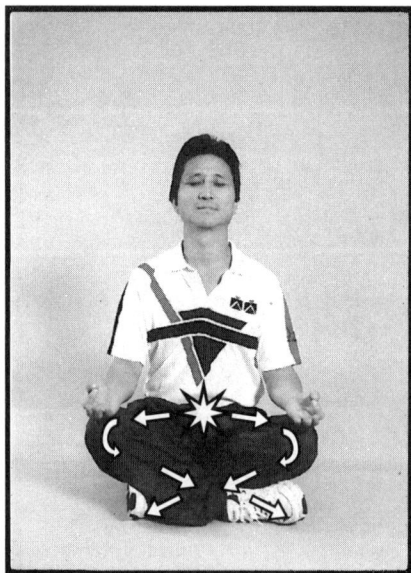

H

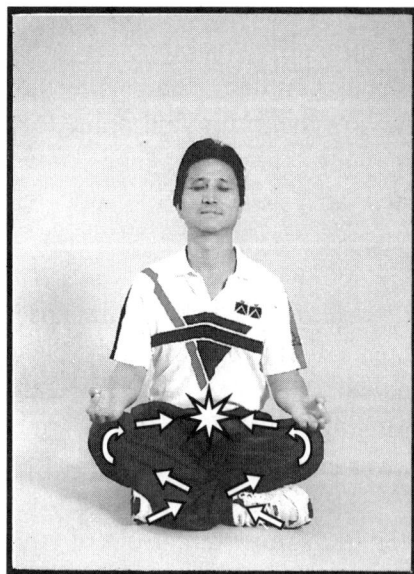

I

Benefits:

Advanced Breathing #2 will give you all the benefits of Advanced Breathing #1, plus it will:

* give you spiritual power.

* help open clogs in the blood circulation or the flow of energy through the power of *ki*.

* improve the five senses: vision, hearing, smell, touch, and taste.

* increase your power to prevent and heal mental and physical problems through *ki*.

The first time you try to feel the flow of *ki* will not be easy. *Ki* moves slowly (at least at first), and it will take you time to get it to flow long distances within your body. The more you concentrate and practice, the easier it will become.

After five to ten days you should be able to feel a strong reaction. After thirty to forty days you should feel more energetic, more confident, and more positive about yourself. After one hundred days you will know how to utilize your own *ki*, and move it around your body. Then, and only then, will you be ready to learn Advanced Breathing #3.

Advanced Breathing #3

Advanced breathing #3 is breathing through the skin. Now, I realize that we are not amphibians, and we can't really exchange enough oxygen through the skin to keep us alive; but we can draw *ki* through our skin. In Advanced Breathing #3 we can direct the *ki* to clean up and strengthen the entire body, or we can direct the *ki* to one area for healing purposes. This is the most advanced Power Breathing exercise in this book, and the best healing exercise.

Preparation:

Prepare the same way you would for Advanced Breathing #1 (see page 85).

How to do it:

A. Exhale smoothly through the nose, intentionally making a clear mental picture that you are expelling all the weak *ki* from your body through your skin, from the bottom of your feet to the top of your head. The weak *ki* will take all of the junk out of your body with it.

B. Inhale deeply through the nose, intentionally making a clear mental picture that you are part of nature, and that you are breathing *ki* from all three natural sources (the earth, the air, and the sun/sky) through your skin and storing it into your lower energy center.

C. Repeat A and B a few times, intentionally making a clear mental picture that you are gathering the *ki* in the storage tank of your lower energy center until it is full. Your body should feel clean and light. You should feel that you are one with nature: that nature is part of you, and that you are part of nature.

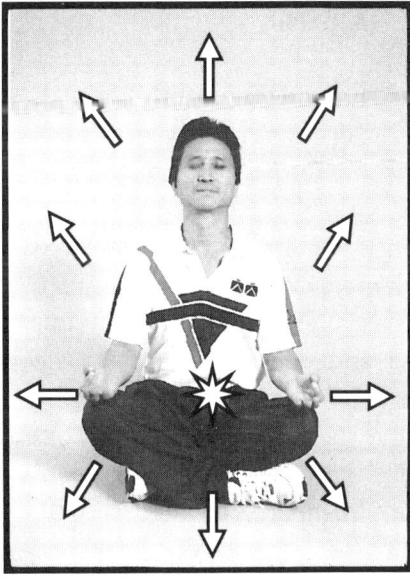

A

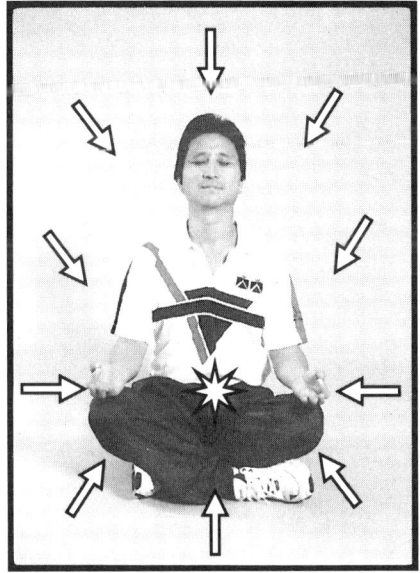

B

From this point on, you will be trying to heal your pains from injuries and diseases using *ki* (for example: lower back pain, headaches, high blood pressure, etc.)

D1. Lower back pain

Exhale very gently through the nose, intentionally making a clear mental picture that you are sending *ki* from your lower energy center to your lower back area. Visualize that you are moving the *ki* all around your lower back, loosening up clogs in the blood circulation or flow of energy. For two to three minutes, continue breathing as in steps A and B, and take away the weak *ki* and replace it with strong *ki*.

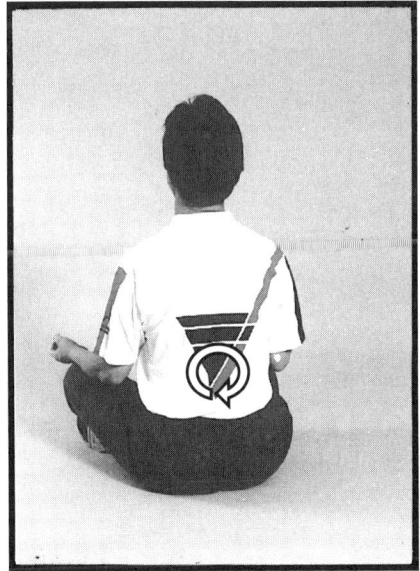

D1

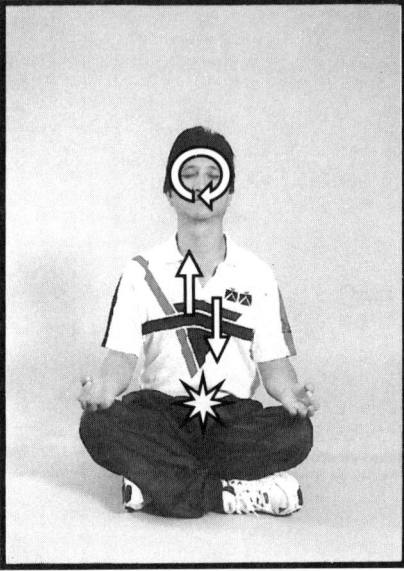

D2

D2. **Headache**

Exhale very gently through the nose, intentionally making a clear mental picture that you are sending *ki* from your lower energy center to your head and neck area. Visualize that you are moving the *ki* all around your head and neck, opening up the veins and intentionally removing all the stale blood and toxins out of the head and replacing them with fresh, oxygenated blood. For two to three minutes, continue breathing as in steps A and B, and take away the weak *ki* and replace it with strong *ki*.

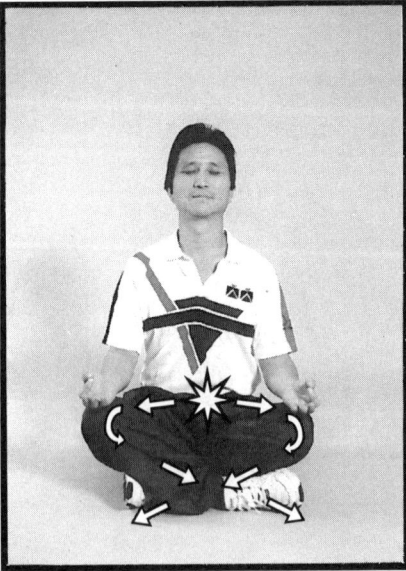

D3

D3. **High blood pressure.**

Exhale very gently through the nose, intentionally making a clear mental picture that you are sending *ki* from your lower energy center to the bottom of your feet. Visualize that you are moving the stress out of your body through your feet. For two to three minutes, continue breathing as in steps A and B, and take away the weak *ki* and replace it with strong *ki*. Your blood pressure will go down.

D4. **Liver infection**

Exhale very gently through the nose, intentionally making a clear mental picture that you are sending *ki* from your lower energy center to your liver. Visualize that you are moving the *ki* all around your abdomen, mobilizing the white blood cells to attack and destroy any germs, viruses, or other foreign bodies infecting the liver. For two to three minutes, continue breathing as in steps A and B, and take away the weak *ki* and replace it with strong *ki*.

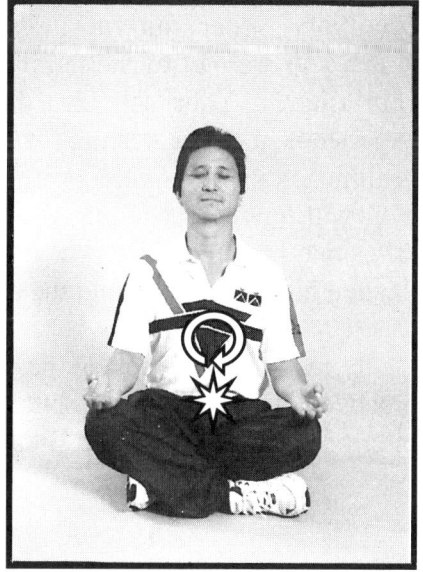

D4

E. Repeat steps A and B a few more times to clean all of the weak *ki* out of your system and to refill your lower energy center with strong *ki*.

Benefits:

You will gain all the benefits of Advanced Breathing #2, plus Advanced Breathing #3 will:

* help you to understand how you are one with nature.

* heal and cure a lot of painful injuries and diseases.

* be the best prevention against diseases.

* develop your sixth sense, the one that will allow you to see the future consequences of present actions.

* enliven your *ki* to increase the energy available to your body, mind, and spirit.

Practice for ten to twenty minutes at least one time a day and whenever else you need it. After five to ten days you will feel much lighter, and you will begin to notice an improvement in your physical condition. After thirty to forty days you will feel that you are not alone -- that you are part of the family of nature and that every part of nature is your friend. Your pain and discomfort should be all gone. You will experience a great feeling of harmony and belonging. You will be healthier, stronger, more energetic, more confident, and more positive. You will have the winning feeling that comes along with healthy living. After one hundred days you will really want to share with everyone else this feeling of harmony and the other health benefits you have received.

Always go back to basic breathing to re-learn and continue to practice. It will help you better understand and better perform all of the Intermediate and Advanced Breathing.

Summary of Power Breathing:

Basic Breathing: learn to breathe with the lower abdomen.

Intermediate Breathing: learn to relax the solar plexus and tighten the lower abdomen, close the rectum, and tighten the legs, in order to clean out the entire body.

Advanced Breathing: learn to visualize the movement of *ki*, and direct it to areas that need energy for healing purposes.

I truly appreciate your persistence and dedication to get this far. I feel I did not waste my time writing this book. If you are confident in what you have learned and achieved, share your knowledge with others. For even more advanced training, you can use Power Breathing in special situations as outlined in the next section.

SPECIAL APPLICATIONS OF POWER BREATHING

Rhythm Power Breathing

Rhythm Power Breathing is a self-massage. It is an excellent way to release tension and stress, and to strengthen your spine, including your connective disks. It is the best exercise for digestive problems, and can stop diarrhea or constipation almost immediately. It will especially help you release gas that may cause stomach aches. By improving digestion, it will strengthen all of your muscles and organs, including the heart and lungs.

Rhythm Power Breathing is absolutely necessary for anyone who sits for long hours doing office work. It will release your tension and enliven you so that you can work more efficiently.

Preparation:

When Power Breathing, you can practice lying down, seated on the floor or in a chair, or standing. However, Rhythm Power breathing can only be performed effectively in the seated position, either on the floor or in a chair. You may sit however you are comfortable, as long as your back remains straight. If you sit on the floor, cross your legs in what we call *jung ja*. If you are flexible, you can put one leg on top of the other in the half-lotus, or *ban ka bu ja* position. If you are very flexible, you can put both legs on top of each other in the full lotus or *ka bu ja* position (see p. 86 for illustrations.)

1. Sit in a comfortable position, either on the floor or in a chair. Place both hands over your lower energy center, or place the palms on the knees.

2. Loosen up your whole body and mind, including your muscles, joints, and mental tension. (This step is even more important than learning how to breathe).

3. Straighten your body, so that you are equal and balanced from left to right, front to back, and top to bottom. Your center of balance should be your lower energy center, but be careful not to tense any part of your body.

4. Slightly close your eyes so that you can barely see. Because your attention will be naturally drawn to things that you see, try not to see anything, so that your mind can go blank without going to sleep.

5. Maintain a pleasant smile. It will loosen up your face muscles and give you peace of mind.

How to do it:

A. Place both hands on your lower abdomen (or on your knees). Inhale through the nose as deeply as possible, pulling the energy all the way to the bottom of your body.

B. Exhale through the mouth as long as possible (practicing either Basic or Intermediate breathing). Keep your head still and rock your lower abdomen and hips left to right and back again. Continue rocking until you have exhaled all the way.

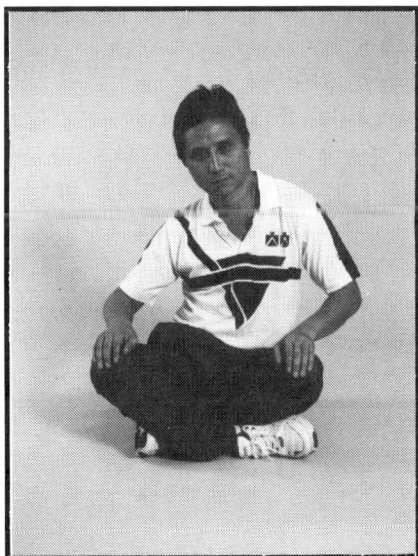

A on the Floor

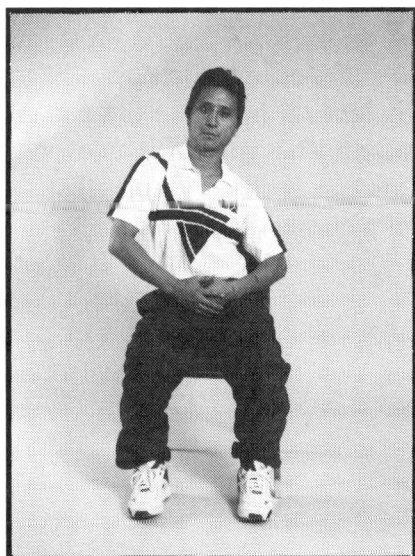

A in a chair

C. Repeat A and B from five to ten times, whenever you feel indigestion, sleepy, stress, or tension.

Benefits:

Rhythm Power Breathing will:

* release stress and tension.

* adjust the spine and strengthen the lower back.

* improve digestion.

* heal diarrhea, constipation, and stomach aches.

* clean out internal organs.

* increase blood circulation.

* strengthen the heart and lungs.

You can do this self-massage at the office, in the car, on an airplane, at home, in the park, virtually any time, any where. I strongly recommend you do it two or three times a day. Don't worry if your stomach starts to gurgle, that is completely normal. It is also normal to burp during this exercise.

Bending Power Breathing

Bending Power Breathing is the key to developing deeper and longer breathing for the cleansing breath. It will give you a healthier and happier long life.

Ordinary people use approximately one-third of their lung capacity as they breathe with their chest. Through Power Breathing they can use their full normal lung capacity, and through Bending Power Breathing even extend their lung capacity a little beyond normal. By bending the body, they can compress the internal organs to force even more stale air and stomach gasses out. This will allow them more room to draw fresh air in. It will also allow a deeper cleansing action with the cleansing breath.

Preparation:

When Power Breathing, you can practice lying down, seated on the floor or in a chair, or standing. However, Bending Power Breathing can not be performed effectively when lying down; you must be either in the seated or standing position, either on the floor or in a chair. You may sit however you are comfortable, as long as your back remains straight.

The other preparations are the same as those for Rhythm Power Breathing on pages 100-101.

How to do it:

A. Inhale through the nose as deeply as possible, drawing the energy all the way down into the feet.

B. Exhale through a slightly opened mouth while massaging the solar plexus with both hands and bending the abdomen forward.

C. Straighten your body up and inhale through the nose as deeply as possible, drawing the energy all the way down into the feet.

D. Exhale through a slightly opened mouth and move your hands down to your lower abdomen. Exhale as long as possible, cleaning out your entire body like a vacuum cleaner, all the way from the bottom of your feet to the top of your head.

E. Repeat A through D between five and ten times.

Benefits:

Bending Power Breathing will:

* get all of the stale gasses out of your body's systems.

* release tension and stress.

* make the body feel light and refreshed.

You can do this exercise any time, any where that you need to relieve stress and tension. I recommend you do it at least two or three times a day.

Bending Power Breathing while Standing

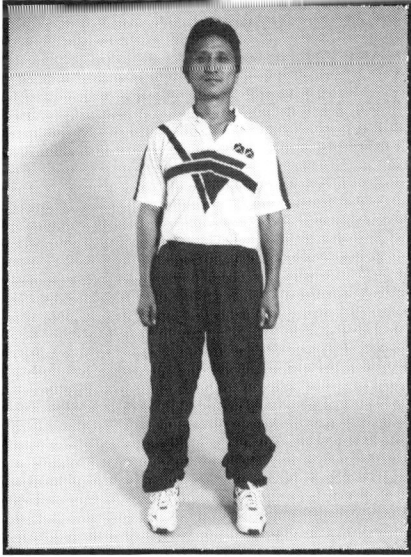

A, C

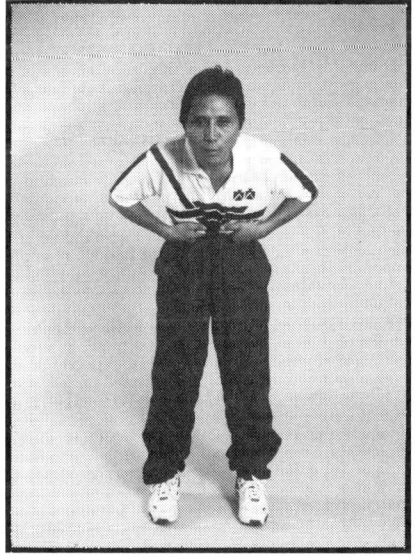

B

Bending Power Breathing while Sitting

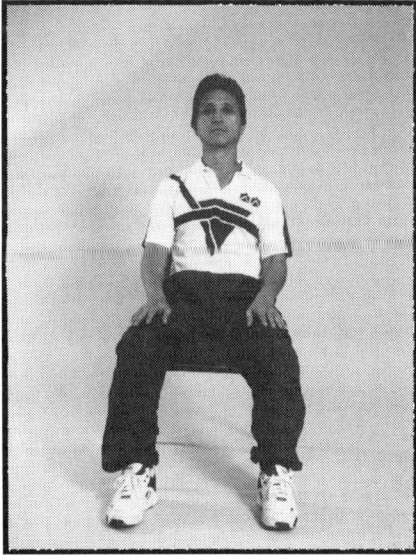

A, C

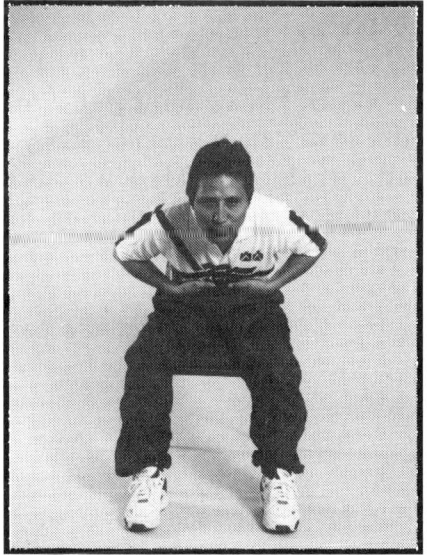

D

Massage Power Breathing

Massage Power Breathing is a laundry system for your internal organs. It will enliven them and increase their function greatly. Your lungs and heart will feel like dancing, and your brain will feel refreshed. If you have any weakness in your internal organs, you will discover them before they have a chance to seriously hurt you.

Preparation:

When Power Breathing, you can practice lying down, seated on the floor or in a chair, or standing. Massage Power Breathing can be practiced any of these ways, but most effectively in the seated or standing position, either on the floor or in a chair. You may sit however you are comfortable, as long as your back remains straight.

The other preparations are the same as those for Rhythm Power Breathing on pages 100-101.

How to do it:

A. Inhale through the nose all the way down deep into your lower abdomen.

B. Exhale through the mouth while placing your left palm against your lower energy center and your right palm over your left hand. Roll your hands up and down about one inch, alternately applying more pressure with the thumbs on the top, and then more pressure with the pinkies on the bottom.

C. Inhale through the nose all the way down deep into your lower abdomen.

D. Exhale through the mouth while placing your right palm against your lower energy center and your left palm over your right hand. Roll your hands up and down about one inch, alternately applying more pressure with the thumbs on the top, and then more pressure with the pinkies on the bottom.

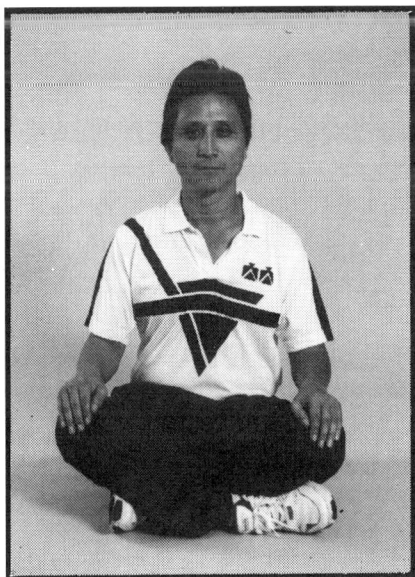

A, C, E, G, I, K

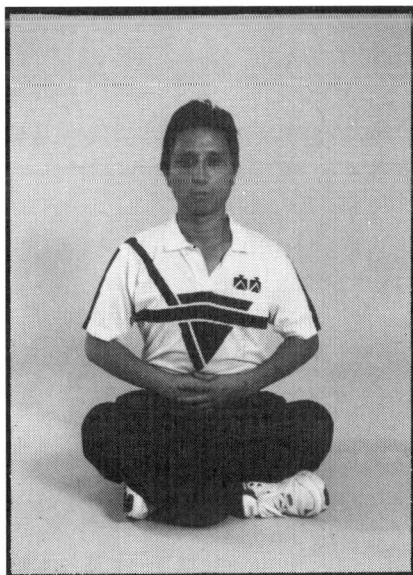

B, D

E. Inhale through the nose all the way down deep into your lower abdomen.

F. Exhale through the mouth and pat yourself down the center of the chest from collar bone to groin with the right hand.

G. Inhale through the nose all the way down deep into your lower abdomen.

H. Exhale through the mouth and pat yourself down the center of the chest from the collar bone to the groin with the left hand.

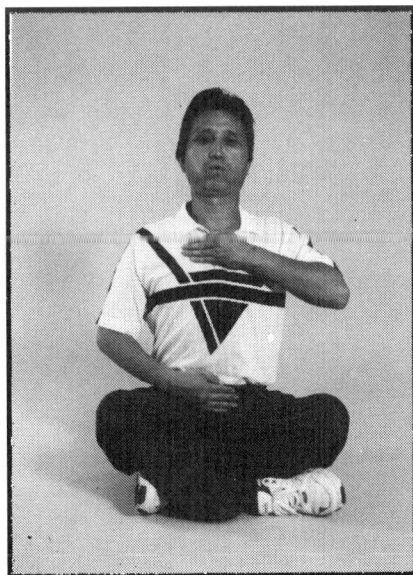

H

I. Inhale through the nose all the way down deep into your lower abdomen.

J. Exhale through the mouth while using all ten finger tips to tap all around your face and head.

K. Inhale through the nose all the way down deep into your lower abdomen.

L. Exhale through the mouth while washing your face and hair with air.

M. Repeat A through L from five to ten times.

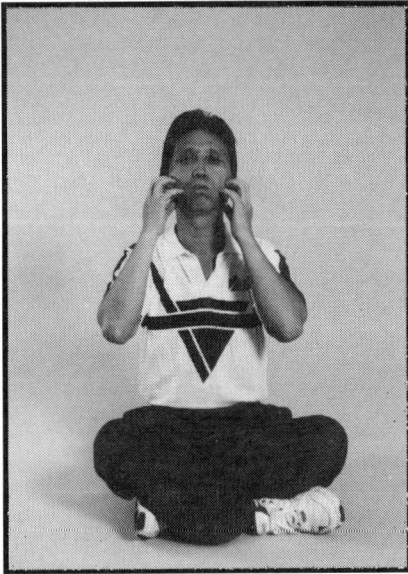

J

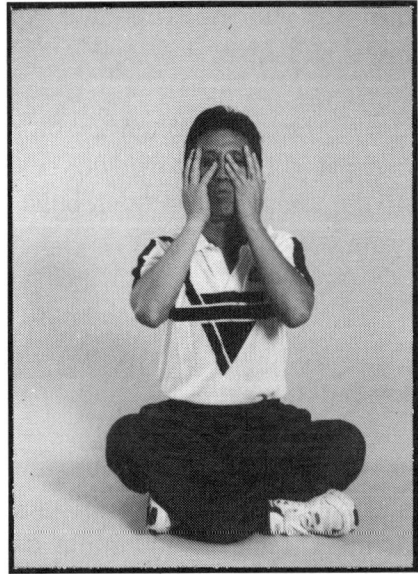

L

Benefits:

Massage Power Breathing will.

* release stress and tension.

* freshen up the inside of your lungs, stomach, and brain.

* expel all stale gas from the body.

* aid digestion.

Do not worry if you burp or "break wind" during this exercise; that is a normal reaction to cleaning your digestive system by releasing trapped gasses. I recommend that you do this exercise at least two times a day, any where, any time.

Natural Power Breathing

Power Breathing is not a new technique. It is a great gift from nature for human beings everywhere. Power Breathing occurs naturally in many instances, and can be specially applied in other circumstances.

All human beings breathe Power Breathing from birth. Babies breathe from their abdomen naturally. When a baby cries, if you touch his lower abdomen, you will find it is tightened as hard as a rock. This is natural Power Breathing.

Laughing

We all naturally return to Power Breathing from time to time.

Do you know why a smile makes us happy? Laughing is an excellent health exercise for the body and the mind. Physically, you naturally return to Power Breathing. The next time you laugh, touch your lower abdomen to feel how tight it becomes. Also, your body and mind feel better due to the release of "endorphins", a natural morphine-like substance that your body produces to cover pain that also works to elevate your mood.

Besides, nobody likes to see an ugly face. A smile makes for happiness. It makes you and others happy. Smiling is one of the great natural forms of Power Breathing for health. Many comedians live longer than their more serious contemporaries.

Yelling

Yelling is a natural form of Power Breathing. I am not talking about yelling at someone out of anger. The anger will make you sick. I mean yelling in a loud voice to spontaneously release a strong emotion. For example, someone who has just accomplished something he is proud of -- like reaching the top of a mountain after a long climb -- might let out a "Ya-Hoo" kind of yell. It represents a feeling that all of the world is his, and his body feels great. Other examples of spontaneous yells might be cheers for great performances, yells of pain, or martial arts yells. If you feel your lower abdomen during such a yell, you will find that it is tight.

Yelling is a form of Power Breathing because it represents a moment when your body and mind are one. There is a sudden build up of emotion that must be released, and the yell releases the emotion. It shows that we are in harmony with nature.

Yelling develops a good voice. It also is a great exercise for health because it is Power Breathing. Yelling helps create concentration, and is a strong weapon for self-defense.

Climbing

Ever wonder why mountain people are so healthy? Climbing is healthy because it is a form of Power Breathing, there is a lot of fresh air, and it clears your mind. When you lift your foot to climb, your thigh comes up as if to touch your abdomen. When you push your foot down, your stomach naturally tightens, causing Power Breathing. (Other natural forms of Power Breathing due to manual labor include lifting -- when done properly -- and swinging a tool like a pickax).

In our modern culture, we do not get the opportunity to climb many mountains. We drive instead of walk, and even tall buildings have elevators. This makes life very easy and comfortable, but it also makes life unhealthy. We need to re-create this natural exercise to maintain our health.

Whenever possible, if you live or work upstairs, walk up and down the stairs instead of taking the elevator. If you work or live above the fifth floor, take the elevator most of the way, and walk two or three flights of stairs. Don't be one of those people who pays good money to a health club so he can use its stair-climber, yet will not walk up a flight of real stairs.

Martial Arts Power Breathing

Power Breathing with meditation will clear your mind (see Chapter 7 for more about meditation). It will help you build inner strength so that you can get the maximum benefit from the discipline and training of the martial arts.

Power Breathing when combined with meditation will allow you to focus your power to any part of your body or mind. It is especially good for development of balance, as well as speed, power, and accuracy. It will improve your basics, forms, sparring, self-defense, and especially breaking technique. How?

To develop proper technique, practice slowly: inhale, kick or punch slowly and exhale, inhale as your foot or hand returns to ready position. When you go at normal speed, just breathe naturally, trying to exhale on the strike or block. When you practice continuous actions over a long period of time, you will need more oxygen, so you should breathe through your nose and mouth at the same time.

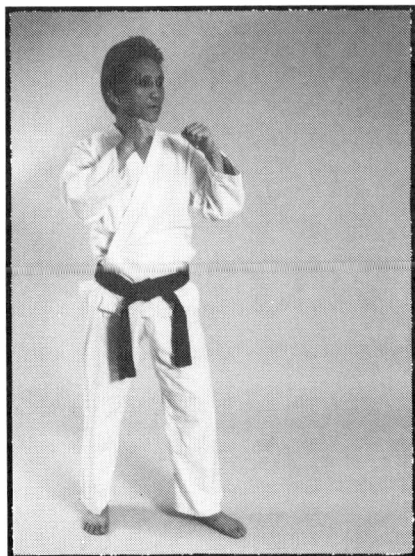

Punch: inhale
through the nose

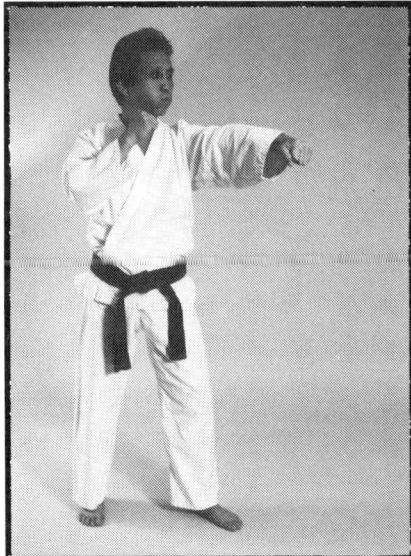

Punch: exhale
through the mouth

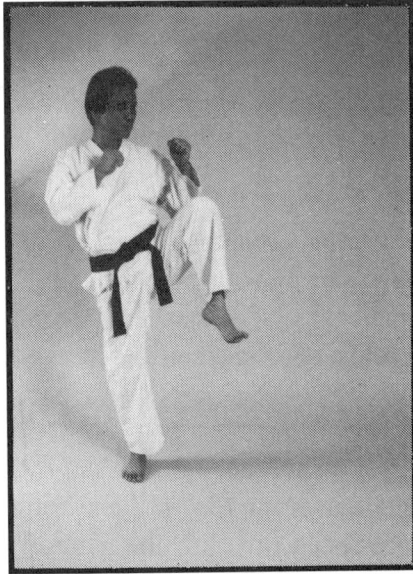

Kick: inhale and
lift knee

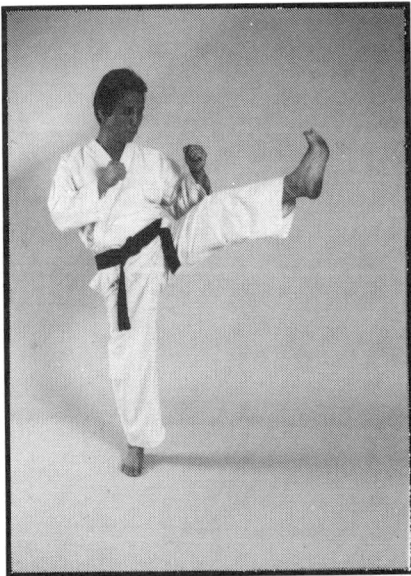

Kick: exhale and
extend kick

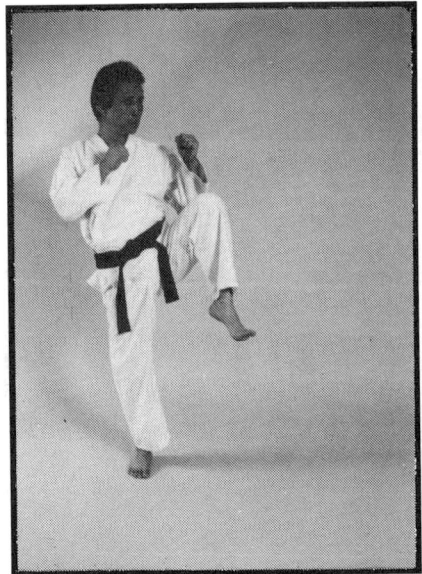

Kick: inhale and
withdraw kick

Martial Arts Breaking Technique

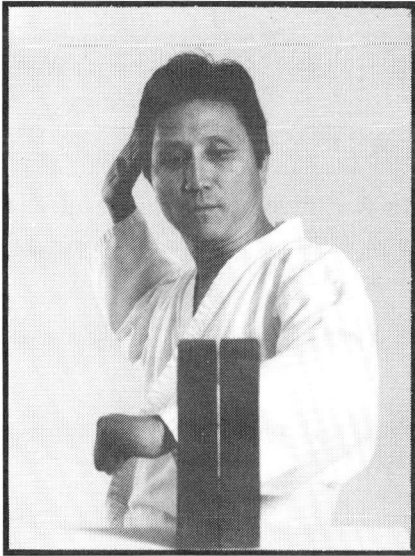

Knife-hand Strike:
inhale

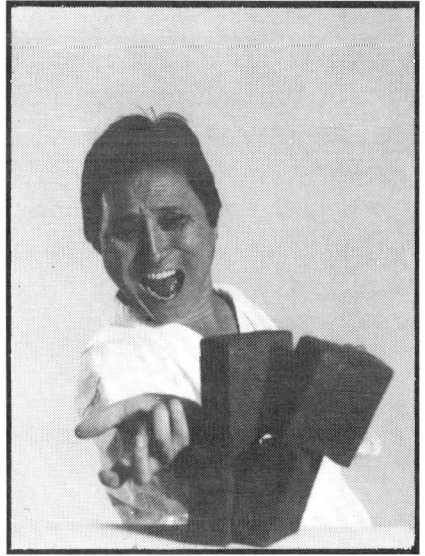

Knife-hand Strike:
hold breath or exhale
and break

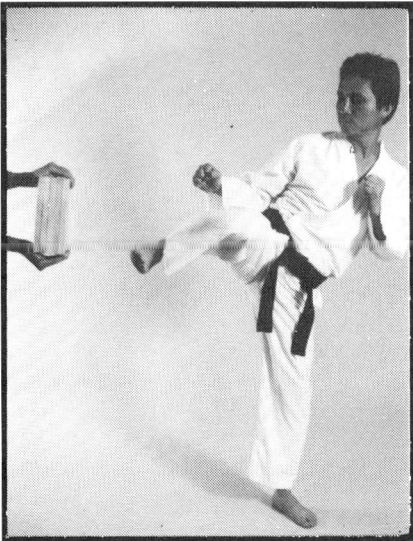

Side Kick:
Inhale and lift

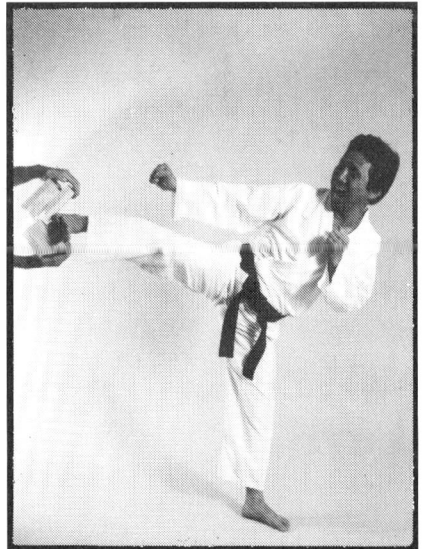

Side Kick:
hold breath or exhale
and break

When you attempt to break bricks or concrete with a knife-hand strike, you must focus your mind on your knife-hand and move all of your power and *ki* to your hand. With Power Breathing and practice, it will happen. This is mind control of your body, or mind over matter. With practice, you can improve your control.

In the martial arts, Power Breathing will give you better results in your training, you will have more fun, and you will not hurt yourself. Martial arts training is a great exercise for body, mind, and spirit.

Exercise Power Breathing

Exercise with Power Breathing is real exercise, because the purpose of exercise is health. Health must be developed from the inside out, not the other way around. If you want to be healthy, you need good blood circulation, which will give you good digestion, a strong immune system, and a fresh mind. In order to have good blood circulation, you need strong internal organs. What makes the internal organs strong? Power Breathing. If you practice Power Breathing while exercising, you will get better health benefits and better results from your training.

Running

Running is a great natural exercise as long as you run a distance within your physical limitations. Be sure to wear good, protective footwear to cushion your joints from the unnatural asphalt and concrete surfaces.

Running requires more oxygen than walking or just jogging, so you will almost certainly need to breathe through your mouth. Other than these differences, you can follow the same basic procedures as in walking (see pages 406-408). You can also intentionally send *ki*, or energy, to your legs through visualization as described in Advanced Breathing (pp. 83-98).

Weight Lifting

Weight lifting is not really a natural exercise, but most of the movements are natural, and, when combined with Power Breathing, it can be very beneficial. Generally speaking, breathe according to your chest cavity. For any action that opens your chest (pulling), breathe in; for any action that closes your chest (pushing), breathe out. Let's look at a common example for bench pressing a free weight barbell:

Grasp the weight with your hands and lift it off of the supports (A). Inhale and lower the weights to your chest (B: chest expanding). Exhale as you press the weights (A: chest contracting.) Repeat for a full set, then return the weights to the supports.

Weight machines are usually designed so that you should exhale when you lift the weight, and inhale as you lower the weights. Let's look at the lat. pull down:

Grasp the bar firmly and inhale (C: chest expanded.) Exhale as you pull the bar down to lift the weights (D: chest contracted.) Inhale as you lower the weights by allowing the bar to go up (C: chest expanded.) Repeat for a full set, then release the bar.

Free Weights

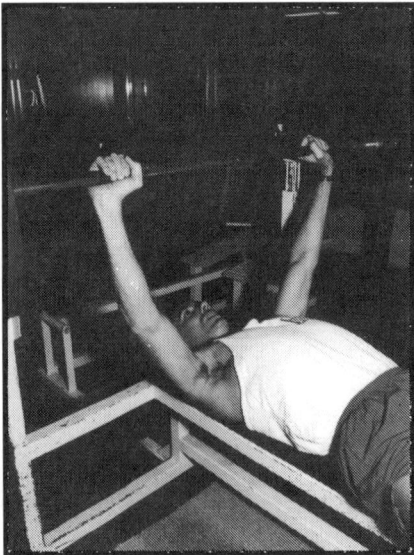
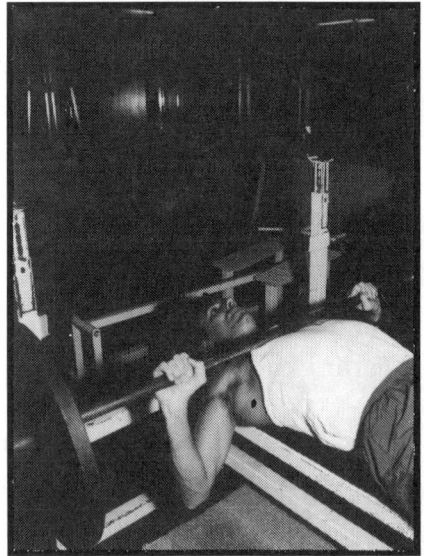

A   B

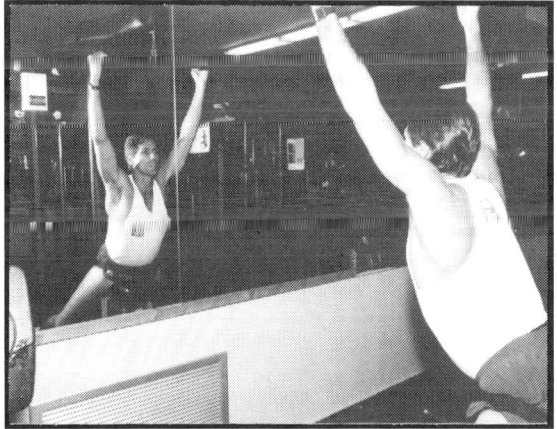

C

D

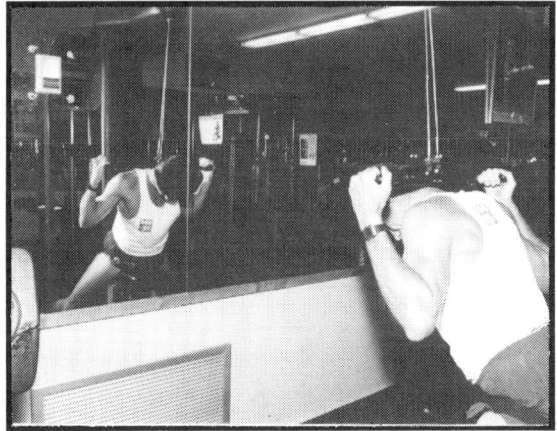

Whether using free weights or machines, be sure to move the weights slowly. Quick, explosive motions are dangerous for the joints. Remember: you are lifting to increase your strength (and health), not to demonstrate your strength (except in competitions). Weight lifting, when done properly with energy breathing, can improve your strength and health. When done improperly, it can cripple you.

Calisthenics

Calisthenics are exercises without equipment: jumping jacks, push ups, sit-ups, etc. The effect of calisthenics can be greatly improved with Power Breathing. In fact, there is an entire section of this book about calisthenic exercises combined with Power Breathing called "Power Exercises" (see Chapter 8). Here are some general guidelines:

When moving slowly, breathe in when the action causes the chest or abdomen to open, and breathe out when the action causes the chest or abdomen to close, or the waist to bend. If your chest does not open or close, breathe in for pulling motions, breathe out for pushing motions.

When moving at normal speed, breathe normally. When performing hard exercise, breathe through the mouth and nose combined to get more oxygen.

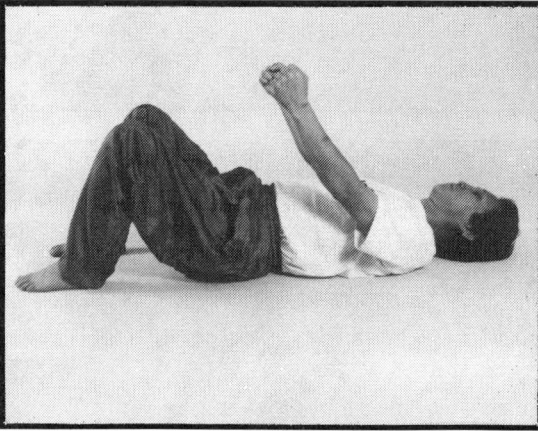

Sit-up: inhale when flat

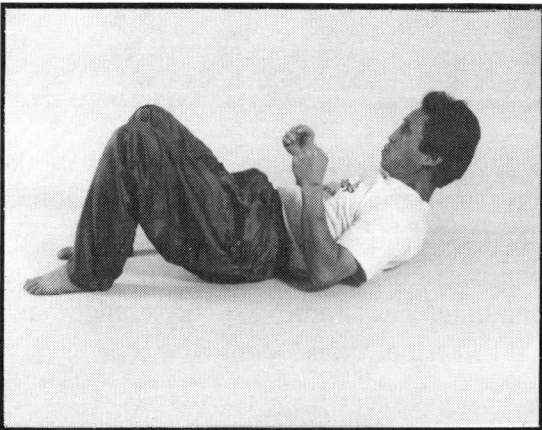

Sit-up: exhale when bent

You have to breathe wherever you go. All day, all night, all the time, you never stop breathing as long as you are alive. If you breathe properly, you will be healthy. If you breathe improperly, you will get sick and suffer unnecessarily during your life. Always breathe Power Breathing, and make yourself healthy.

NATURAL, NUTRITIONAL FOOD

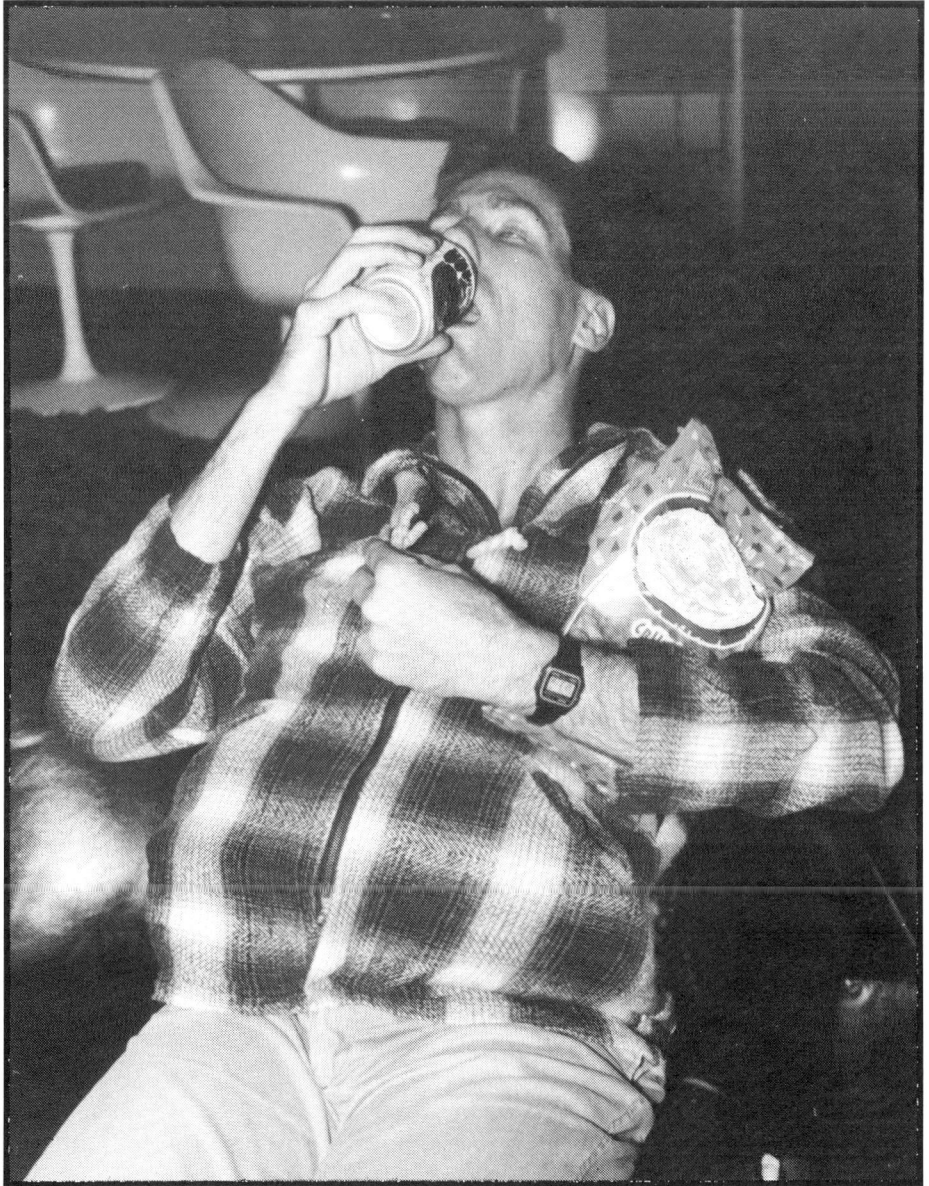

Throw away junk food and get in shape.

Everywhere you look: in every book store, on every talk show, in every newspaper and magazine, someone is promoting a new diet. Everyone from celebrities to athletes to scientists has his own opinions on what works for him, and therefore what will work for everyone else.

I do not have a "new" diet. I am not privy to some new research, nor do I have a revolutionary new concept. I have already stated that proper nutrition is one of the four corner supports of the foundation for healthy living.

What do I mean by proper nutrition?

Real food.

Good food.

Whole, natural, nutritional food as designed by nature.

I keep going back to the same cause to find the same solution: the reason we have so many modern sicknesses that we cannot cure is that we have gotten too far away from nature.

1. We do not have a healthy mental attitude toward the stresses in our lives.

2. We do not breathe the way we were intended to breathe.

3. We do not eat the foods nature has provided for us.

4. We do not move and exercise the way our bodies were intended to move.

Instead, we adulterate and pervert nature's masterpieces, thinking we are improving them. I have always believed that a little knowledge is dangerous. I believe that we (the human race) have reached a point with our scientific technology where we are beginning to understand some of the chemicals and processes involved in nutrition. We do not yet completely understand anything, and anyone who tells you that he does is far more ignorant than he himself imagines. I believe our technology is good enough to identify some of the mistakes we have made, but certainly not good enough to improve on nature.

For example, let's look at sugar. Sugar in its natural form is a necessary part of a healthy diet. The sugars you find in nature, though, are far different than the sugar you find in our grocery stores. Our wonderful technology has enabled us to grind and beat and strip and bleach nature's energy source into pretty white crystals of pure carbon-hydrogen-oxygen, devoid of the vitamins and minerals necessary for their proper digestion. Therefore, whenever we eat processed sugar, our bodies take vitamins and minerals already present and re-appropriate them to digesting the sugar. So instead of giving us nutrition, the sugar takes away nutrition as it gives us energy. Doesn't it make more sense to eat a peach or a banana which contains natural sugar AND the necessary vitamins and minerals needed to digest it? Doesn't it make more sense to eat natural foods that give nutrition and energy at the same time instead of processed foods that take away nutrition to give us calories?

As a second example, let's look at some grains. Natural whole grains like rice and wheat have been staples of human nutrition for centuries. One day, someone decided that these grains could be improved upon by taking away some pieces of the grains, and polishing them. The resultant foods (white rice and white flour) were pleasing to the eye, but not nearly as nutritious as the natural grains. As science developed, we discovered chemical ways to put back some of the nutrients we had taken out. We call these new foods "enriched".

Does it make sense to you that we should take a grain, polish away some of the nutrients, then put chemical substitutes for the nutrients back in? It seems to me that nature knew enough to put the right nutrients there in the first place, and we should leave well enough alone. It goes back to my basic belief that we should cooperate with nature, not try to conquer it.

Now let's look at a practical example: Mr. Blimpie is grossly overweight because he eats too much greasy food, candy, cakes, and virtually anything else that he can put in his mouth. He is unhealthy because he is not eating natural foods in natural quantities. Do you think he should go on a special diet on which he drinks only "great tasting shakes" of chemical powder? Or should he eat special foods in neat, frozen packages, with low calories and reduced fat made with food substitutes?

If the problem is that he is eating unnatural food in unnatural quantities, the solution is not to give him more unnatural foods in equally unnatural quantities. Those diets have a history of not working over the long run. The participants lose fifty pounds and then gain their weight back. That kind of weight fluctuation is dangerous.

If Mr. Blimpie could just eat natural foods in natural quantities, perhaps reducing his fat intake to correct his grossly overweight condition, he would begin to lose weight and gain health at the same time. He does not need to starve. He does not need to take additives and supplements. He needs to change the bad habits that created the unhealthy conditions in the first place. If he ever returns to those bad habits, the unhealthy conditions will return as well.

So good nutrition is just cooperating with nature. When you fight against nature, you will lose because you are fighting against yourself. Fortunately, nature has a way of giving you warning signs that you are off the path. If you pay attention to your body, it will show you the right way to go. You will regain the natural strength and health that is your birthright.

Here are some practical applications of the general principal "cooperate with nature":

1. Do not eat too much.

2. Do not eat junk food.

3. Eat natural, nutritional foods.

124

I will explain what I mean by each of these in greater detail:

1. Do not eat too much.

Everything is relative. Any natural substance can kill you if you take a large enough quantity. Very small amounts of arsenic (a natural substance) will kill you, so it is considered a deadly poison. Water is considered the source of life, yet thousands of people die each year of drowning because they ingest too much water.

No one will tell you vitamins are bad for you, yet you can get sick from taking too high a dosage of vitamins!

Fortunately, you will not get an overdose of vitamins from eating natural foods. Natural foods contain proper amounts of vitamins and other nutrients, and you will not normally be able to eat enough to make you sick from the vitamins. However, if you drink large quantities of juice (you would not eat thirty oranges, but you could drink the juice of thirty oranges) or take too many vitamin pills, you can overdose to the point of getting diarrhea and other problems. Do I have to tell you vitamin pills are not a natural food?

Eating too much is not good for you. Even natural, nutritional food can be overeaten, and you will get stomach aches, indigestion, and excess weight. If you eat sensible amounts -- basically, eat when you are hungry and stop eating before you feel full -- you will be healthy. It is not as easy to eat too much good food as it is to eat too much junk food, but it is possible.

The opposite is also true: do not eat too little.

Modern society and the pressure to look beautiful have created some strange starvation diseases like Anorexia Nervosa and Bulimia. I'm not saying that you should never miss a meal. Occasionally, fasting is good to clean out your system. However, fasting is not a healthy way of life. Your body needs nutrition to stay healthy. Eating natural, nutritional food is the best way to maintain health.

2. Do not eat junk foods.

What, exactly, are junk foods? There is an old saying, "One man's junk is another man's treasure." This saying is also true of food. Is chocolate a treasure or trash? Many people consider it a treasure, and use it as a reward for good behavior. I consider it junk, and here's why:

Junk food is anything that is eaten as if it were a food, but has nutrients taken away or additives put in to it to change its usefulness to the body. Because their food value has been altered, junk foods might be non-nutritional, or even anti-nutritional. Let's look at a few examples to help you understand what I mean:

Alcohol - is regularly consumed as if it were a food (beverage). I consider alcohol a poison; it is used as a disinfectant to kill germs in medical situations. As long as we don't drink too much, we do not die of poisoning, we just suffer some of the symptoms of poisoning: dizziness, loss of balance, loss of mental faculties. Because the human body can metabolize alcohol, we can purify our systems in a few hours or a day.

Alcohol is not a nutrient. It contains lots of calories that are not balanced with vitamins and minerals. People who drink a lot get fat (beer bellies). Alcohol kills brain cells, and it puts a strain on the liver and kidneys to purify the bloodstream. The liver and kidneys would not be strained if you drank maybe one or two drinks a week. However, when you drink large amounts of alcohol at one sitting, or consistent amounts every day, your organs get strained, and cannot function properly.

Caffeine - Caffeine is a stimulant, not a nutrient. Although it is derived from natural substances, most of the caffeine in the American diet is no longer natural. It is a chemical additive to some high sugar/low-nutrient beverages and snacks. Does that sound healthy to you?

In addition, most people who use caffeine drink four or more cups of coffee, cola, or other sources of caffeine in a day. Think about it: caffeine is a stimulant, and we stimulate ourselves, then re-stimulate, then re-stimulate again. We get to the point where we depend on the stimulant to feel "normal". This is more an addiction than nutrition.

126

Sugar - is believed by some to be the leading cause of disease in America today. The use of refined sugar (don't let the sugar pushers try to confuse you: refined sugar is very different from natural sugar) has risen sharply but steadily over the past few hundred years. The increase in incidence (cases per 1,000) of diseases like diabetes and cancer seems suspiciously parallel.

Sugar rots your teeth.

Sugar goes into the bloodstream very quickly, almost without digestion. When it enters the blood stream, which has already established a careful balance between the amount of sugar and oxygen, your body finds itself in a chemical crisis: too much sugar. You feel a burst of energy, and then the pancreas produces insulin and the adrenal cortex produce other hormones to deal with this emergency condition of too much sugar in the blood. In a few minutes all the sugar has been dealt with, and there is a slight excess of insulin, and a general lack of energy. What is the natural response? More sugar for more energy. The cycle repeats itself, depleting your supply of insulin and your ability to deal with the sugars. In the mean time, valuable vitamins and minerals have been used up to digest the sugar, depleting your system. This roller coaster ride of sugar rushes followed by sugar blues creates a very real addiction to the sugar.

Sugar is everywhere. Look at the ingredients of ANY prepared food -- canned, packaged, or frozen -- and you will probably find sugar as one of the foremost ingredients. It's in peanut butter, bread, catsup, fruit *drinks*, soup, everywhere. Restaurant cooks use sugar to flavor almost everything. It has gotten to the point that it is hard to eat if you refuse to eat sugar. You can forget fast food. You either have to prepare all of your own foods, eat raw foods (like salads without sugared dressing), or specially prepared foods.

So what do you do?

- Prepare some of your own foods.

- Read labels and buy low sugar or no sugar foods.

- Eat lots of salads and meals without sweet sauces.

127

The only reason cooks and food companies put sugar in everything is because it increases sales. The day after we all stop buying sugar coated doughnuts is the day they will stop making them in massive quantities.

Most "soft drinks" that we drink every day contain both sugar and caffeine. Is it any surprise that we feel "up" after drinking one? We are addicting ourselves to stimulants and sugar. Yet the "up" doesn't last long, and we soon reach for another . . . and another.

Red Meat - I do not recommend red meat for the average person because I do not believe our bodies were designed to digest it efficiently. If we look at our teeth, we have teeth more like herbivores than carnivores. Flesh-eating animals have long canine teeth or fangs for tearing the flesh and swallowing it in chunks. Grazing animals have grinding teeth that are designed to mash the vegetables into a pulp.

Man's teeth are not really suited to tearing flesh. His digestive tract does not deal with meats efficiently. Red meat can stay in the intestines for a week or more being digested. Fruits are digested usually within an hour, and vegetables and starches are digested in several hours. Why would you want to make your system work for a week on a job it could do in a few hours?

As a second consideration, red meats contain a higher percentage of cholesterol and fats than is ideal for the average person. In other words, if you eat meat, you increase your likelihood of arterial sclerosis and of just getting fat.

Salt - is a broad name given to a group of chemical compounds found naturally in our bodies. They are necessary for life and healthy in their natural quantities. We lose salts whenever we sweat, and need to replace them. We should get enough salts in natural foods to maintain a healthy balance.

One specific salt is table salt, or sodium chloride. It is not bad in its naturally occurring quantities, but dangerous when it becomes too concentrated (This is the same salt that will melt ice on the road and rust your car). The problem is that people put salt as a flavoring in everything (like sugar). It is in your soup, bread, peanut butter, etc. Plus, people will put additional salt right on their food as a seasoning. It is "normal" to place a salt shaker on the table so that each person can salt the food to his taste. Is it any wonder some of us get too much salt? Too much salt leads to high blood pressure and hypertension.

What can we do? Leave the salt shaker on the table; do not pick it up and sprinkle it on your food. It will not take a whole week for your taste buds to adjust, and food will taste fine without salt. Do not add salt unnecessarily as a flavoring when cooking. Eat foods with natural salts other than sodium chloride: for example, bananas and tomatoes are high in potassium chloride, a necessary salt.

The answer, once again, is that natural, nutritional foods contain more than enough salts and any other nutrients our bodies need, in the proper quantities. Even those in exceptionally hot climates doing exceptionally heavy, sweaty exercise can get enough salts from the local natural foods.

Additives We add everything from preservatives to food color to sugar substitutes to our modern foods. Some food preservation is necessary, but we do not need foods with the shelf-life of neutronium. When we put these preservatives into our digestive system, it just doesn't know what to do with them. The more chemicals we add to our food, the more unnatural substances we put into our bodies, and the less healthy we become. Try to eat as many fresh foods as possible, and use refrigeration and pasteurization as your main preservatives.

Food coloring makes sense from a sales standpoint, because most people will buy the food that looks better. It does not make sense from a nutritional standpoint, though, because our systems were not designed to digest dye. Some dyes have already been linked to cancer; I believe it is just a matter of time before the harmful effects of the other dyes are established. Avoid foods with color added.

Sugar substitutes are other unnecessary food additives. Saccharine was the first sugar substitute, so it has been around long enough to be researched. What did they find? Read the label of a popular sugarless gum: "Use of this product may be hazardous to your health. This product contains saccharin which has been determined to cause cancer in laboratory animals." Yum.

I believe it will only be a matter of time before we find out what the other artificial sweeteners cause. One thing is for certain: they are not natural, nutritional foods.

3. Eat natural, nutritional foods

There is not one good set of foods to be eaten by everyone, everywhere. People who live at the equator have grossly different needs than those who live in the arctic circle. They should eat different foods. The foods they need are locally supplied by nature. Americans do not need to eat more Japanese mushrooms, or Korean ginseng. Americans need to eat locally grown foods. Floridians need to eat lots of fresh fruits and vegetables, which grow year-round, because of the heat. Alaskans need to eat fat to keep warm. Florida oranges will not keep an Alaskan warm, and seal blubber will make a Floridian uncomfortably fat.

Another important aspect to take into account is your lifestyle. An accountant probably does not need a high-energy, high protein diet. He spends the majority of his day sitting and figuring, and only a small part of his day exercising. On the other hand, a valet parking attendant might spend the major part of a night running. He definitely needs some high energy, low fat foods. A professional bodybuilder or football player needs size and strength. He requires a relatively high protein diet to replace the tissues damaged during his exercises. Everyone must take the general principals and apply them to his particular situation, including physical, professional, and emotional environment. People who travel a lot should not worry too much about the local foods. As long as the traveller is healthy, he should be able to eat local natural foods safely.

The need for water varies with the environment. People who eat a lot of fresh fruits and vegetables, which contain a lot of water, need very little additional water. People who eat a lot of meats, which require extra water to digest, need more water. People who live in hot climates or whose work involves a lot of sweat, need to replace the sweat with fresh water. People who are burning fat (losing weight) need lots of water to wash away the waste products of the fat burning process.

The best foods are fresh fruits and vegetables. These are nature's packages of nutrition, whole and complete. Fruits and vegetables contain almost no fat, so they can be eaten in relatively large quantities without making you gain weight. Only when fatty butter and cream sauces are added to vegetables do they become fattening.

Fruits have a cleansing effect on the system, and some fruits contain enzymes that aid in digestion of proteins and fats. Fruits are an excellent food for breakfast and for snacks. Any time you feel you have overeaten, especially when you have eaten too much fatty food, you can start to clean out your digestive system by eating only fruit the following day for breakfast and/or lunch.

Because cooking destroys some nutrients, especially vitamins, it is better to eat fruits and vegetables raw whenever possible. Some vegetables are difficult or impossible to digest when they are raw, though, so they must be cooked. The best way to cook vegetables to retain their nutrients is to steam them. Baking is the next best possibility, followed by boiling last because boiling washes away too many nutrients.

Grains are also very healthy foods. Grains must be cooked to be easily digested, and can be made into pastas, breads, and other enjoyable foods. The key is to cook or buy foods made with the whole grain, not an adulterated version, even if it has been enriched with other chemicals. Rice, cereals, breads, and pastas are excellent sources of energy, which also contain protein without much fat. Again, the butters and creams we put on our grains is what makes them fattening.

Beans and nuts are high protein vegetable foods. Nuts should be eaten raw whenever possible, because cooking can destroy the lecithin, which helps the body properly digest the oils (fats) in the nuts. Beans must be cooked to be easily digested, and are natural combinations of proteins and carbohydrates. Beans and grains have different mixtures of the essential amino acids (proteins) and combining them improves the food value of both.

Seafood and poultry are the most digestible of the animal fleshes. They are relatively low in fat and high in protein. I do not personally advocate strict vegetarianism. I think moderate amounts of seafood and poultry are part of a balanced diet.

Dairy products are basically difficult to digest (more difficult than vegetables, but less difficult than meats). Cow's milk is designed to be digested by little cows. Our stomachs are not the same as those of cows -- if they were, we could get big and beefy eating grass.

However, since American children have been drinking milk, they have been growing taller and stronger than their parents. Milk seems to be healthy for children, whose bones and teeth are growing. Because adults are no longer growing, they do not need as much milk or other dairy products.

Dairy products are high in calcium, protein, and fats. Adults do not need the calcium (in fact, they can get too much, which leads to problems). The protein can be useful to active people, but the fats usually are not needed by the average person. Skim and low-fat milks are high protein and low fat, but not natural. They may be used for short terms by people trying to lose weight, but I do not recommend them as a steady diet.

Food Intolerance and Allergies

A significant percentage of the population is allergic to various foods. Some estimates say that over 50% of the world's population is lactose intolerant to one degree or another, and that as many as 30 million Americans suffer from the same problem[1]. Lactose is a sugar present in milk. This means that one out of two people could be allergic to milk or milk products.

Signs of food allergy are headaches (especially migraines), diarrhea, arthritis, asthma, and specific food cravings. It does not surprise me that people have allergies to chocolate, caffeine, or other unnatural foods. What did surprise me was that there are some people who are allergic to foods that are natural and nutritional to the rest of the population. As I just said, a large percentage of people are allergic to milk or milk products. Another significant allergy is coeliac disease, or gluten intolerance. Gluten is an ingredient in grain products like wheat, rye, and oats. This means that some people are allergic to grains, even natural whole grains like whole wheat or oats. Other common foods which significant segments of the population may be allergic to include: eggs, yeast, chocolate, oranges, benzoic acid, tomatoes, fish, pork, beef, corn, soy, tea, goat's milk, coffee, peanuts, bacon, potatoes, and nuts[2].

If you suspect you have a food intolerance or allergy, consult an allergist to determine which foods, if any, you are allergic to. Because of allergies, one man's nutrition may be another man's poison.

How to Lose Weight

Your image of yourself affects the self you become. If you think you are stupid, you never try to learn things, and remain ignorant. If you think you are smart, you are always interested in learning something new, and increase your knowledge. This "self-fulfilling prophesy" has been proven in experiments with young children many times. Likewise, if you think you are slim and attractive, you will do the things that help keep you slim and attractive. If you think you will always be fat, you will always do the things to keep you fat. If you want to lose weight, the first thing you need to change is your mind.

Losing weight is so easy, it's a piece of cake:

If you want to lose weight, you will already start losing.
If you don't want to lose weight, you will stay fat.
If you are afraid to change, you will keep your bad habits and you will get fatter and fatter.

What could be simpler than that?

Being fat costs you extra money, time, and energy.

When you eat too much you pay more for grocery, restaurant, and convenience store bills. Fatty foods often cost more than healthy foods. A diet of natural, nutritional foods in proper amounts actually costs less money than a diet of junk food.

When you are a slave to your stomach, you spend more time eating and digesting, and less time working, playing, and enjoying life.

Because it takes more energy to move a body with fatty tissue, you end up moving less and running out of energy a lot sooner.

Is it worth it?

The second thing you need to change is your habits. Your current bad habits have gotten you into this condition. If you change your eating habits to lose weight, then go back to your old habits, you will regain your old weight. If you want to change, you have to change your habits forever. If you always do what you always did, you'll always get what you always got.

In order to Lose Weight:

1. Begin eating natural, nutritional foods in reasonable quantities.
2. Reduce your weight by reducing your fat intake, forcing your body to burn the fat you have stored.

3. Begin an exercise program that incorporates aerobic activity.

Natural, nutritional foods provide the proper balance of vitamins, minerals, proteins, fats, and carbohydrates to restore your body to balance. When you eat foods that have been prepared with unnaturally large amounts of sugars and fats, and missing vitamins and minerals, your body gets thrown out of balance. Your digestive system does not work properly, your fat storage mechanisms do not work properly, and your tastes get perverted.

Reduce your fat intake to reduce fat. If you eat fat, you will get fat. It is difficult for your body to turn protein and carbohydrate into fat (it can be done if you eat large amounts, but it is an inefficient process.) It is extremely easy for your body to turn fat into fat. If you eat enough carbohydrates to fuel your movement, all the fat you eat will be stored as fat. On the other hand, if you do not eat enough carbohydrates to fuel your movement, your body must turn to fats and proteins to find fuel. If the fats are not present in your diet, it must go to your stored fat to find the energy.

Exercise does two things to reduce fat: it burns more energy than sitting still, and it changes your metabolism from a fat storing process to a fat burning process. If you have ever looked at calorie charts, you would find that you could go out and run two miles in fifteen minutes (pretty

135

fast), then come back and eat one candy bar and get more calories than you burned (230)[3]. How can anyone lose weight at that rate? The answer is that because your body is exercising, it changes the way it deals with the foods you eat. It is less prone to store them as fat, and more prone to use them for energy. This is one reason why people who exercise are able to eat a lot more and still stay slim.

I have had many Tae Kwon Do students lose weight because of the exercise and self-discipline involved in martial arts training. I believe the most any one student of mine has lost is 110 pounds. On the other hand, I have had several students gain enough weight to become fat during their Tae Kwon Do training. I never used to understand how this could happen. Then one day I realized that these students would train very hard and work up a big appetite. They would go home, usually late at night, and eat everything they could stuff in their mouths, and then go to bed. Little by little the food they ate (most of it not very natural or nutritious) would be turned into fat. Even a great exercise program cannot overcome bad habits like those.

If you want to change the result, you have to find the cause and change it. In my personal opinion being overweight is a totally unnecessary health problem in the U.S.A. today. Actually, being physically fat is not the real problem; the real problem is that people have too much mental fat. A strong and lean mind can change a body quite easily. A fat and lazy mind cannot control itself, let alone a hungry body.

I have seen so many overweight people around me, and the reason they are overweight is that they cannot control themselves or their minds. They are overweight simply because they allow themselves to eat too much fat and do not exercise. If they would trim off some of their mental fat, they could be a little tougher on themselves and change their bad habits.

Let's look at some simple choices:

1. If you want to be lazy, sickly, and dumpy-looking, then do not even read this book. Just stay on your couch and eat junk food.

1) If you want to be energetic, healthy, and attractive, eat natural, nutritional food.

2. If you want to be controlled by mental fat, then let your body match your mind and eat more fatty food.

2) If you want to be strong, disciplined, and self-confident, take Tae Kwon Do classes and eat healthy food.

3. If you hate yourself and do not like the people who care about you like your family and friends, then don't exercise at all and eat a lot.

3) If you love yourself, and love your family and friends, and want to spend a long time with them, balance the four corners of the foundation of your health.

4. If you want to continue having difficulty moving around, chafing the insides of your legs and feeling awkward when you try any physical activity, then keep your thunder thighs.

4) If you want to feel lighter, with more spring in your step and more confidence in your physical abilities, then do Aerobic Self-Defense.

5. If you want to strain your heart and damage it so that you may die young, or if you live to grow old, you will be unhealthy, then keep eating those greasy, fatty foods.

5) If you want to keep a healthy heart that will allow you to stay active well past the age of 70, then start to lose weight.

6. If you enjoy lower back pain from carrying around that belly, then keep your spare tire.

6) If you want to be free from unnecessary pain, then start shedding those pounds today.

7. If you want to keep your blood vessels clogged up and reduce the circulation to your whole body, and suffer from headaches all the time, then keep eating those cookies, candies, and cakes.

7) If you want good, clear circulation that will keep your entire body healthy and free from disease, then eat natural, nutritional foods.

I was never overweight physically, but I was overweight mentally. My mental fat did not express itself in a fat body, but it did express itself in pain and suffering. I did not realize I had a problem until it hit me hard enough to get my attention, and then I paid a high price. I am on a healthy diet now and I will continue to eat natural and nutritional foods as long as I live on this beautiful earth, because I love myself and I love the people who care about me. I want to take care of my body, so my body will take care of me, and I will be able to give to the people I love.

I strongly believe that if you love, respect, and believe in yourself, you can start now to begin taking better care of yourself. You can become proud of yourself and your appearance. You will find out who you truly are: a person of health, confidence, energy, and natural beauty. You will be in good shape.

More specifically, to lose weight you should:

1. Create a clear mental picture of yourself as you would like to be. Imprint this image on your unconscious mind.

2. Set a measurable goal as to how much you will lose. Set a long term goal (e.g., thirty pounds in six months), and a short term goal (e.g., one or two pounds a week). Be careful not to overestimate yourself. If you lose more than one or two pounds a week you are probably not losing just fat.

3. Do not eat too much at one time.

4. Do not eat fatty foods, especially red meat (beef and pork). Plan with your doctor or nutritionist a diet that will limit your daily fat grams to approximately 20 to 40 (eating too little fat is also dangerous, but usually not a realistic problem.)

5. Eat natural and nutritional foods. Natural foods help your body to regain its natural regulation and balance.

6. Exercise. Moderate exercise helps burn fat and helps improve your health and shape. Power Exercise is the best exercise to improve health, and Tae Kwon Do is the best overall exercise for body, mind, and spirit.

7. Tell yourself and tell as many people as possible, especially those who care about you, that you will lose weight. Get your pride involved, so that you will be ashamed to have these people see you unless you are losing weight.

Say things like,

"I can tell I am losing weight."
"I feel slim and trim since I improved my diet."

Think of all the negative things about being overweight and say them out loud. Then say positive things about the future like,

"I am so happy I am losing weight."
"I am a winner and can do whatever I believe in. I am strong."

Losing weight is an exciting opportunity to compete with yourself. You should not compare or compete with others, because no one has your body. Also, no one else controls whether or not you gain weight. It is something that is completely within your control.

When you lose weight and get into better shape, you will find out who you truly are. You will feel like you are born again and a true winner. Nothing contributes to success like success. When you succeed in losing weight, you will feel that no one and nothing can stop you. Your future will be brighter than ever and you will have confidence that you can achieve whatever you set out to do.

Even if I knew I were going to die tomorrow, I would want to be healthy today. As long as I live, I want to be healthy. The worst thing we can have in this life is bad health. Do you remember the news stories of the controversial medical doctor who invented the suicide machine for patients who were suffering from terminal illnesses? Bad health is worse than death. Make a decision now to throw away all your fat, both physical and mental, and become healthy. The longest journey begins with a single step. Take that step. Lose weight and get in shape. Build a healthier and happier life.

Foods that are low in fat

Most people become fat because they eat too much fat. (Everything is relative to the individual, so I will speak in generalizations and averages. One ounce of fat may be too much for you, whereas four ounces of fat may not be too much for someone else.) If you are fat, you are eating too much fat for you. You are what you eat. Your body can only build tissue with the materials you supply. If you supply fat, you will build fat. If you eat too little fat, you will lose your fat.

The problem is that fat is not always in the form of white spongy stuff on the side of a steak. Fats and oils are usually hidden where you cannot see them. Unfortunately, fats are usually what makes food taste good to the average person.

How much fat is too much? An average man can lose weight eating between 30 and 60 grams of fat per day, and the average woman can lose weight eating between 20 and 40 grams of fat per day. Under certain circumstances, people can eat only 10 grams of fat or less without hurting themselves, but it is dangerous.

Any general principle must be qualified because your body could have different requirements than the "average". Your body today could also have different requirements than your body six months from now. It is always wise to consult a physician or nutritionist when applying general principles to your specific situation.

It is also wise to bring about change with patience. Losing more than a couple of pounds a week is dangerous, because you can only burn a couple of pounds of fat in a week. Weight losses of five or more pounds in one week (sometimes even one day) indicate that something else besides fat is being lost: water, muscle, something. If you greatly reduce your intake of sodium, you could lose some water weight. If you take meats out of your diet, you could lose the weight of waste products in your intestines. You might lose a few large chunks of weight at the beginning, but a healthy weight loss program involves losing only a couple pounds per week.

Now, let's look at some common foods so you can better understand where you are getting too much fat. Here are some fast food items from popular restaurants:

Food	Fat grams[4]
Cheeseburger	17 g.
reg. french fries	11 g.
Vanilla shake	11 g.
Total	39 g. in 1 meal!
Fried chicken leg and thigh dinner	35 g.
Filet of fish sandwich	25 g.
Burrito Supreme	22 g.
Double cheeseburger	48 g.
1 slice cheese pizza	10 g.

Fast foods usually contain more than enough fats for a whole day in one meal. Large meals like two double cheeseburgers, fries, and a shake can contain a whole week's worth of fat in one meal.

Where do all these fat grams come from? The meat, the grease, and the sauces. Let me show you something:

Food	Fat grams
Baked Potato (8 oz.)	0.5 g
Fast food French fries (2.4 oz.)	11.0 g (8 oz. = 33 g.)
Bag of Potato chips (2 oz.)	20.0 g (8 oz. = 80 g.)
4 oz. roasted chicken	
skinless white	4.6 g.
skinless dark	9.9 g.
dark with skin	15.2 g.
Apple (whole)	0.4 g
Apple pie (1 slice)	11.9 g.
chocolate (1 oz.)	9.0 g.
8 oz. whole milk	8.0 g.
8 oz. 2% fat milk	4.7 g.
8 oz. skim milk	0.4 g.
Lobster cooked plain (7 oz.)	2.0 g.
Lobster with butter (2 tsp.)	10.0 g.
Lobster Newbury (7 oz.)	21.2 g.
Tuna canned in water (6 1/2 oz.)	1.7 g.
Tuna canned in oil (6 1/2 oz.)	22.1 g.
Garden vegetable salad	2.0 g.
Garden vegetable salad with oil and	
vinegar dressing (3 tbsp.)	24.5 g.

I hope you can see that you don't have to give up food to lose fat. You just have to give up eating fats. Baked potatoes are fine, but greasy fries or chips are out. Tuna can be low fat or high fat, depending on how it is packaged and prepared. Salads can become fattening if you use the wrong dressing. The packaging and preparation make a world of difference.

For example: a raw or baked potato (8 oz.) has less than one gram of fat. If you put four teaspoons of butter on that potato, you will eat 16.4 grams of fat. If you take that same potato and turn it into a small order of french fries (only 2.4 oz.) in a popular fast food chain, you could eat 11 grams of fat (33 g. for the whole 8 oz. potato). That same potato in a small bag of chips (only 2 oz.) could give you 20 grams of fat (80 g. for 8 oz.) The potato itself is not fat, but the way it is prepared can make it fattening

Similarly, a garden salad has virtually no fat in it. Put on three tablespoons of dressing, and the same salad has more fat grams (24) than a cheeseburger. Once you realize this, you can eat many of your favorite foods as long as you prepare them with low-fat flavorings.

Start reading labels and boxes. Plan your meals with low fat foods, and keep a running count of the fat grams you have eaten daily. You can lose weight eating three meals a day and snacks, if you eat the right foods (see pages 145-160).

Of course, there are some foods that are just no-no's while you are losing weight, no matter how they are packaged or prepared : butter, mayonnaise, miracle whip, margarine, oils (cooking and salad dressing), nuts, olives, and avocados. These are many of the preparations that turn low fat foods into high fat foods. Once you have lost your weight, you can eat the natural foods in this list on a weight maintenance program.

You can eat three meals a day and lose weight. You can even eat snacks, if they are the right snacks. You need not be hungry. Just think positive, watch your fat intake, drink a lot of water, and do some form of aerobic exercise like Tae Kwon Do training. The pounds will slowly and evenly melt away.

I strongly recommend that you drink a lot of water (six to eight glasses per day) while you are losing weight. Do not drink water before going to bed (going to the bathroom will disturb your sleep) or when you will not be able to go to the bathroom for a long while (for example, on a long drive). Do drink at least one glass first thing in the morning, before every meal, with snacks, and between meals. Drink a lot of water after an exercise session. First of all, water gives your stomach a full feeling. You will be less likely to eat too much food when your stomach feels full. Second, it will help wash away the by-products of fat digestion. When you are burning fat, you will be cleaning out a lot of junk stored in your body. The water will help wash it away without clogging anything up. You do not need to drink nearly so much water once you have reached your healthy weight, and you are maintaining health. However, some doctors recommend that everyone drink eight glasses of water a day.

During weight loss you may also want to take some transition measures to help you adapt. For example, if you are accustomed to the taste of butter, you may have to use fat-free butter flavoring on your popcorn or baked potatoes to make them edible. You might also use skim or low-fat milks and milk products. These flavors and foods are not natural, so I do not recommend them as part of a healthy diet. However, it is better to eat small amounts of unnatural food if they will help you enjoy natural food enough to eat it, until your taste buds adjust to the subtle tastes of natural foods. When you have lost your excess weight, you can eat reasonable amounts of real butter and real milk products in proper balance.

Sample weight loss menus

Breakfast

Breakfast is probably the most important meal of the day. If you do not eat breakfast, your body thinks it is starving, and slows down the metabolic processes so that you can survive starvation. If you eat breakfast, your body gears up to digest the food, and maintains a higher metabolic rate. When you are trying to lose weight, you want a high metabolism. You will burn more fat and feel more energetic.

You can keep your basic breakfast habits, or you can change them radically and still maintain low fat meals. You can eat cold cereal, hot cereal, eggs, fruit, or a shake. Below are some sample menus for low-fat breakfasts that include a different range of tastes. Many people eat the same or virtually the same breakfast every day. You may do that, or change it on the weekends, or rotate two different breakfasts every other day, or eat a different breakfast every day. I do not want to set up a strict diet for you to follow, meal-by-meal, day-by-day. I want to show you some examples of the good foods available, so you can mix and match them to your tastes and be happy while you are losing weight. You can even find foods on a restaurant menu that are close to these, and low in fat.

Sample Breakfast menus: Fat grams

#1 Cold cereal

1 glass water	0.0
1 glass fruit juice/herbal tea	0.0
1 banana or other fresh fruit	0.6
1 cup whole grain cold cereal	0.6
with fruit juice instead of milk	0.0
total fat grams	1.2

#2 Hot cereal

1 glass water	0.0
1 glass fruit juice/herbal tea	0.0
1/4 cup raisins or other fruit	0.2
1 cup whole grain oat meal (hot cereal)	2.5
with water or apple juice	0.0
total fat grams	2.7

#3 Fruit

1 glass water	0.0
1 glass fruit juice/herbal tea	0.0
1 bagel	1.0
(with fruit preserves)	0.0
1/2 cantaloupe filled with	0.7
1 cup low fat yogurt (with fruit)	3.0
total fat grams	4.7

#4 Eggs

1 glass water	0.0
1 glass fruit juice/herbal tea	0.0
1 slice whole grain toast or english muffin	2.5
with fruit preserves	0.0
4 boiled egg whites	0.0
total fat grams	2.5

#5 Energy shake

Energy shake (put all in blender)

6 ice cubes	0.0
1 cup low fat yogurt with fruit	3.0
3 bananas	1.8
fruit juice	0.0
total fat grams	4.8

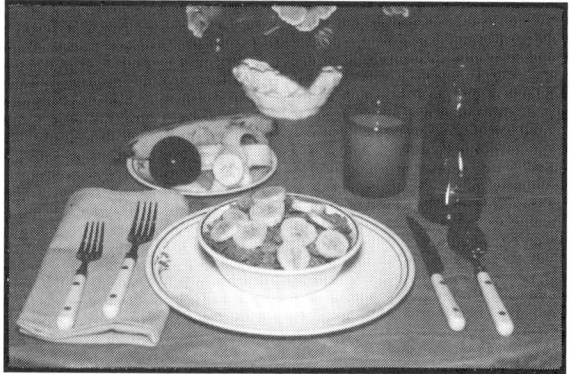

#1. The cold cereal meal suggests a whole grain cereal. This does not include frosted anything. You can eat wheat, bran, oats, rice, any grain or mixture of grains, as long as they are whole grains. I suggest fruit juice instead of milk to keep the fat content down. Fruit juices are naturally sweet, and will make the cereal sweeter. Try it; I think you'll like it. You may also substitute skim milk at a cost of 0.4 g. per cup, or low fat (1%) milk at a cost of 2.6 g. per cup, without going over 5 g. for the meal. The fresh banana or other seasonal fruit like peaches, strawberries, or cherries will also sweeten and enliven the taste. If you find one bowl is just not enough, eat extra fruit or try two bowls, as long as your fat content stays near 5 g. for the meal.

Notice I haven't included coffee in the beverage option. Remember, caffeine is not a desirable part of a nutritious diet. That is why I only suggest herbal tea. If you cannot do without your coffee, drink one cup of black coffee without any increase in fat content. Do not add sugar or milk, and especially do not use chemical imitations of sugar or milk.

#2. The hot cereal option is basically the same as the cold cereal option, but better suited to cold winter days. Again, it doesn't have to be oat meal; it could be wheat, bran, etc. The fruit juice works well with hot cereals, too.

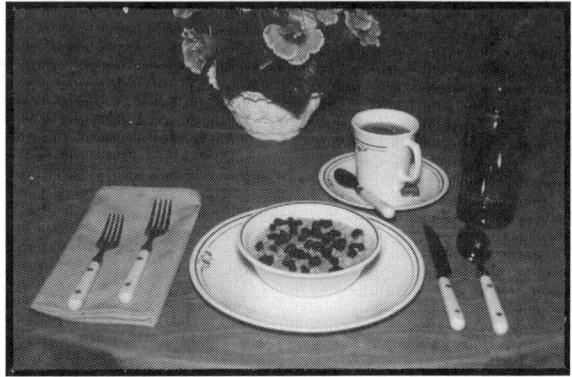

#3. The fruit option is really that: eat fruit. You can choose whatever is in season: melon, citrus, plums, apples, bananas, pineapple, grapes, etc. Fruit contains almost no protein, but it is a good breakfast. To increase the protein content, add

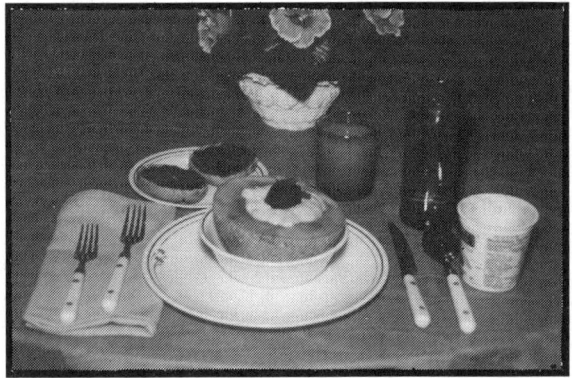

yogurt. While you are reducing fat, you may have to use low-fat yogurt to stay within your fat gram limits. Once you reach your proper weight, only eat whole milk yogurt (7.4 g. per cup) to maintain the best health. You can dip the fruit in the yogurt, or dip the yogurt into the center of your melon. It is delicious. If you find that you need more than fruit to feel full, eat a bagel for more substance.

#4. Eggs are high in fat. One egg contains over 5 g. of fat, but all the fat is in the yolk. If you really want to eat eggs, you can get high quality protein from the egg whites with virtually no fats. Just do not scramble or fry the eggs in oil or fat. Boil or poach the egg whites, or microwave them. Without the yolks, the eggs are much smaller, so you may need to eat twice as many to get the same volume. I do not really recommend splitting up a natural food like the egg. Eating only the white is a short-term fat loss measure. A healthy natural diet would include the whole egg, or none at all.

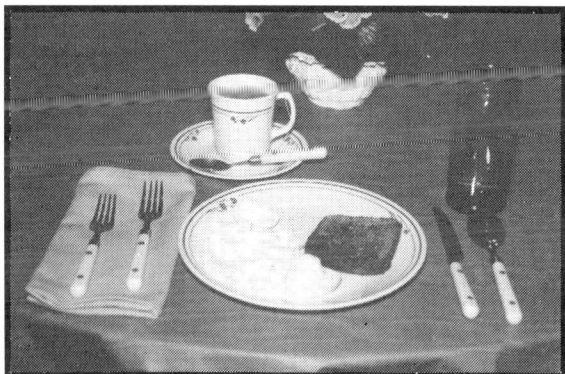

#5. The fruit shake is your chance for creativity. Utilize whatever fruits you can find, but the best starting point is two or three bananas and some fresh juice. You can add frozen or fresh fruit. The ice cubes are there to make it cold. Just like eating only fruit, the shake has almost no protein unless you add something like low-fat yogurt. You will find it satisfying and a lot healthier than a shake made from powder.

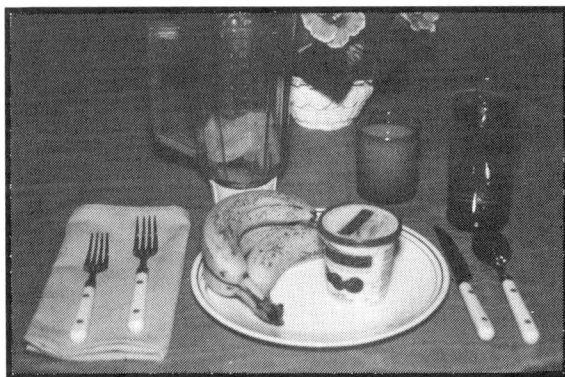

Noticeably missing from the breakfast selections are pancakes, waffles, and French toast. All three can be natural, nutritional foods when made with whole grain flour. Unfortunately, the butter, eggs, and milk involved in the preparation add too much fat for a weight loss menu. Once you have achieved your healthy weight, feel free to eat these whole grain options.

Snacks:

Snacks are not taboo. It is O.K. to eat between meals to keep your metabolism high and your appetite under control. Just be sure to eat no- or low-fat snacks. The best snacks are raw fruits and vegetables. You can alternate your snacks according to what you are eating for your meals. You probably do not want to eat a bagel for breakfast, two snacks, and lunch. A variety like an apple at breakfast, a bagel for a snack, some vegetables for lunch, and some popcorn in the afternoon is much more enjoyable and healthy.

Low-fat snacks:	**Fat grams**
1 glass water	0.0 g.
plus any one of the following:	
fresh fruit (whatever is in season)	1.0 g.
raisins or other dried fruit	1.0 g.
fresh raw vegetables (broccoli, carrots, etc.)	1.0 g.
graham or other crackers, ea. (with fruit preserves)	0.7 g.
English muffin or bagel (with fruit preserves)	2.0 g.
Low fat yogurt (with fruit)	3.0 g.
4 cups air popped popcorn (no butter, no salt)	2.0 g.

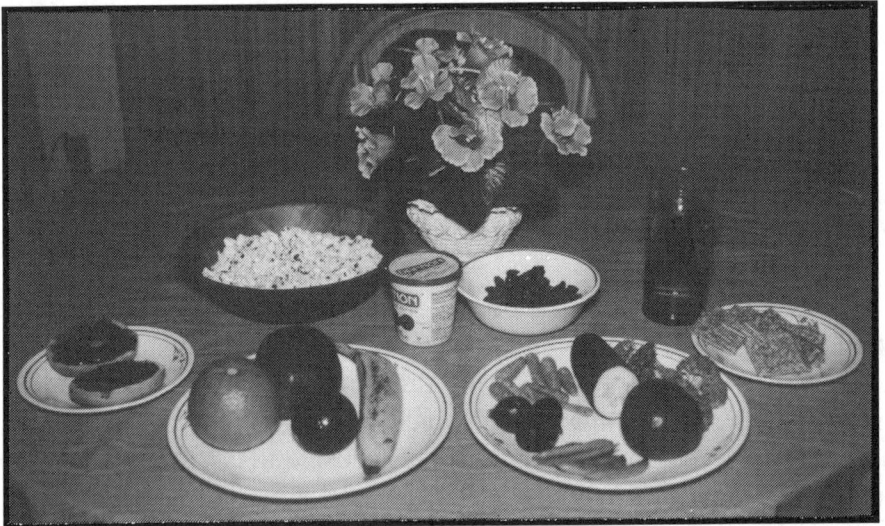

Lunches:

The quality of your lunch will determine the quality of your afternoon. A heavy lunch will make you sleepy. Overeating will give you indigestion. A low-fat, high energy lunch will give you the vitality to do your best.

You should have two meals that contain protein during the day. Do not eat all fruit or all vegetables for both breakfast and lunch. Alternate, so that either breakfast or lunch contains adequate protein.

There are lots of options for lunch, with options within options. You can eat similar lunches to those you eat now, or you can make some radical changes. There are plenty of low-fat lunches including soups, salads, sandwiches, and hot meals. Whether you prepare your own lunches or eat at restaurants, you can try the following sample menus:

Sample Lunch menus:	Fat grams
#1 Soup	
1 glass water	0.0 g
1 bowl soup (black bean, vegetable, chicken noodle, turkey)	2.5 g.
1 roll or 2 slices whole grain bread	2.0 g.
total	4.5 g.
#2 Salad	
1 glass water	0.0 g.
1 glass herbal iced tea	0.0 g.
vegetable salad	2.0 g.
low cal./low fat dressing	1.0 g.
1/2 cup low fat cottage cheese	3.0 g.
1 roll or 2 slices whole grain bread	2.0 g.
total	8.0 g.

#3 Sandwich

1 glass water	0.0 g.
1 cup herbal tea	0.0 g.
1 sandwich	
2 slices whole grain bread	2.0 g.
2 slices lean chicken, turkey,	
or fish (baked or tuna)	2.0 g.
Lettuce and tomato	0.1 g.
<u>Small salad or fresh vegetables</u>	<u>1.0 g.</u>
total	5.1 g.

#4 Hot lunch

1 glass water	0.0 g.
1 glass fruit juice	0.0 g.
1 cup spaghetti or whole grain pasta	0.7 g.
with 1/2 cup tomato sauce	1.8 g.
<u>steamed vegetables</u>	<u>1.0 g.</u>
total	3.5 g.

#5 baked potato

1 glass water	0.0 g.
1 glass vegetable juice	0.0 g.
1 large baked potato	0.2 g.
<u>2 tbsp. sour cream</u>	<u>5.0 g.</u>
total	5.2 g.

Noticeably absent from each lunch menu is dessert. If you can accept the fact that meals can be enjoyable without dessert, you can lose weight and become healthy. Once you are at your healthy weight, you can indulge yourself occasionally, as a treat, with a dessert. I do not define "occasionally, as a treat" to mean every meal, or even every day. High sugar desserts are unhealthy, and can be tolerated here and there, but not too often. If you can manage to re-define dessert to include fresh fruits and melons, you can eat dessert every meal. If you want high sugar/high fat cookies, candies, and cakes, you will never get healthy.

#1 Soup is a good, warm source of nourishment. You can make your own, open a can or package, or order from a restaurant. When you make your own, you can control how much fat you put in. When you open a can or a package, you can read the label to find your fat content. When you order from a restaurant, you can only guess what you are getting. Generally speaking, vegetable and noodle soups are safe. Cream of anything, hearty beef, or consumes are probably not.

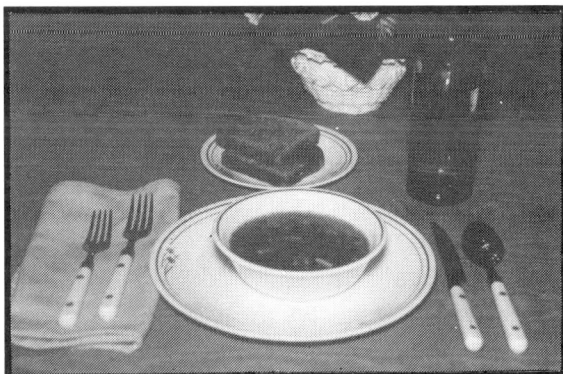

#2 Salads are the best possible meals, because you are eating raw food as nature provides it. Fruit salad is great, if it is fresh. Avoid canned fruits, and especially fruits canned in sugar. Fresh vegetables contain almost no fat (2 g. is an extremely generous estimate, depending on how much of which vegetables you use), but the dressing is where you can gain weight. Use no-oil, no-mayonnaise dressings: usually a lo-cal dressing is low in fat, although it may not be all natural. Vinegars, lemon and other fruit juices, herbs, and mustards all make good dressing ingredients. You can make your own favorite, or you might try taco salsa as a salad dressing. The cottage cheese is added for protein, if there are no beans in your salad. Any restaurant with a good salad bar -- even Wendy's -- makes eating out simple.

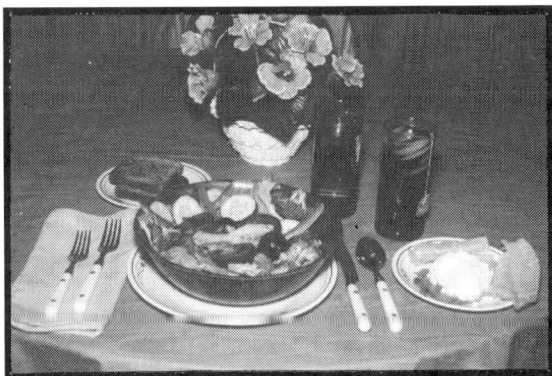

#3 The sandwich is the all-American bag lunch. You can make very healthy and nutritious sandwiches with very little effort. Buy lean sliced chicken or turkey, or slice your own from your leftovers. You can eat tuna or baked fish (re-heat it in a

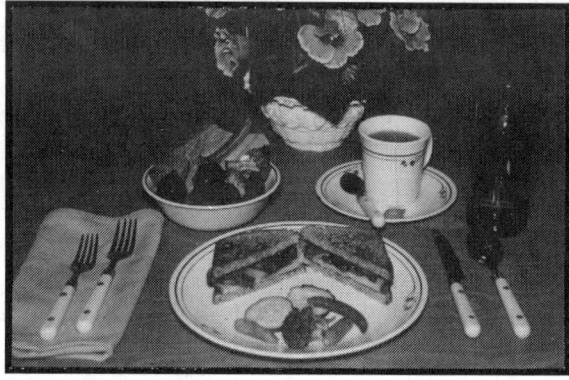

microwave.) Just stay away from breaded or fried fish (or chicken). Dress up and moisten your sandwich with sliced tomato and lettuce, or some sprouts, or cucumber, or whatever fresh vegetable suits your taste.

#4 There are thousands of hot lunches you can prepare or buy in restaurants, as long as you read labels and menus carefully. Watch out for pork and beef, fried anything, cheese, and cream sauces. Pasta and rice are very low in fat, as long as you don't

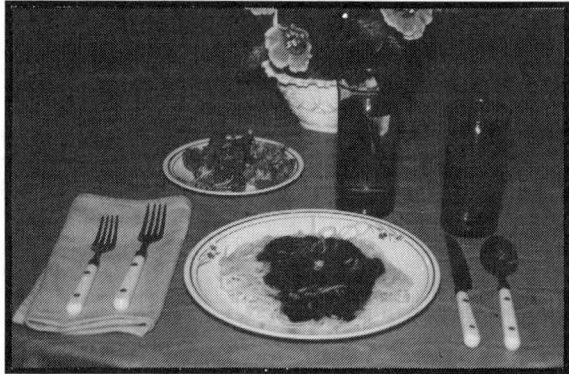

add a fatty sauce. Tomato sauce has a little oil in it, and is excellent unless you add greasy sausage or ground beef. Chicken tastes good in tomato sauce (chicken cacciatore), and would be a good addition to flavor and increase the protein value of the meal. You might even eat frozen "t.v. dinners", providing you read the package for fat content and natural ingredients (no powdered potatoes or fake cheese). See the dinner suggestions for more ideas on hot lunches.

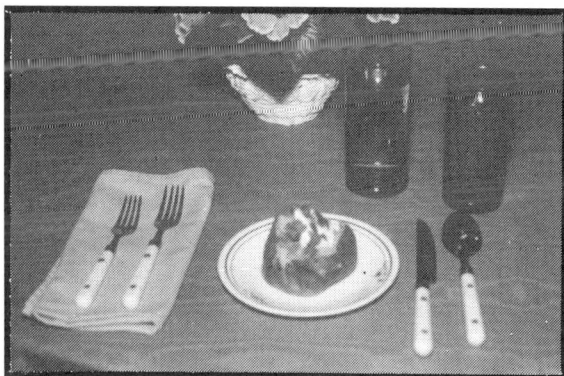

#5 In the past few years people have realized that they need not eat a traditional "meal" in order to get good nutrition. Depending on your appetite, one good baked potato could pass for a meal when you are trying to lose weight. Potatoes have almost no fat, are filling, and very healthy when eaten with the skin. If you cannot enjoy the plain potato, add just a little sour cream and chives. Butter or margarine are too high in fat to be considered, and fake butter flavor is unnatural and unhealthy (but may be used until you have lost your weight). You could add some steamed vegetables without significantly increasing the fat content, if you like (1 g. is a high estimate, depending on the amount and kind of vegetables.)

Dinners

Americans consider dinner the main meal of the day because it is the time the family can gather together and share their day. Unfortunately, we have developed the habit of eating our most fattening foods at dinner and then not doing any exercise. This process contributes to unnecessary weight gain.

We can still maintain the family dinner without the fat by altering the menu. Nutritionally, we should eat our most substantial meals earlier in the day when we can use the fuel for work and play. The evening meal should be lighter, because we will be less active in the evening. Never eat right before going to bed: if you do, your heart and digestive organs will not get a chance to rest -- and they need rest. Here are some lower-fat alternatives for dinner:

Sample Dinner menus:	Fat grams
#1	
1 glass water	0.0 g.
1 glass fruit juice	0.0 g
4 oz. broiled fish	0.4 - 14.0 g.
1/2 cup whole grain rice	0.6 g.
steamed vegetables	1.0 g.
total	2.0 or more g.

#2

1 glass water	0.0 g.
1 glass herbal iced tea	0.0 g.
4 oz. broiled chicken (1/2 breast)	3.1 g.
1 baked potato	0.2 g.
steamed vegetables	1.0 g.
total	4.3 g.

#3

1 glass water	0.0 g.
1 glass fruit juice	0.0 g.
spaghetti or other whole grain pasta	0.7 g.
with tomato sauce	1.7 g.
with chicken or fish	3.1 g.
garden salad	1.0 g.
with dressing	1.0 g.
total	7.5 g.

#4

1 glass water	0.0 g.
1 glass vegetable juice	0.0 g.
black beans and rice (2 cups)	3.0 g.
garden salad	1.0 g.
with dressing	1.0 g.
total	5.0 g.

#5

1 glass water	0.0 g.
1 cup hot herbal tea	0.0 g.
Chicken chow mein (1 cup)	4.0 g.
1 cup whole grain rice	1.2 g.
total	5.2 g.

157

Options #1 and #2 are basically the same: a portion of meat, a portion of carbohydrate, and a portion of vegetable. You can find lots of different kinds of fish to steam, bake, or broil. You can bake or roast your chicken with all sorts of low-fat sauces and herbs. You can exchange rice for potato for pasta. You can steam any fresh vegetable, or use frozen, or even canned vegetables. You can increase your portions of carbohydrate or vegetable without much effect on the fat content. These are traditional three-course American dinners without the fat. You can even find high quality frozen dinners with low fat content -- just look out for the fake foods and chemical additives.

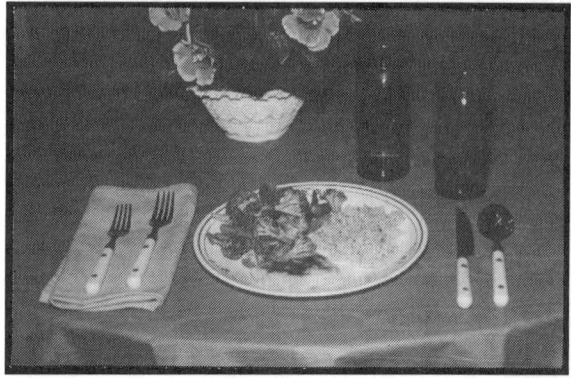

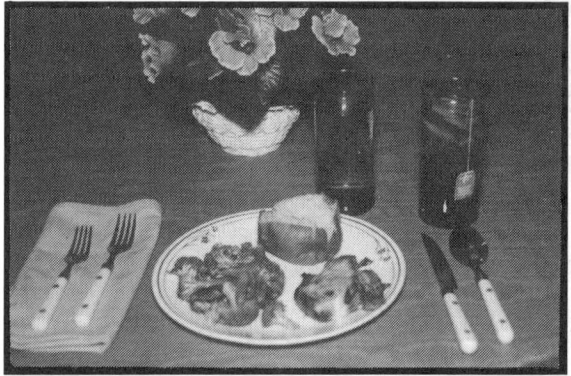

#3 Pasta with tomato sauce is virtually the same as lunch spaghetti. You might exchange the chicken for seafood or beans. Pasta fazool is an Italian dish (really a soup) of pasta and beans. There are enough different pastas, beans, and fish to offer a lot of variety for this dinner.

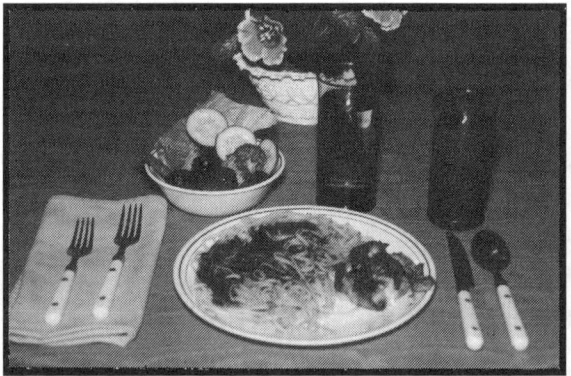

#4 Beans and rice has been a staple of human diet for centuries. Whether it's Cuban black bean, Jamaican red peas, Mexican pinto beans, garbanzo beans, lentils, butter beans or black-eyed peas; human beings have been mixing the local legumes with rice to improve the protein value of each. Although some people consider this inexpensive, simple food to be the food of "poor folks", it seems to me that the poor folks are a lot healthier than the rich, beef-eaters who look down on them. Letting this specific kind of "soul food" (without the fat and grease) into our diets occasionally would improve the quality and the variety.

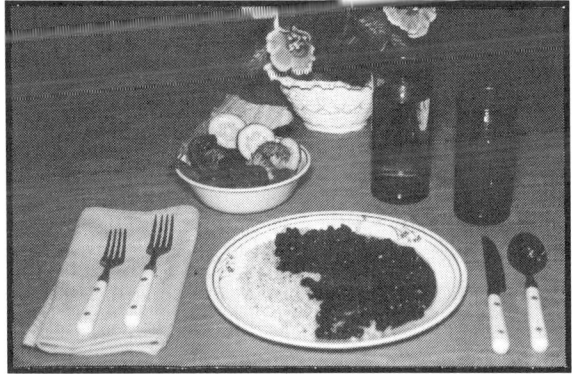

#5 Oriental foods, it seems, are naturally healthy. Stir-frying vegetables is a good way to cook them without getting much oil all over them. Any meal with rice, vegetables, and chicken or fish is a good, healthy meal unless you ruin it with a fattening or unhealthy sauce. Soy sauce is good in moderation, but m.s.g. is a definite no-no. Oriental food is delicious and healthy as long as you cook your own, read your package, or request "no m.s.g." at the restaurant.

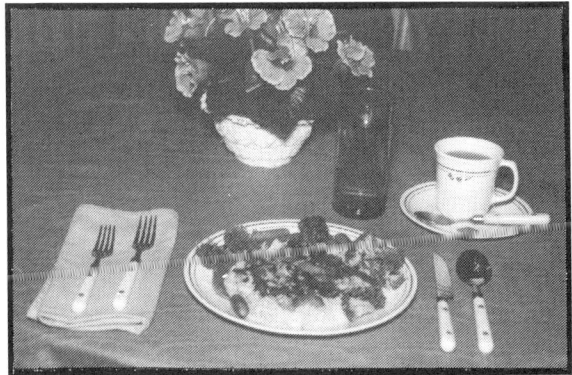

Summary:

You can eat good food and lose weight and improve your health at the same time. You could easily eat three meals and two snacks a day (Breakfast and Dinner #1, Lunch #4) and still be under ten grams of fat per day. Remember, I said that a low fat intake could be unhealthy, but that is an extreme. You can add a couple of grams of fat here and there for flavor and still stay within your recommendation (20 - 40 g. for a woman, 30 - 60 g. for a man). Just eat natural foods that are low in fat, and get rid of the high fat, high sugar junk foods. Once you reach your desired weight, you can stop counting fat grams and just eat natural foods. Cookies, candies, and cakes are not good for even a healthy body. You really have to make a life-long choice between junk and health. Once the decision is made, it's just a question of forming new, good habits. You won't regret it.

How to Gain weight

There are some people who really have trouble gaining weight. They are usually nervous young people with a high metabolism. There are three steps to gaining weight:

1. Slow down your metabolism.
2. Eat more nutritious food.
3. Exercise.

The best way to slow down your metabolism is to do Power Breathing. Even basic Power Breathing slows down your heart rate and helps you relax. Once you can begin to relax, your hormones can start to return to their natural state of balance, and you won't burn everything you eat for nervous energy.

Second, you simply must eat more nutritious food. Eating more junk will not help you gain useful weight. You may gain fat, but even a thin person does not need to gain excess fat. To increase your muscle, eat proteins and especially carbohydrates (natural grains). Your body must have excess calories present before it can build muscle, so high protein isn't enough by itself. Eat more often: five or six meals a day. I do not recommend protein powders and other supplements: they seem to work over the short run (body builders gain muscle), but they are not natural foods, so the side effects on the internal organs will not always show up right away. If your goal is to get big at any cost, use powders and even steroids. If your goal is to be healthier, eat natural foods.

Exercise stimulates the body to grow. If you ask your body to do something new, it will try to accommodate you. You can play ball, do heavy physical labor, do exercises, lift weights, or practice Tae Kwon Do. Your muscles will be stimulated, and if you feed them properly, they will grow. It is possible to over-stimulate them by working them harder than they can rebuild, or stimulate them the wrong way by doing an exercise like long distance running that stimulates them to remain thin. Within these simple guidelines you should be able to gradually adjust yourself to achieve a healthy weight. I do not mean you will be able to compete for Mr. Olympia; I mean you will achieve a healthy weight for your body.

Summary:

We are each born as human beings with a common chemistry on the same planet. We are also individuals, having minor physiological differences and living in different climates. If we can apply the general rules to our specific situation, we should be able to cope successfully with this wonderful adventure we call life.

The general rule is simple: nature provides the necessary nutrients for all our needs. When we pervert the foods nature provides for us, we create our own problems. Nature will usually give us a sign that we are doing something wrong, and we can figure it out by paying attention to the signs. When we ignore the signs and maintain our wrong behavior, we are the ones who suffer. Nature continues, and the smartest survive.

Be one of the smart ones. Whether you live a day or a century, live healthy. Don't stuff your body with unnatural substances; it will only rebel. Eat natural, nutritional foods and allow your body to work the way it was designed. Don't try to conquer nature; cooperate with it. If you take care of your body, it will take care of you.

MEDITATION

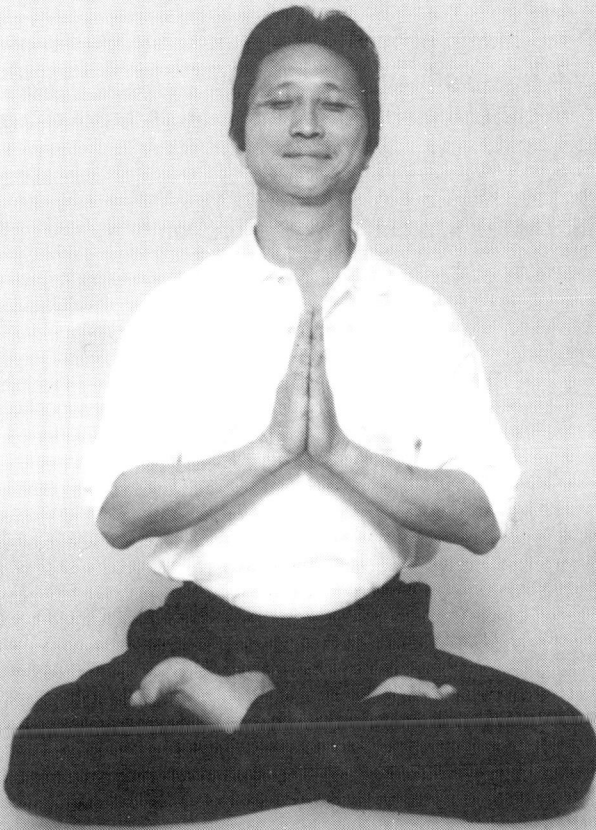

"Meditation is natural, nutritional __mental__ food."

-- Y. K. Kim

Meditation creates a healthy mental attitude.

Meditation will empty your mind and clear your thought processes. It will give you peace of mind and positive mental energy. Meditation will release stress and tension. It will help you generate strength for your body, mind, and spirit.

I think that many people have a misconception of meditation. Some people think that meditation is something that is mystical, spiritual, and/or religious. Although meditation can be all of those things and more, it doesn't have to be any of them.

Meditation is the most inexpensive and most valuable daily mini-vacation.

There are 5 kinds of meditation:

1. Concentration Meditation

2. Reflective Meditation

3. Relaxation Meditation

4. Power Meditation

5. Self-Mastery Meditation.

Hand Positions for Meditation

Hap jang kwan (two hands together) represents neutrality -- neither positive nor negative, *um* or *yang*. This posture will help you appreciate yourself and your place in nature. It will calm your mind and body.
Posture: *jung ja, ban ka bu ja, ka bu ja,* or free.

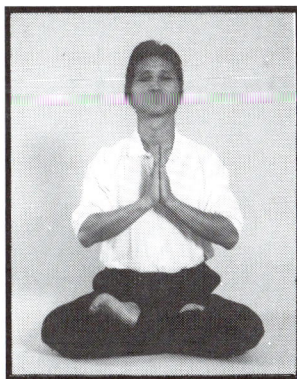

Ki cho kwan (one hand on the other, thumbs interlocked) represents the foundation of the body and mind. This posture will strengthen your body and mind.
Posture: *jung ja, ban ka bu ja, ka bu ja,* or free.

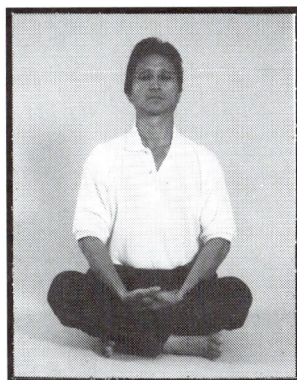

Wan sung kwan (thumb and index finger form a circle, with backs of hands on knees) represents complete achievement. This posture will allow you to receive natural *ki*. It will help you feel oneness with nature.
Posture: *jung ja, ban ka bu ja, ka bu ja,* or free.

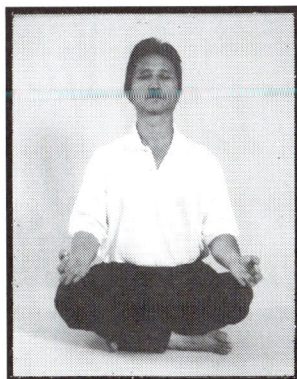

Proper posture will create a healthy body and a clear mind.

Concentration Meditation

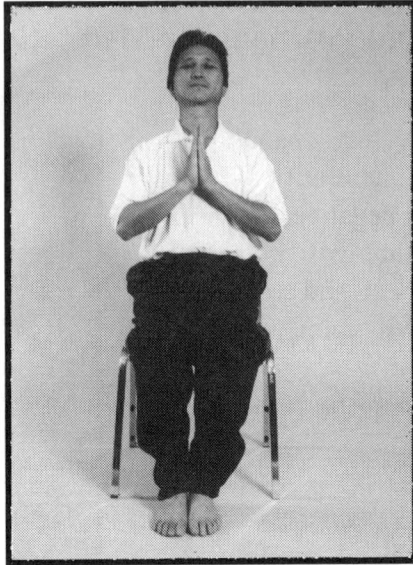

Hap jang kwan in a chair

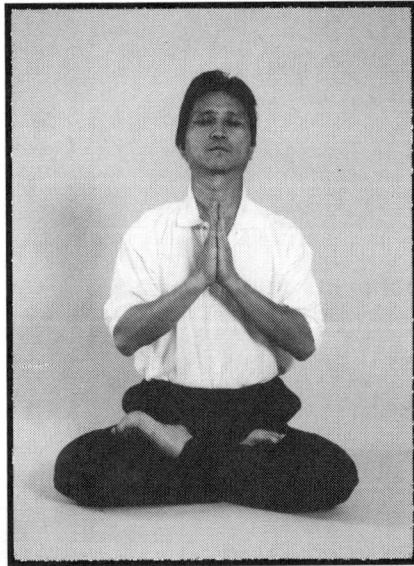

Ka bu ja Hap jang kwan

Concentration is the key to achieve your goals
-- Y. K. Kim

When you concentrate on your ideas and thoughts, or what you are doing, or what you will do, you must focus on one thing at a time. When you have a complete, clear understanding of your words and thoughts, and/or a complete, clear mental picture of what you are doing, or a mental rehearsal of what you are about to do, you can get the maximum benefit from whatever you do because you will have a clear, open mind, improved memory, and more confidence.

How to do it:

A. Sit down with your back and neck straight. If you are sitting on the floor, cross your legs for comfort (and sit on a small pillow if necessary.) Proper posture will create a healthy body and a clear mind.

B. Place your palms together in front of your heart, with your fingers pointing toward your chin, as if praying (*hap jang kwan.*)

C. Inhale through the nose for about one second, then exhale through the mouth for about one second, as deeply as possible within the time frame. Repeat this breathing pattern from three to ten times, depending on your aerobic fitness, in order to clean your mind of unnecessary negative thoughts.

D. Return to normal breathing, as deeply and quietly as possible, in and out through the nose (you may practice Basic or Intermediate Breathing, depending on your development).

E1. To concentrate on your ideas and thoughts, only focus on one idea or thought at a time, and continue to repeat that idea or thought in your mind until you can see a clear mental picture of it. It will help you clarify that idea or thought. Or, you can make a mental picture of your idea or thought and study it: look at each detail and how each detail fits with the others.

167

E2. To concentrate on what you are doing, use steps A through D to clear away distracting thoughts, then focus on the importance of what you are doing. Repeat to yourself the meaning and importance of what you are doing, or make a mental picture of it. When you focus on the importance of what you are doing either with words or a picture (or both), you will clear away all unnecessary distractions, and you can return to the task at hand with confidence and a clear mind.

E3. To concentrate on what you are about to do, think about what you will say or do, one thing at a time, in the proper order, and repeat the words to yourself. Go through a mental rehearsal so that you have a clear mental picture, and concentrate on that picture. You will be confident in your speech or actions. If you are approaching a learning situation, you cannot predict what will happen one thing at a time, so you can only prepare yourself to open your mind to learn as much as possible.

Benefits:

* When you have a clear mind, you will not be distracted by any extraneous thoughts.

* When you have a clear mental picture and you mentally rehearse what you will say or do, you will have more confidence, and your performance will be easier and more accurate.

* When you open your mind and really want to learn, listening, concentrating, and studying will be much easier and more enjoyable.

Preparation is the key to success.

Cautions:

If you have a bad knee or ankle, be careful about crossing your legs to sit on the floor. You might be more comfortable in a chair.

It is possible to do this meditation in the car, sometimes even if you are driving, but don't ever close your eyes while driving.

If you cannot sit down anywhere, you can do this meditation while standing. Just open your legs about shoulder width apart, and maintain the same hand position as in the seated meditation, or you can put your hands at your side.

If you are sick in bed or cannot straighten your back, you may have to try this meditation lying down, but you may easily fall asleep.

Reflective Meditation

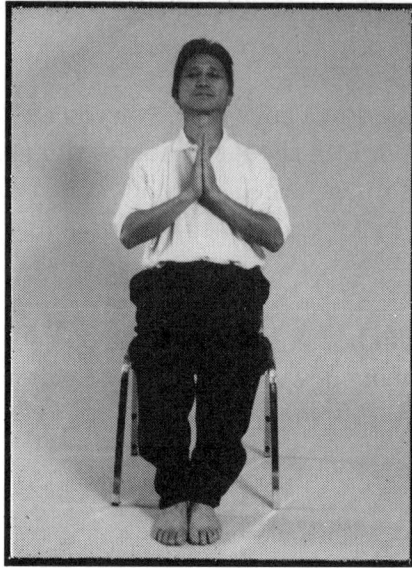

Hap jang kwan in a chair

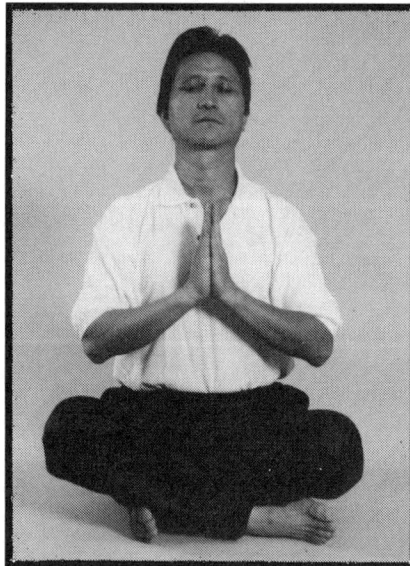

Jung ja hap jang kwan

Reflection will develop the winning habit.
-- Y. K. Kim

When you mentally review what happened during a class, an event, a day, a year, or your entire lifetime, you are engaging in Reflective Meditation. During reflection you should not only remember what happened, but evaluate it. You can learn from your mistakes and your successes so that you can reduce the number of future mistakes and increase the number of future successes. It will help you develop the winning habit.

How to do it:

A. Sit down with your back and neck straight. If you are sitting on the floor, cross your legs for comfort (and sit on a small pillow if necessary.) Proper posture will create a healthy body and a clear mind.

B. Place your palms together in front of your heart, with your fingers pointing toward your chin, as if praying (*hap jang kwan*).

C. Inhale through the nose for about one second, then exhale through the mouth for about one second, as deeply as possible within the time frame. Repeat this breathing pattern from three to ten times, depending on your aerobic fitness, in order to clean your mind of unnecessary negative thoughts.

D. Return to Basic Breathing #3, as deeply and quietly as possible, breathing in and out through the nose (or through the mouth quietly).

E. Concentrate on what you have done (closing meditation) at the end of a workout or at the end of the day. Say to yourself,

"I did _____ and _____ today. First I did _____, and next I did _____ (think about what you did, one thing at a time, in the proper order.)

"I remember I made a mistake when I did _____ wrong, and also _____. I know I can improve by doing _____ and _____ next time.

"I did do _____ and _____ very well today, and I feel proud of myself. All in all, it was a good workout/day, and I know tomorrow will be even better."

Closing meditation is important for peace of mind, because you will have a clear idea of how to proceed next time.

Benefits:

* By reviewing what happened, you will improve your memory.

* By reviewing facts and figures, and new concepts, you will increase your chances of remembering and using them.

* By reviewing your successes, you will have more confidence and better knowledge of yourself.

* By reviewing your mistakes, you will have better knowledge of yourself and identify a course of self-improvement.

Relaxation Meditation

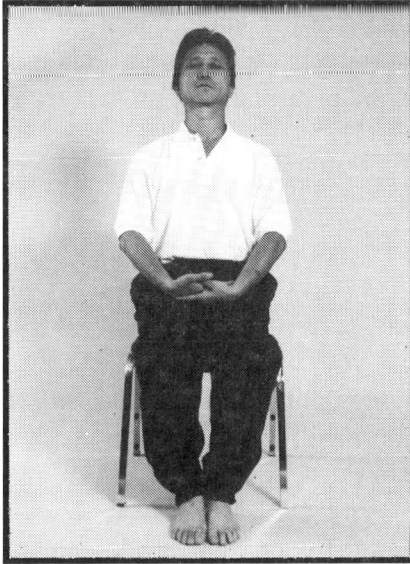

Ki cho kwan in a chair

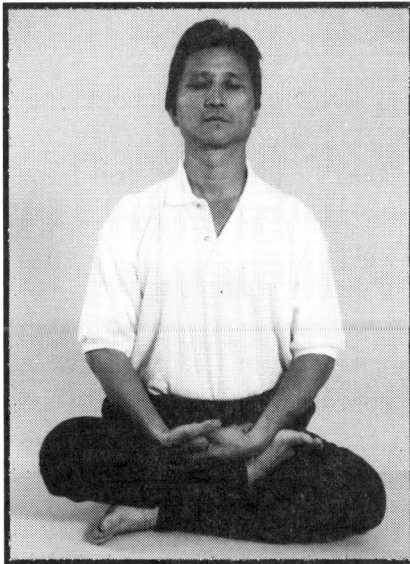

Ban ka bu ja Ki cho kwan

Relaxation will recharge your energy for healthy living.
-- Y. K. Kim

Relaxation meditation is good for your muscles as well as your major organs, especially the heart, lungs, and brain. Your body will become physically stronger at the same time it releases stress and tension, and disposes of waste products. You can do this meditation at the office or at home, in your car, on an airplane, or anywhere, almost any time.

How to do it:

A. Sit down with your back and neck straight. If you are sitting on the floor, cross your legs for comfort (and sit on a small pillow if necessary.) Proper posture will create a healthy body and a clear mind.

B. Place the palm of your right hand against the back of your left hand and extend both arms so that the backs of your wrists touch your thighs.

C. Inhale through the nose for about one second, then exhale through the mouth for about one second, as deeply as possible within the time frame. Repeat this breathing pattern from three to ten times, depending on your aerobic fitness, in order to clean your mind of unnecessary negative thoughts.

D. Start with your left arm. Make a fist. As you inhale through your nose as slowly as possible, tighten your grip and your entire arm up to the shoulder. As you exhale through the mouth as slowly as possible, relax your fist and arm. Say to yourself,

"My arm feels warm and heavy. My arm is loose and relaxed, and I feel great."

E. Next, feel your right arm. Make a fist. As you inhale through your nose as slowly as possible, tighten your grip and your entire arm up to the shoulder. As you exhale through the mouth as slowly as possible, relax your fist and arm. Say to yourself,

"My arm feels warm and heavy. My arm is loose and relaxed, and I feel great."

F. Next, tighten your left leg as you breathe in through your nose as slowly as possible. As you exhale through the mouth, relax your leg. Say to yourself,

"My leg feels warm and heavy. My leg is limber and relaxed, and I feel great."

G. Next tighten your right leg as you breathe in through your nose as slowly as possible. As you exhale through the mouth, relax your leg. Say to yourself,

"My leg feels warm and heavy. My leg is limber and relaxed, and I feel great."

H. Next, tuck your chin to touch your chest, inhale through the nose as slowly as possible and tighten your back muscles and spine. As you exhale through the mouth, relax all over. Say to yourself,

"My back feels warm. It is loose and relaxed, and I feel great."

I. Next, tighten your abdomen and chest muscles as you inhale as slowly as possible. As you exhale through the mouth, relax all over (including your lower abdomen). Say to yourself,

"My abdomen and chest feel warm. My body feels loose and relaxed, and my heart feels great."

J. Next, tighten your entire face, neck, and head, including all your face muscles, as you inhale as slowly as possible. As you exhale through the mouth, relax. Say to yourself,

"My head feels warm. My face and neck feel loose and relaxed. My mind feels great."

K. Next, relax your mind. Your mind is an organ, not a striated muscle. Like your stomach or liver, and unlike your arms or legs, you do not exercise your mind by tensing or relaxing it. You need to move it indirectly. The best way to move the mind indirectly is through vibration . . . specifically humming.

Rock your head gently from side to side and hum in a deep tone as you exhale. Vary the tone slightly, so that the vibrations can relax your brain as they resonate through it.

L. Relax and return to Basic Breathing #3 (or Advanced Breathing #3), as deeply and quietly as possible, imagining that you are breathing all over your body through your skin. Your whole body feels wonderful. Say to yourself,

"I feel wonderful. I feel great. My body is relaxed and peaceful."

Benefits:

Relaxation Meditation will:

* build up your muscular strength through dynamic tension.

* strengthen and refresh your heart, while the deep, controlled breathing will clean your lungs.

* massage the abdominal organs -- the liver, kidneys, spleen, pancreas, intestines, and gall bladder -- by the downward movement of the diaphragm during deep breathing.

* empty the lungs and stomach of old, stale air (carbon dioxide).

* release a lot of pent-up stress.

* open the blood vessels to allow better circulation. The improved circulation will help clean toxins out of your muscles and organs, and deliver fresh oxygen and nutrients.

* allow the heart to work with less resistance because the blood flow is less restricted and more efficient.

* improve the immune system, make it stronger, and give it more reserve resistance to prevent disease.

* relax your mind while the circulation is chemically cleaning and refreshing the brain. This combination chemical/psychological revitalization will improve your mental capabilities.

* help you sleep better. This meditation is good for insomnia.

* make your stronger, healthier, and happier, both physically and mentally.

Caution:

Do not hold your breath between inhalation and exhalation -- it puts undue pressure on the heart, nervous system, and hormonal regulators.

Power Meditation

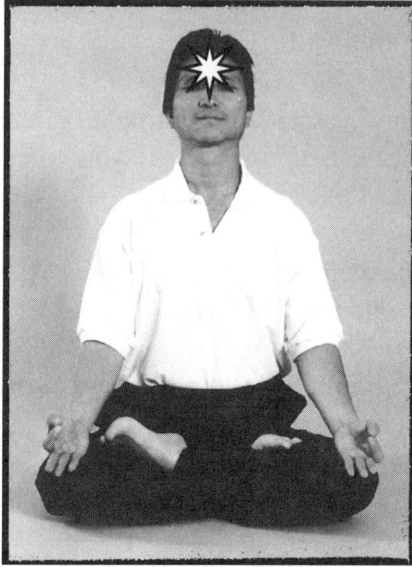

the high energy center
Wan sung kwan, Ka bu Ja

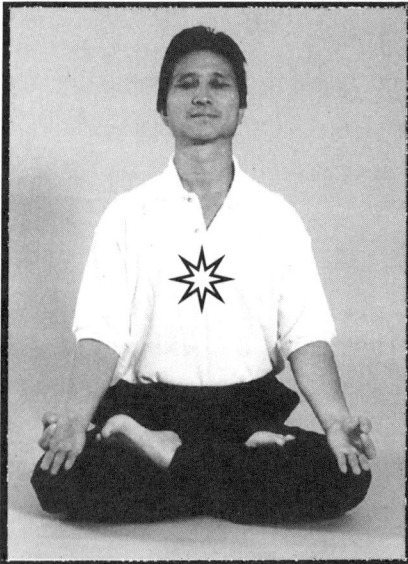

the middle energy center
Wan sung kwan, Ka bu ja

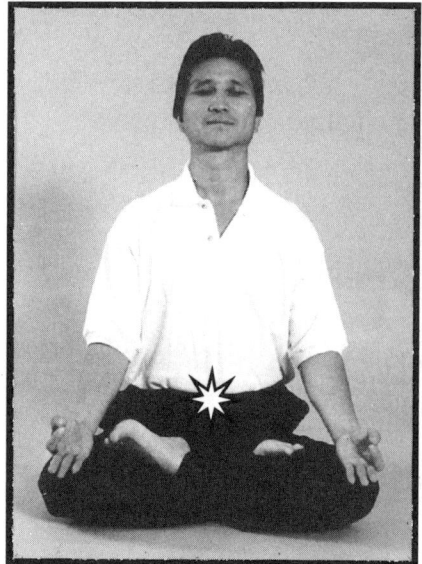

the lower energy center
Wan sung kwan, Ka bu ja

"Power Meditation will give you more energy and a long, healthy life. "   *-- Y. K. Kim*

Power meditation can give you power by getting you in touch with universal energy, or *ki*. By universal energy I mean natural energy, or, as I refer to it when dealing with living beings, internal energy. In order to do this meditation you must first understand the three external sources of *ki*: the sun or sky (*chun ki*), the air (*dae ki*), and the earth (*chi ki*.) Let me illustrate what I mean with this example: plants combine the energy of the sun (through photosynthesis) with chemicals from the air (carbon dioxide), and nutrients from the earth (including water). When the three sources are combined, the plant can flourish; take away any one source, and the plant will die.

Second, you must understand that Eastern medicine is not based on chemical reactions alone, but on the natural medicine of energy flow or *ki*. According to this theory, health is the result of proper energy flow, and disease is the result of a block in the energy flow.

In the West we have a materialistic culture, and tend to believe only what can be seen or touched. In the East we have a spiritual culture, and we believe in things that we can feel, even if we cannot see or touch them. Western scientists cannot locate *ki*, and therefore do not accept its existence. Eastern doctors utilize *ki* to heal their patients.

As I mentioned earlier, energy or *ki* flows along channels (sometimes called meridians), and gathers around centers (sometimes called chakras). Most authorities identify many energy centers (usually seven), but I find that depth unnecessary for the average person. I will only concentrate on the three main energy centers, which, for simplicity, I will call the lower, middle, and high centers.

The **lower energy center** *(ha dan jun)* is located one hand's width below and behind your navel. **It is your foundation**, and the center of your

> **strength** -- which powers your movement in work and play;
>
> **stamina** -- which is your sexual energy that can be re-directed to initiating and consummating any creative or passionate act;
>
> **balance** -- which keeps you centered.

The **middle energy center** *(joong dan jun)* is located about one fist's depth behind your sternum. **It is the home of your emotions**, and the center for your

> **power of communication** -- which develops clear self-expression that helps others to understand whatever point you are trying to make, and builds a positive self-image that inspires others to cooperate with you;

> **power of belief** -- which increases self-esteem and self-respect, and makes you proud of yourself;

> **power of love** -- which creates the loving relationships that will give you enjoyment in your life.

The **high energy center** *(sang dan jun)* is located just behind the middle point between your eyebrows, often called the third eye. **It is the home of your spiritual energy**, and the center for your

> **power of direction** -- which will give you a clear, positive goal in your life and the right direction to follow to achieve your goal,

> **power of the spirit** -- which creates a positive mental attitude and strong mental energy that will give you a sense of justice, passionate leadership, and the winning habit to support success in your life, and

> **peace of mind** -- which leads people from all walks of life to their ultimate dream: happiness.

When you try to get in touch with universal energy or *ki*, you must first of all believe that it exists. If you can clean your mind of all negative thoughts and open yourself to accept what is natural, you will find universal energy within yourself. If you do not have an open mind, or can not clean away all doubts and negative thoughts, you will not be able to utilize *ki*.

Let me remind you again of the example I use to illustrate what I mean by *ki*, so that you may believe it is real. Close your eyes for a minute and engage in a sexual fantasy. When you do, you get excited, or "horny". Your heart rate and respiration increase; your palms begin to sweat; you can feel the energy flowing to your sexual organs. When you get energy from nowhere but your own mind, you are experiencing *ki*, which is universal (or internal) energy.

Similarly, if you can imagine or recall a time when you were afraid, or sad, or angry, and can feel those feelings again, you are experiencing universal energy. *Ki* is real, and we all have experienced it. We just have not learned to control it. This meditation will help you get in touch with *ki* and enable you to use it to help you succeed in life.

How to do it:

A. Sit down with your back and neck straight. If you are sitting on the floor, cross your legs for comfort (and sit on a small pillow if necessary.) Proper posture will create a healthy body and a clear mind.

B. Open your hands and touch the tip of the thumb and index finger on each hand together to form a circle. Rest the backs of your hands on your knees. This posture leaves you open to accept *ki*.

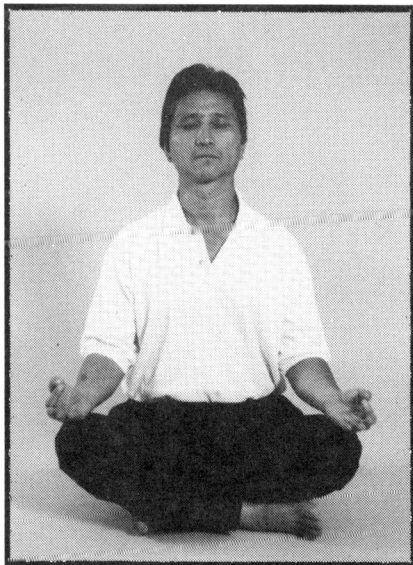

A, B, C, D

181

C. Inhale through the nose for about one second, then exhale through the mouth for about one second, as deeply as possible within the time frame. Repeat this breathing pattern from three to ten times, depending on your aerobic fitness, in order to clean your mind of unnecessary negative thoughts.

D. Return to normal breathing, as deeply and quietly as possible, in and out through the nose.

to develop *ha dan jun*

E1. With each breath, imagine that you are inhaling universal energy all over your whole body, as if through the skin. You must visualize the *ki* moving in a clear mental picture. Intentionally visualize that you are gathering the *ki* into the storage tank of your lower energy center (*ha dan jun*) for a few breaths.

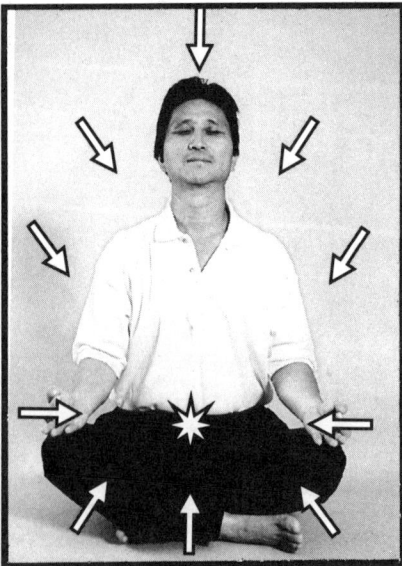

E1

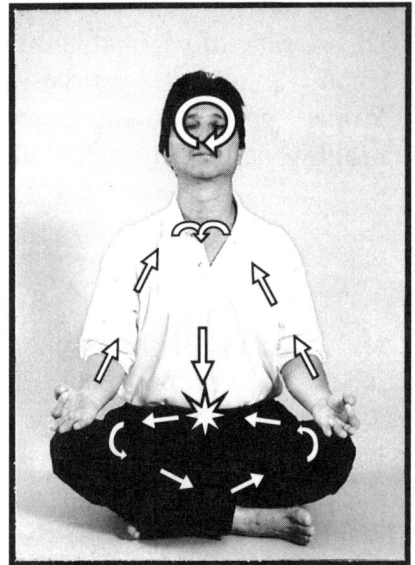

E2

E2. Inhale and draw *ki* from all three sources: the earth (*chi ki*), the air (*dae ki*), and the sun (*chun ki*), and then intentionally move the *ki* around your whole body. As you continue to visualize this movement of *ki*, it will become second nature to you.

Say to yourself,

"The lower energy center is the foundation of my body, mind, and spirit.

"This energy will give me the strength I will need to power my movement in work and play.

"This energy will give me stamina, which is my sexual energy. I can redirect this energy to initiate or consummate any creative or passionate act.

"This energy will give me good balance and keep me centered."

E3. Exhale throughout your whole body, as if through the skin, and expel all the weak *ki*.

E4. Repeat E2 and E3 for several breaths, but while you are saying these things to yourself, breathe almost unconsciously.

E5. Either open your eyes and relax, or continue to F1.

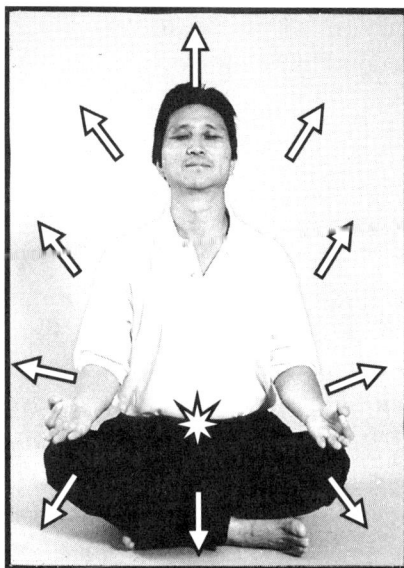

E3

183

to develop *jung dan jun*

F1. With each breath, imagine that you are inhaling universal energy all over your whole body, as if through the skin. You must visualize the *ki* moving in a clear mental picture. Intentionally visualize that you are gathering the *ki* into your middle energy center (*jung dan jun*) for a few breaths.

F2. Inhale and draw *ki* from all three sources: the earth (*chi ki*), the air (*dae ki*), and the sun and sky (*chun ki*), and then intentionally move the *ki* around your whole body. As you continue to visualize this movement of *ki*, it will become second nature to you.

Say to yourself,

"The middle energy center is the home of my emotions.

"This energy will give me the power of communication. I will have a clear self-expression that will build up a positive self-image that will help others to understand me and inspire others to cooperate with me.

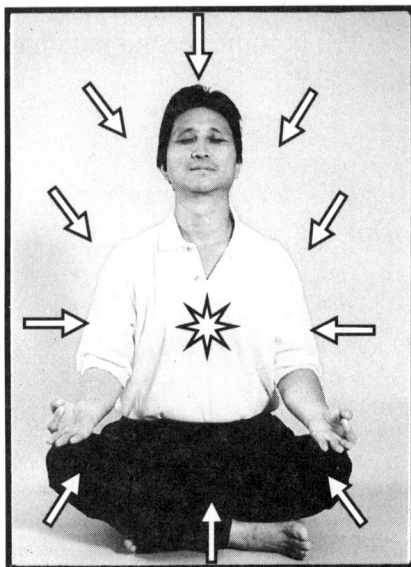

F1

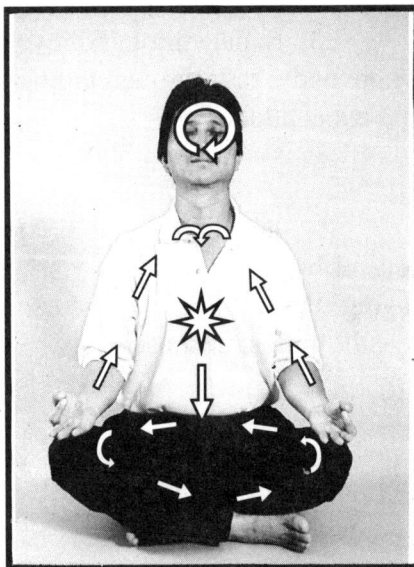

F2

184

"This energy will give me the power of belief, which will increase my self-esteem and self-respect, and make me proud of myself.

"This energy will give me the power of love, which will create the loving relationships that will give me enjoyment in my life."

F3.   Exhale throughout your whole body, as if through the skin, and expel all the weak *ki*.

F4. Repeat F2 and F3 for several breaths, but while you are saying these things to yourself, breathe almost unconsciously.

F5. Either open your eyes and relax, or go on to G1.

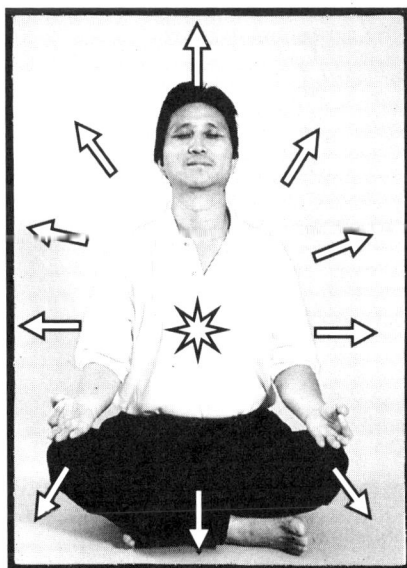

F3

to develop *sang dan jun*

G1. With each breath, imagine that you are inhaling universal energy all over your whole body, as if through the skin. You must visualize the *ki* moving in a clear mental picture. Intentionally visualize that you are gathering the *ki* into your high energy center (*sang dan jun*) for a few breaths.

G2. Inhale and draw *ki* from all three sources: the earth (*chi ki*), the air (*dae ki*), and the sun (*chun ki*), and then intentionally move the *ki* around your whole body. As you continue to visualize this movement of *ki*, it will become second nature to you.

Say to yourself,

"The high energy center is the center of my spiritual energy.

"This energy will give me the power of direction, which will give me a clear, positive goal in my life and the right direction to follow to achieve my goal.

"It will give me the power of the spirit, which will create a positive mental attitude and strong mental energy that will give me a sense of justice, passionate leadership, and the winning habit to support success in my life.

"This energy will give me peace of mind, which leads people from all walks of life to their ultimate dream: happiness."

G3. Exhale throughout your whole body, as if through the skin, and expel all the weak *ki*.

G4. Repeat G2 and G3 for several breaths, but while you are saying these things to yourself, breathe almost unconsciously.

G5. Open your eyes, and relax.

186

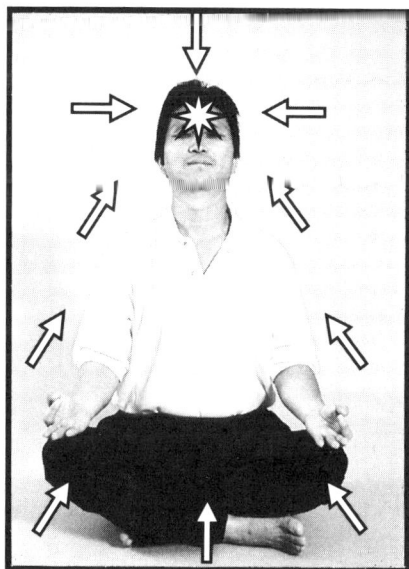

G1

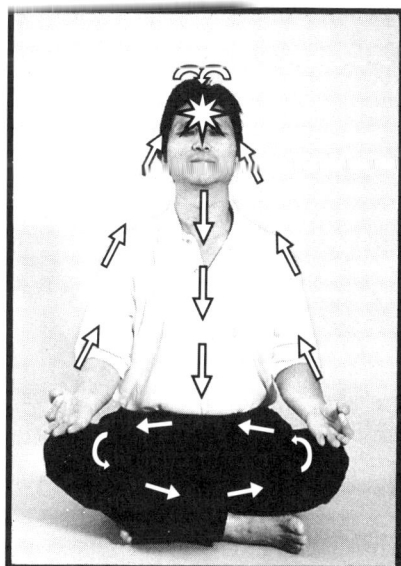

G2

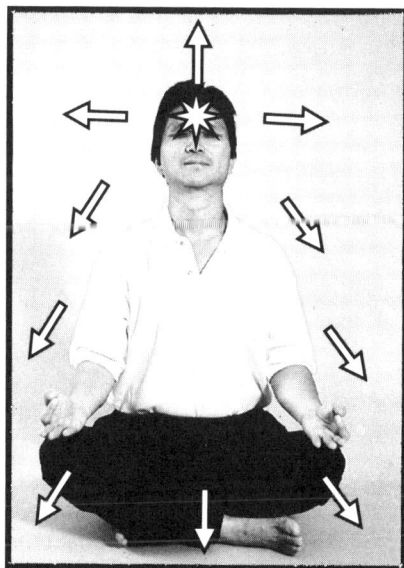

G3

Benefits:

This meditation will:

* increase the amount of *ki* in your body and mind.

* release stress and tension and allow you to become healthier, stronger, and happier.

* give you strength, stamina, and balance.

* improve your power of communication, build your self-esteem, and help you develop loving relationships.

* help you develop a positive attitude, find the right direction for your life, and develop passionate leadership and the winning habit for success in your life.

* give you peace of mind.

Self-Mastery Meditation

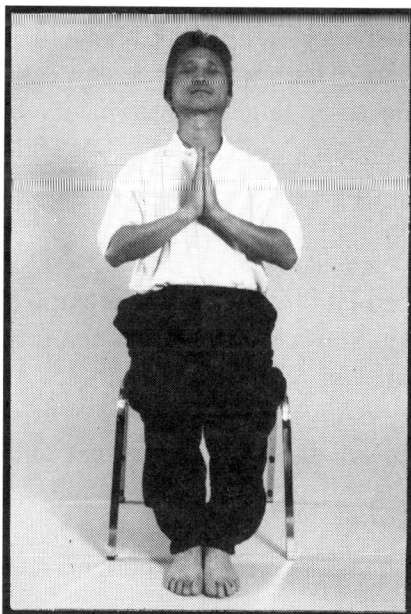

Hap jang kwan in a chair

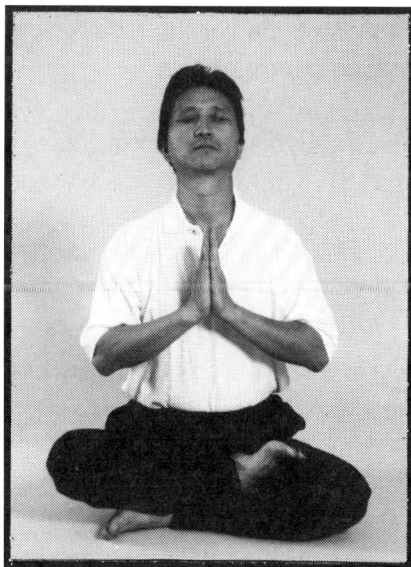

Ban ka bu ja Hap jang kwan

Self-mastery means a healthy mental attitude.

Self-mastery will help you throw away all your negative thoughts and habits, which I call "mental fat." Many people store anger, fear, guilt, depression, laziness, and evil like a time bomb inside themselves. The longer they store this junk, the more the poison eats them up inside. In addition, they continue to indulge in bad habits like drugs, excessive alcohol, smoking, over-eating, eating junk food, and shallow breathing. This meditation will help you find these poisons and dispose of them before they destroy you.

Self-mastery meditation will help you empty your mind and body of this negativity so that you can find out who you truly are. When your mind is clean and clear, you will be hungry to devour natural, nutritional <u>mental</u> food, which is positive mental energy or *ki*. You will develop a healthy mental attitude, which is the foundation of healthy living, and one of the four corners of the foundation of your health.

Let's take a look at some negative thoughts and habits:

Emotions

1. Anger - you hate someone or yourself, or even a situation that you feel you have no control over.

2. Fear - you are afraid you will be attacked, or that you will lose your job, your spouse, your health, or anything else.

3. Guilt - you have done something to hurt someone else or yourself, and you regret it.

4. Depression - you treat yourself as if you were weak or dumb, or otherwise unworthy.

Attitudes

5. Narrow mind - you only look at the world from one perspective, and cannot see things any other way.

6. Closed mind - you refuse to see anything but what you want to see.

190

7. Dumb mind - you do not even know enough to tell right from wrong.

8. Evil mind - you are selfish; you do not care if you hurt other people, as long as you can get something for yourself.

9. Negative mind - you only see the negative side of everything.

10. Twisted mind - you think, speak, and act the wrong way.

11. Violent mind - you try to solve problems through violence.

12. Arrogant mind - you ignore others because you think you are superior.

Habits

13. Bad temper - you do not control yourself and show your anger any time and any where.

14. Laziness - you have no desire, no energy, no activity. You are out of shape because you do not exercise.

15. Addictions - you are hooked on drugs; you are an alcoholic; or you smoke.

16. Overeating - you eat too much, or you eat too much junk food.

17. Shallow breathing - you breathe only in your chest, not from your lower abdomen.

To get rid of negative thoughts and habits:

If you want to throw them away, they will go away.
If you do not want to throw them away, they will stay with you forever.
If you are afraid to throw them away, they will get worse.

How to do it:

A. Sit down with your back and neck straight. If you are sitting on the floor, cross your legs for comfort (and sit on a small pillow if necessary.) Proper posture will create a healthy body and a clear mind.

B. Place your palms together in front of your heart, with your fingers pointing toward your chin, as if praying (*hap jang kwan*).

C. Inhale through the nose for about one second, then exhale through the mouth for about one second, as deeply as possible within the time frame.   Repeat this breathing pattern from three to ten times, depending on your aerobic fitness, in order to focus your mind.

D. Return to Basic Breathing #3, as deeply and quietly as possible, in and out through the nose (or exhale quietly through the mouth).

E. Begin to review yourself and your situation:

- Who or what is trying to hurt you?

- What is bothering you?

- What is restricting you?

F. Find the cause of your anger, fear, guilt, or depression, and cure the cause.

For anger, say to yourself:

"I really hate _____ (person).

"But, if I keep this hatred in my heart, can I hurt him? Not really. I actually end up hurting myself.

"What benefit will I get by keeping my anger? Nothing good. The more anger I keep inside, the worse it is for my health and my emotional well-being.

"What comes around, goes around. Somebody else will repay him for the bad things he has done, or he will eventually hurt himself. It is not my responsibility.

"I need to throw away my anger. I do not need to hate anybody. I like people.

"I forgive him and myself for any bad we have done.

"I feel much better already. I feel relieved. I feel peace.

"Nothing can bother me, and nothing can stop me. My unnecessary obstacles are gone. I feel strong. I feel great."

For fear, say to yourself:

"I am afraid I will be attacked by _____.

"I will do my best to avoid _____. I will stay away from the places where _____ is. I will try to walk away or talk my way out of a confrontation.

"I want to be peaceful, but if _____ tries to hurt me, I will have to defend myself. I will certainly pay _____ back double or triple, if necessary.

"If my life is threatened, I will use any weapon I can to defend myself. I will be prepared to take care of the situation.

"I feel confident that I can defend myself. If I worry too much, I will scare myself. I do not want to become my own enemy. I will not spend my life being afraid of what might happen. I will face life and reality, not some horror movie that only exists in my imagination.

"I am confident that I can defend myself. No one will bother me, and no one will hurt me. My best weapon is self-confidence."

-- or --

"I am afraid I will lose _____ (my job, my spouse, etc.)

"I will do my best, no matter what happens. If I work hard, I have nothing to worry about. Even if I am laid off or the company closes, I can find another job. I have special talents. I can do a good job for any company. Any company that hires me will be very lucky, because I am such a good worker.

"What else can I do but try my best? If I sit around and worry, will that help? If I drink and smoke a lot, will that help? Those things will only hurt and depress me.

"I am not going to treat myself that way. If I don't treat myself with respect, who will? There is only one person like me in the whole world. I need to be my own best friend, not my own worst enemy. I love, trust, respect, and believe in myself. I feel very confident. I feel great."

For guilt, say to yourself:

"I did _____ (bad thing) to _____ (person), and hurt him. I feel very bad about it, and I will try to do _____ to change it/make up for it.

"I am not proud of myself, but no one is perfect. I am only a human being, and the most important thing is that I learn from this mistake.

"I know that everyone makes mistakes. Losers live with their mistakes, and repeat them. Winners learn from their mistakes and do not repeat them. I will be a winner, and learn my lesson.

"Everyone has some kind of guilt, because everyone has made mistakes. Guilt is good when it teaches me not to make the same mistake twice. Guilt becomes bad when I have already learned the lesson, and I still beat myself up for the same mistake. From now on I will forget the past, and do only right and positive things in the future.

"I forgive myself for my mistakes, and I am positive about the future. I feel much better. I have a peaceful mind."

For depression, say to yourself:

"I am lucky to have _____ and _____. When I think of all the people who are less fortunate than me, I realize all that I have. I need to concentrate on the positive, not the negative.

"If I wallow in my depression, I will feel terrible about myself and never have the confidence to try to do anything.

"I have lots of goals to achieve. Some day I want to _____ and _____. I have no time to be depressed, if I want to achieve these goals. I must get busy right away.

"I have _____ (person) and _____ (person) who care about me. I would like to achieve my goals and do something good for them."

G. Review yourself and your attitudes to discover what kind of mental fat you have.

Ask yourself:

"Do I have a narrow or closed mind? Can I appreciate the other person's point of view? If not, what good does this do me? It will lead to nothing but trouble, because I will not be able to see problems before they arise. Starting now, I will have an open mind, and consider other possibilities and other points of view. I will see things more clearly and understand the situation much better.

"Do I have a dumb mind? Do I know enough to make good decisions? If not, what will happen to me? I will end up destroying myself out of ignorance. I must make a serious effort to learn more. I must read and study, and talk to wise people, and think carefully about every important decision. If I can do that, I will have a wonderful life.

"Do I have an evil mind? Do I cheat other people to gain an advantage for myself? If so, when I die, can I take these material things with me? How do I feel when someone else tries to cheat me or my family? It is not too late to change. What comes around, goes around, and it will be my turn soon. I do not want to live with my heart in jail, even if my body is free. I want to change my lifestyle for the better. If I start helping others, they will help me. I will live fairly, and happily.

"Do I have a negative mind? Do I always look at the negative aspects of everything? Do I concentrate on what I don't have instead of what I do have? What good will this do me? I tell myself I will never be disappointed, but the truth is that I am always disappointed, and never happy. Negative thinking leads to depression. The key to happiness is in learning to appreciate all that I have. If I expect the worst, I will help it come true. If I expect the best, I will help it come true. From now on I will look on the positive side. I will count my blessings, and expect an even better tomorrow.

"Do I have a twisted mind? Do I see things differently than other people do? Do I act differently than others do? What will I get if I follow my twisted understanding? Other people will not understand me or what I do. They will reject me rather than accept me. I must pay special attention to how other people act and how they think. I must make a conscious effort to fit it better. I will choose a "mentor" -- someone whom I admire and would like to be like. I will learn to ask myself how my mentor would react to a certain situation, and act accordingly. I will learn to flow with the traffic, rather than crashing and burning. I will start making better decisions and have a better future.

196

"Do I have a violent mind? Do I throw temper tantrums to get my own way? Do I try to overpower people rather than understand them? Do I solve problems physically rather than mentally? What advantage do I get from my violence? I end up breaking things rather than fixing them. I make enemies instead of friends. Even the people I overpower hold a grudge, and just wait for the chance to get even. He who lives by the sword eventually dies by the sword. I would do much better to learn to cooperate rather than to conquer. Peaceful solutions last longer than violent ones, and create a peaceful future. I want peace in my life. I will stop my violent tendencies and react to people with love.

"Do I have an arrogant mind? Do I think my way is better than anyone else's? Do I think I am smarter than everyone else? How do I feel when others treat me like they are better than me? Everyone has strong points and weak points. I have some very strong points, but I also have some weak points. I can learn a lot from other people. I will genuinely try to learn something new from everyone I meet. I will continue to learn more and more, and become a better, more lovable, and happier person."

H. Take an inventory of your bad habits, so you can see what you have to improve.

Say to yourself,

"Do I have a bad temper? Do I blow up at people and situations way out of proportion to their importance? No one deserves to be hurt by my temper but me. What benefit does my temper get me? People may be afraid of me, but they certainly do not love or respect me when I act that way. Temper tantrums are bad for my heart and give me emotional trouble when I try to repair the damage I've done to other people. Starting right now I will control myself, instead of letting other things control me. More people will like me and will want to get close to me, and I will feel much better about myself.

197

"Am I lazy? Would I rather do nothing than get something useful done? Would I rather do something the easy way than the right way? Laziness creates negativity. It is health's enemy, success's enemy, and my enemy. It usually takes as much energy to do something wrong as it takes to do it right, so why not do it right? I am proud of myself whenever I accomplish something. I like to be busy and hate to be bored. Exercise is fun, and makes me feel more energetic and confident in myself. From now on I will develop positive habits in order to keep myself healthy and achieve my goals. I will be healthier and happier with my life.

"Do I take drugs, drink too much, or smoke? If I keep these bad habits, what good will they do me? I feel a little better for a short time, then I feel bad again. I know they are not good for my health, so why do I do it? I have to look at the future, and not just at the temporary good feeling. I have to clearly see myself dead some day with an overdose, or shaking and miserable; I have to see myself dying of cirrhosis of the liver, or lung cancer; or maybe I'll have part of my throat and lungs cut out to save my life. I don't want these things to happen. I need to quit right now. I am glad I stopped taking drugs. I am happy I don't get drunk any more. I am proud that I don't smoke any more. I will be healthy and happy.

"Do I eat too much, or eat junk food? Do I enjoy being fat and unhealthy? Why do I create more problems and discomfort for myself, when I could change so easily? I am not a pig, and I don't need to eat so much. I can eat healthy foods that taste just as good as junk foods, and leave me feeling more energetic. I will be slim and attractive and healthy.

"Do I breathe only in my chest? Do I need only one third as much oxygen as I can get, or do I want to utilize my whole lungs? I have to breathe anyway, so I might as well get the most out of each breath. I just need to pay attention to breathing into my abdomen for a little while until it becomes a habit. I will have healthier organs and a good immune system. "

9. Once your mind is empty of all negative thoughts, begin to fill it with positive thoughts. Say to yourself:

"I am open to positive direction.

"I will balance the four corners of the foundation of my health with a healthy mental attitude, Power Breathing, natural, nutritional food, and Power Exercises.

"I will develop the positive habits of the nine steps to health.

"I am a good person, and I am getting better every day.

"I will set my clear, purposeful, positive goals, and be persistent until I achieve those goals, and strive to become a true winner in my life.

"I deserve to succeed."

"I feel stronger, healthier, more confident, more energetic, more positive, and more passionate every day of my life.

"I can see a bright future.

"I will help millions of other people.

"I am proud of myself, and I will live a healthy and happy life."

No matter what your worst habit is, if you want to solve it, you will. If you do not want to solve it, you never will. If you are not sure, you will keep traveling the path of least resistance: you will follow along in the same rut, and never change.

When you are in a relaxed meditative state, drawing in positive *ki* and expelling weak *ki*, your mind is open to positive change. When you imprint the new you on your unconscious mind by repeating words and images of the new you, you will begin to believe in your new world, and make it happen. For example, when you really believe that you don't smoke, you will stop smoking. Your unconscious habits will be controlled by your unconscious mind, which is beginning to believe that you do not smoke. You will not unconsciously reach for the cigarette out of habit. You will not unconsciously want to smoke. You are literally going to change your brain chemistry to change your behavior.

As you strip away your bad habits, you will begin to find out who you really are. Deep inside, we are all good people. We have all made some bad choices and developed some bad habits -- some have made more bad choices than others -- but bad choices and habits can be changed. We just have to breathe out all of that weak *ki*. As long as you know that you are a good person, you can change your bad habits to good habits, and be proud of yourself once again. Self-mastery meditation is the way to utilize *ki* to change your bad habits to good habits, and change your life.

Solve the big problems first. Once you have changed all of your obvious physical problems like drugs, alcohol, smoking, and over-eating (see the Nutrition section for more details on losing weight), you can work on mental and spiritual problems like bad temper or laziness. The process is the same, just meditate specifically on whatever bad habit you are currently improving.

People who are naturally positive don't need much practice to develop positive habits, and may acquire their new habit in about four days. The average person, on the other hand, requires from twenty to thirty days to develop a good habit. Some people take much longer. Just remember: it is not a race to see who can change the fastest. When we are talking about a one hundred year lifetime, four days or four months are not a long time to develop a good habit the will be around for the rest of your life. The important thing is that you start NOW, TODAY and keep trying until you have changed your bad habits into good ones.

Benefits:

This meditation will supply your whole body with natural universal energy. It will free you of negative thoughts and the limitations you put on yourself. When you replace these thoughts with positive ones, your potential is unlimited. You can have strength and power along with peace of mind. You will be healthy, with clear goals you can use as tools to build a successful life.

SUMMARY:

Meditation is a mini-vacation. It is a daily opportunity to rest, relax, and refresh.

Concentration meditation will help you concentrate on your thoughts and ideas, on what you are doing, or on what you are about to do.

Reflective meditation will help you put the events of the day into focus, so that you can better understand them and formulate a plan for tomorrow.

Relaxation meditation will help you build strength and relax.

Power meditation will help you get in touch with universal energy, or *ki*, to give you personal power.

Self-mastery meditation will help you turn your bad habits into good habits and discover the positive person that you truly are.

POWER EXERCISES

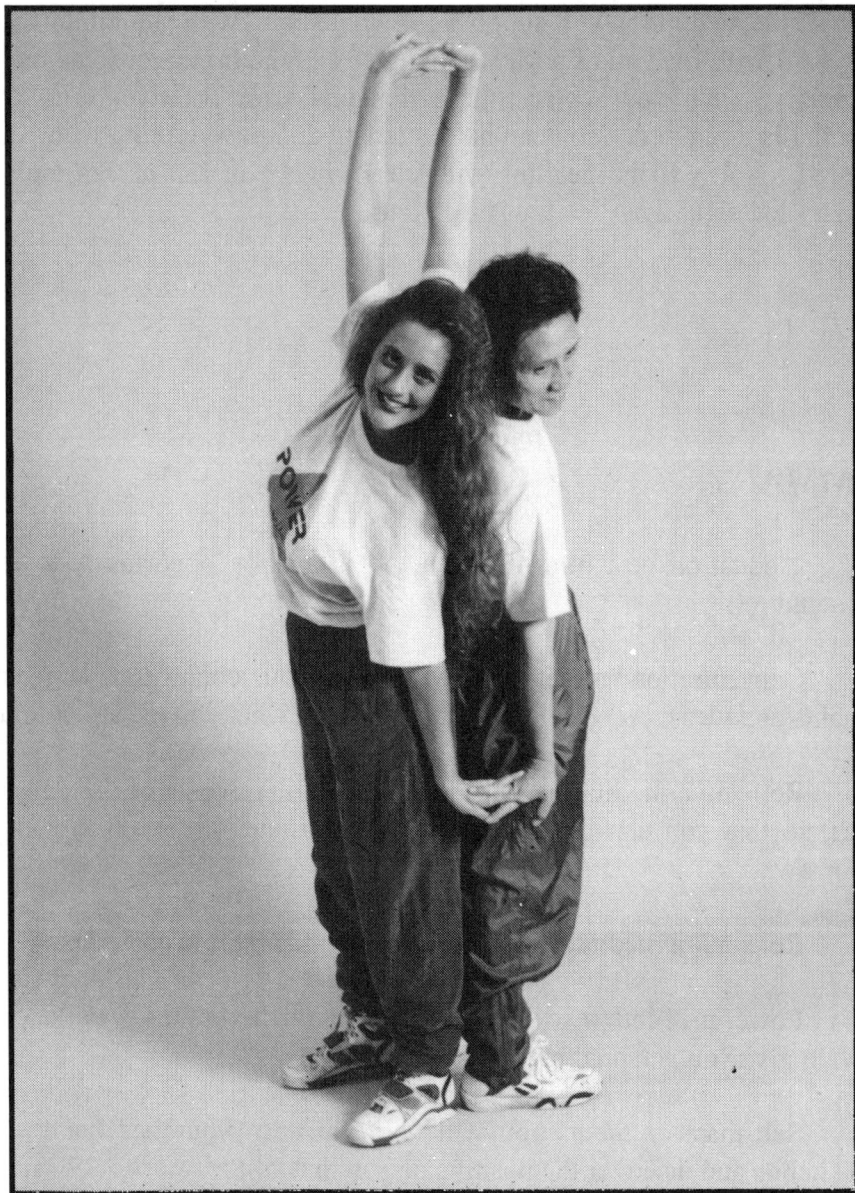

Power Exercises will give you personal power.

Power Exercises are a complete body exercise program using Power Breathing. Power Exercises were designed to loosen up, adjust, and strengthen your entire body; all the joints from fingers to toes, all the muscles from face to feet, and all the internal organs in the body. Power Breathing was also specially designed to release stress and tension, improve digestion, increase the supply of oxygen, increase the blood circulation, open all clogged veins and arteries, and build a strong immune system. It will relieve lower back pain, upper back and neck pain, minor headaches, stomach aches, asthma, high blood pressure, and arthritis. Together, they will prevent you from getting many diseases and injuries, and help you heal the ones you already have. You will be able to sleep deeply and peacefully and wake up feeling great, with lots of energy. You will be healthier, stronger, more confident, more positive, more enthusiastic, and you will feel more lively both physically and mentally every day of your life.

The exercises themselves are divided into different groups (standing, seated, lying down, with a partner, and aerobic self-defense). I do not recommend you try to do all the exercises in one stretch. Begin with the standing exercises only, and learn them for about a week. Then, move on to the seated exercises, using only a few of the standing exercises and all of the seated for about a week. Use different exercises every time, emphasizing the benefits you desire. This way the exercises will never go stale. The third week, use a few standing, a few seated, and all of the lying down exercises. Once you have progressed all the way through the curriculum, you can use whichever group suits your location, time, and needs. I have also identified some appropriate exercises for different situations like: Office Energy Exercises (pp. 379-396), Airplane Energy Exercises (pp. 397-400), Driving Energy Exercises (pp. 401-404), Walking Energy Exercises (pp. 405-408), Morning Energy Exercises (pp. 409-413), and Night Relaxation Exercises just before going to sleep (pp. 414-417). Power Exercises were designed for everybody: young and old, male and female, strong and weak. They are easy to learn and practice, so that everyone can get the maximum benefit.

During Power Exercises always breathe in through the nose and breathe out through the mouth. Breathe deeply into your lower abdomen to utilize Power Breathing whenever you do Power Exercises.

After one week you will notice that aches and pains are starting to go away. You will have more energy at the end of the work day, be able to energize yourself at will, and sleep better at night. After thirty to forty days you can feel that your whole body and mind are in better condition. After one hundred days they will be your second nature. Your improved energy level will make you more attractive to the people around you, because you will be more positive and have more energy to give them.

The bad habits that rob you of your power: shallow breathing, poor posture, poor diet, and lack of exercise have become a way of life to most of us. If you continue these bad habits, you will have to continue to use Power Exercises every day. Should you stop doing Power Exercises, your backaches, headaches, and lack of energy will slowly return to you, just as if you stop eating, your hunger will return. You must replace these bad habits with good habits. The best way to make Power Breathing and Power Exercises your own natural habit is to continue to practice every day. Every day you need to eat, you need to sleep, and you need to do some form of exercise. Power Exercises are the best possible exercises you can do.

Power Exercises are my best friend. They are a part of my daily life. They make me feel younger than ever, stronger than ever, and healthier than ever. I am more energetic, more positive, and more confident in myself, and I am happier than ever. In fact, I am doing Power Exercises right now as I am writing this part of the book at 11:05 p.m., Saturday, Feb. 27th, 1993. You, too, can do these exercises any time of the day, any place, whenever you need energy. Do not worry if people look at you, or what they say about you. Your health is the most important and valuable thing in your life.

Since I designed Power Breathing and Power Exercises, I have been practicing two times a day, plus whenever I need more energy or less tension. I practice any time, any place, as long as I will not bother someone else. I do not worry what others think about me. I remember one time I was in an informal meeting that lasted all day. We were sitting and talking for six hours straight. A few of the others commented that I could not sit still -- that I should have more discipline and self-control. A little while later I saw one of these people taking a aspirin and another taking something to settle his stomach. On the outside, they may have looked more disciplined than I, but I think my way of controlling my health was much better than theirs. What do you think?

I have seen so many people take a pill instead of exercising when they have a headache, stomach ache, back pain, or any other minor problem. I know there is nothing legally or morally wrong with taking these pills, but the side effects will eventually hurt you, and therefore your family, your friends, and even your company. Power Exercises are so easy to learn and so much fun to practice, that I really cannot understand why someone would want to put those strange chemicals in his body when he could feel so much better so easily.

I hope you can master these Power Exercises, and teach your family, friends, and anybody else around you. Then we can have more healthy and happy people around us. Remember: when you teach others, you motivate yourself.

You can do Power Exercises any time, any where, as long as you don't bother someone else. Do not worry what other people say or think about you, because your health is the most important asset in your life. Some day the others will follow you, and learn from you.

I would like to hear from you. If you have any special comments or unique experiences concerning Power Exercises and your own improvements, please write to me and tell me about them.

STANDING POWER EXERCISES

The standing exercises were designed to loosen, adjust, and strengthen all your internal organs, joints, and muscles. You may practice indoors or outdoors, and you do not need any special equipment or a lot of space. All you need is your body. It is a great way to warm up the entire body in preparation for more intense exercise or activity like aerobics, martial arts, swimming, or any sport: football, basketball, baseball, golf, etc., from amateur to pro level.

Caution:

Consult your doctor before beginning this or any exercise program. Read any cautions at the end of each exercise before attempting the exercise.

Standing Exercises

1. Deep Breathing
2. Finger and Wrist Exercises
3. Shoulder Exercises
4. Neck Exercises
5. Face Exercises
6. Chest and Back Exercises
7. Hip and Abdominal Exercises
8. Knee and Thigh Exercise
9. Ankle and Shoulder Exercise
10. Elbow and Hip Exercise
11. Finger Chain Stretch
12. Pull Down Exercise and Loosen up
13. Abdomen and Back Exercises
14. Shoulder and Lower Back Exercises
15. Hamstring and Back Stretch
16. Balance Stretch
17. Internal Organ Massage
18. Skin Massage
19. Body Bouncing

1. Deep Breathing

Deep breathing is good for all internal organs, especially the heart, lungs, liver, kidney, spleen, and brain. The increased oxygen and circulation will enliven the whole body, while the combination of motion and breathing will focus and calm the mind.

How to do it:

A.   Bend your knees slightly, with your feet approximately shoulder width apart.

B. Open your hands, cross your arms in front of you and slowly circle your arms up and over your head as you inhale through your nose into your lower abdomen.

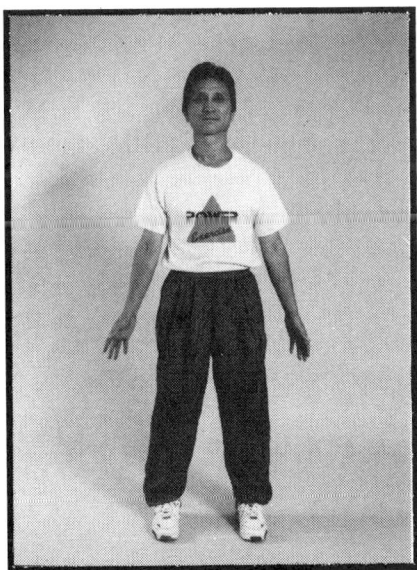

A

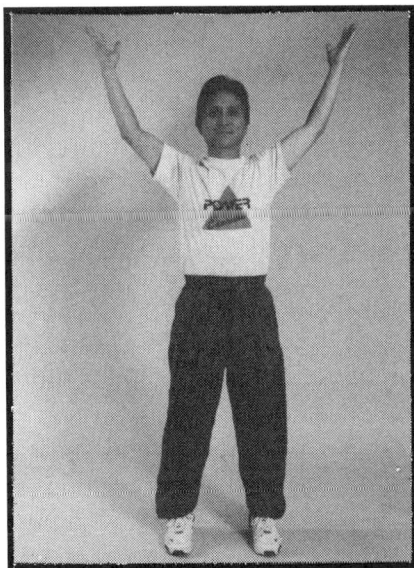

B

C. Continue the circles outward and backward as you continue to inhale and expand the chest.

D. Slowly exhale through your slightly opened mouth as your hands move downward and inward. Bend slightly forward while pulling in or tightening your stomach and stretching your back to push out all the remaining carbon dioxide and stale gas.

E. When your hands come together at the bottom, slowly inhale through your nose again, but this time keep your hands at waist height and open them outward and backward in a half circle.

F. When you have circled outward as far as is comfortable, slowly exhale through the mouth and bring your hands inward. Bend slightly forward while pulling in or tightening your stomach and stretching your back to push out all the carbon dioxide.

G. Repeat A through F.

Benefits:

The deep breathing exercise will:

* increase circulation to the shoulders and chest, and help to loosen up the shoulder joint.

* release pent-up tension and stress.

* open up the chest, enabling the lungs to expand farther and draw in more oxygen. Deep breathing can increase your lung capacity.

* compress and massage the organs of the abdomen when the diaphragm presses down on them.

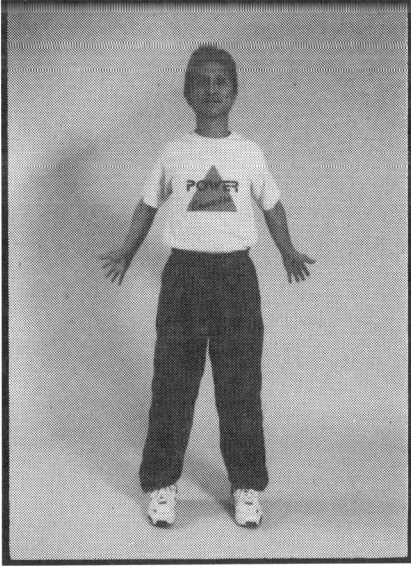

C

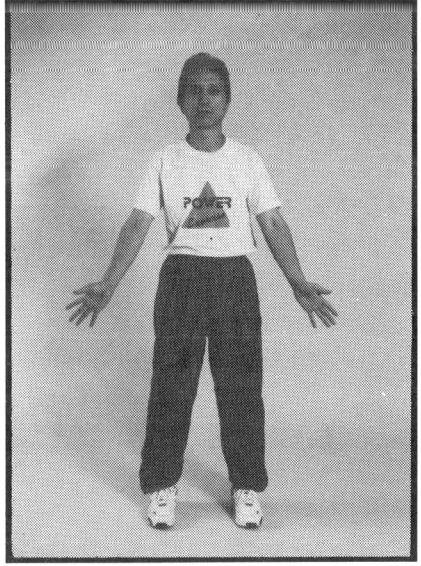

D

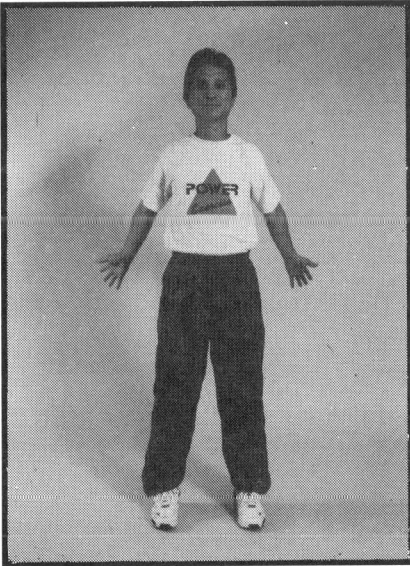

E

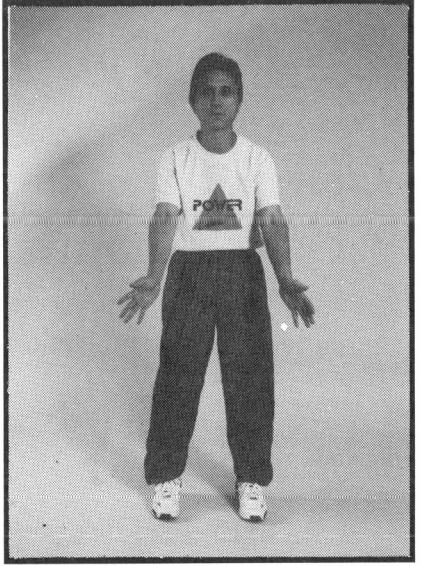

F

* open the chest and release pressure on the lungs and heart when the diaphragm presses downward, so that the heart can work less due to the reduced pressure and increased oxygen in the system.

* strengthen your immune system and make it more resistant to colds, fever, and other diseases.

* deliver oxygen to the brain so that it will be chemically "cleaner", and the mind will be calmer. Deep breathing will also relieve minor headaches.

* regulate both high and low blood pressure by returning the body to its natural state of health and balance.

2. Finger and Wrist Exercises

Each of the five fingers is attached to one of the five major solid organs (heart, liver, pancreas, spleen, and kidneys.) In fact, according to the science of reflexology, the entire body is connected through the nerves to the hands. When you stimulate the fingers, you stimulate the corresponding organ. When you increase the circulation to the hand, you increase the flow of energy to the entire body.

How to do it:

A. Maintain same stance as #1. (Bend your knees slightly, with your feet approximately shoulder width apart).

B. Inhale and join your hands together so that your fingers interlock into a "finger chain".

C. Exhale and turn your palms downward and push down (count 1-4), then inhale and turn your palms forward and outward, and exhale and push them downward and forward (count 5-8).

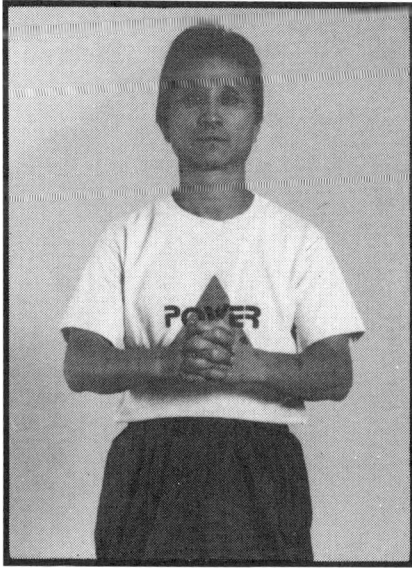

B

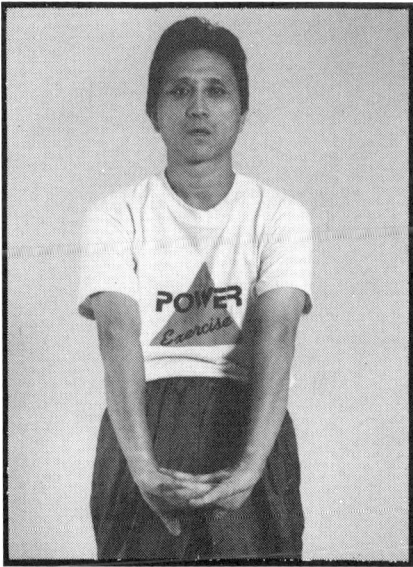

C (down)

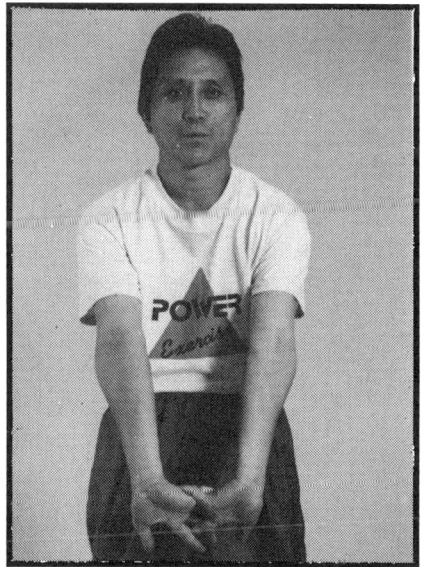

C (out)

D. Release the finger chain and place your right palm on the back of your left hand and grasp the left hand in the right.

E. Stretch the wrist by moving both hands upward toward the chin (4 times).

F. Release the left hand and place the left palm on the back of your right hand and stretch the right wrist in the same manner (4 times).

G. Hold your both wrists in front of your shoulders. Grasp the air with both hands (8 times).

H. Shake your wrists up and down and side to side (count 1-8).

If you cannot remember the exact order at first, don't worry. Doing the exercises in the wrong order is still better than not doing the exercises at all.

Benefits:

The finger and wrist exercises will:

* stimulate the five major solid organs.

* loosen the wrist and finger joints.

* reduce minor headaches by increasing blood circulation.

* reduce high blood pressure by increasing blood circulation.

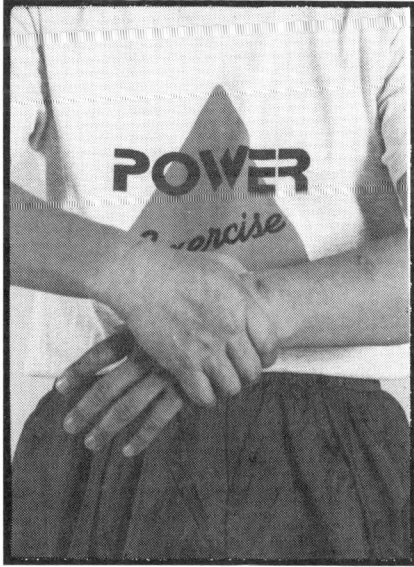

D

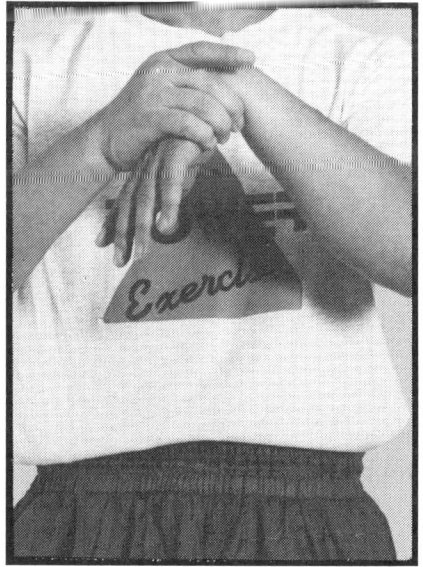

E

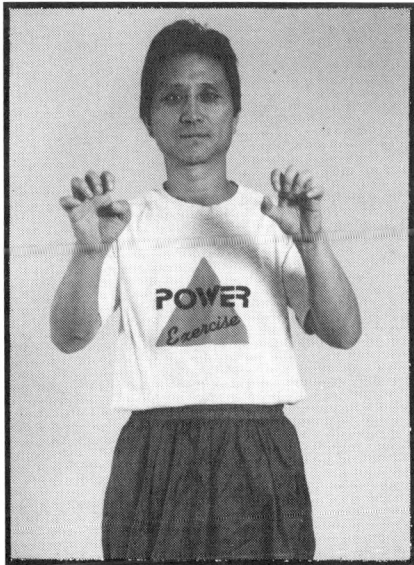

G

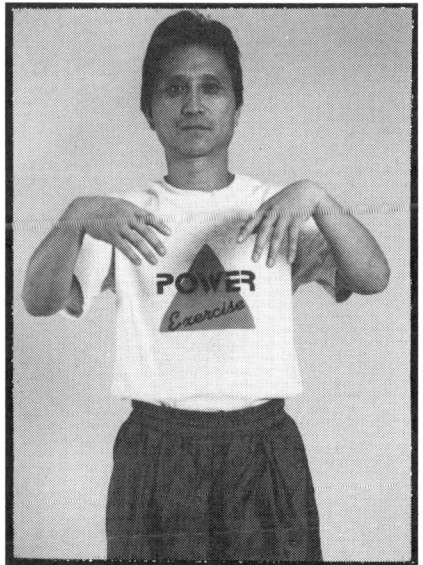

H

213

3. Shoulder Exercises

The shoulders and neck are a sticking point for stress and tension. When we feel stress, we tense the muscles of the shoulders and neck, restricting the flow of blood to the head. These exercises are good for the shoulders, neck, and brain, and can relieve minor stress headaches.

How to do it:

A. Maintain same stance as #2. (Bend your knees slightly, with your feet approximately shoulder width apart).

B. Inhale and shrug your shoulders all the way up to your ears, then exhale and let them drop down and relax (8 repetitions).

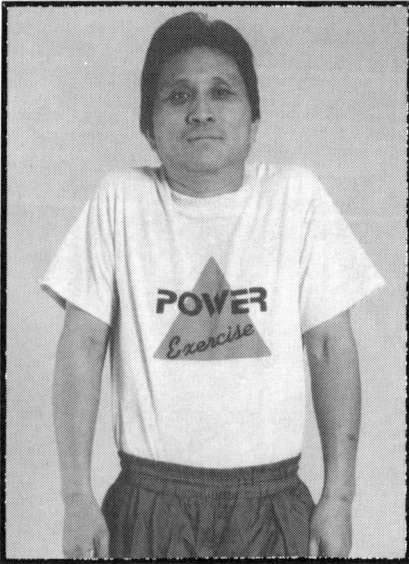

B (up)

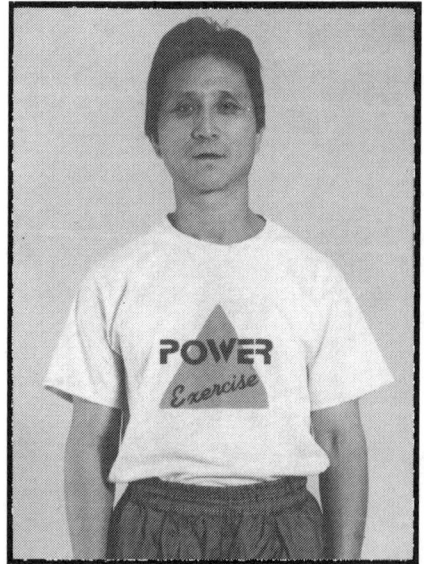

B (relax)

C. Alternately roll your shoulders back and up, then front and down -- first roll the left shoulder forward, then the right (4 ea.)

D. Alternately roll your shoulders front and up, then back and down -- first roll the left shoulder backward, then the right (4 ea.)

Benefits:

The shoulder exercises will:

* increase circulation to shoulders (deltoids and trapezius), chest, and back.

* increase circulation to brain, which can reduce minor headaches.

* release stress and tension by relaxing shoulder and neck muscles.

Caution:

Do not tighten the muscles during B; it will stop the circulation and increase the blood pressure.

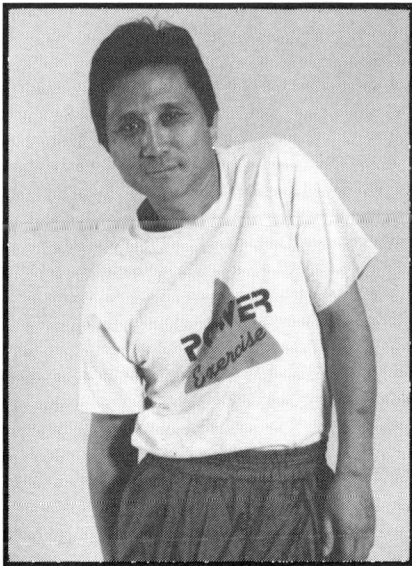

C & D

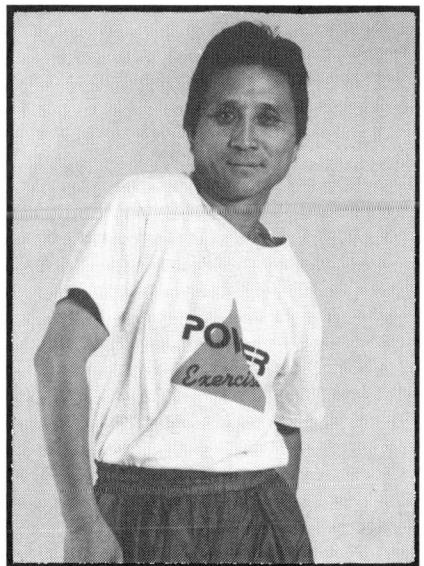

C & D (alternate)

215

4. Neck Exercises

The shoulders and neck are a sticking point for stress and tension. These exercises are good to loosen up the neck muscles and increase circulation to the brain, and can relieve minor stress headaches.

How to do it:

A. Maintain same stance as #3. (Bend your knees slightly, with your feet approximately shoulder width apart). Inhale.

B. Exhale and bend the head forward. Inhale as you bring head back up.

C. Exhale and turn the neck to look left. Inhale and turn the head to face front.

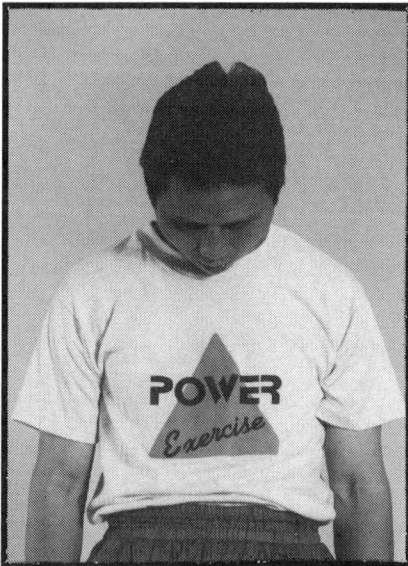

B

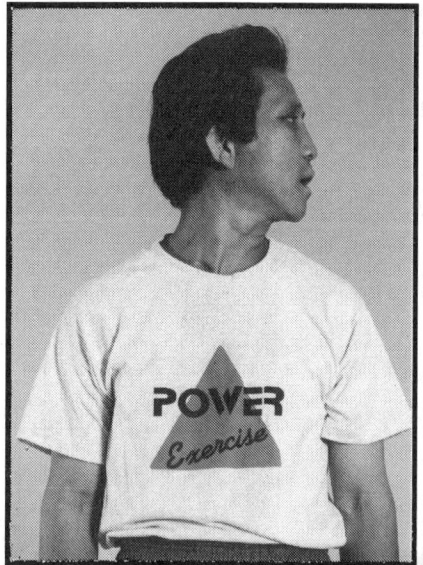

C

D. Exhale and turn the neck to look right. Inhale and turn the head to face front.

E. Exhale and lean the head to the left shoulder. Inhale and bring head back up.

F. Exhale and lean the head to right shoulder. Inhale and bring head back up.

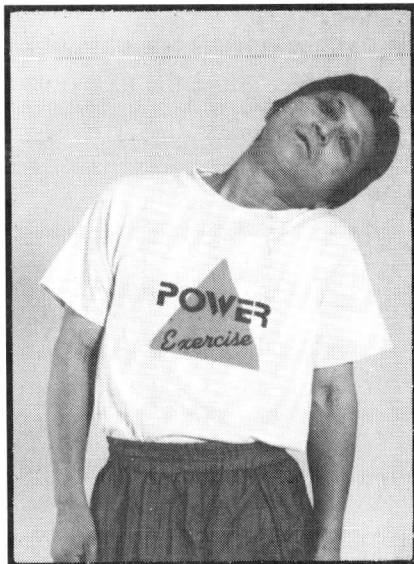

Benefits:

The neck exercises will:

E

* release stress and tension by loosening up the neck muscles.

* increase circulation to the brain, which will freshen your thought processes and reduce minor headaches.

* diagnose and quickly locate problem areas where tension and fatigue have gathered, so that you can prevent the problem from getting worse.

* prevent diseases connected with spinal vertebrae 1, 2, 3, and 4.

Caution:

Neck exercises should be done very slowly.

5. Face Exercises

The muscles of our entire body were designed to be exercised, but most people ignore the face muscles when it is time to exercise.

How to do it:

A. Maintain same stance as #4. (Bend your knees slightly, with your feet approximately shoulder width apart).

B. Tighten all your different face muscles by:

> 1) moving your tongue over each gum, inside and outside the teeth, top and bottom,
> 2) blinking,
> 3) chewing,
> 4) moving your nose and ears, separately and together in random sequence.

C. While making faces, rub your palms together to build up some friction/heat in your hands.

D. Stop making faces and massage the trapezius muscles and the back of your neck with your hands.

E. Continue to move your hands to grasp your ears between your thumb and index finger, pull lightly and massage them.

F. Rub your palms together again to build up heat, press the heel of your palms to your eyes, cheeks and nose.

G. Wash your face with air, while breathing in and out through the mouth very quickly.

H. Continue to massage and wash your scalp while breathing in and out through the mouth very quickly.

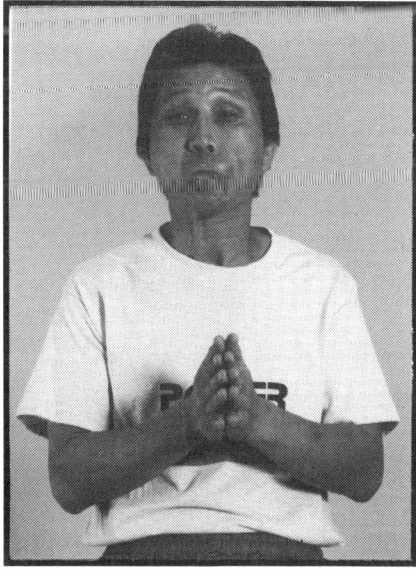

B & C

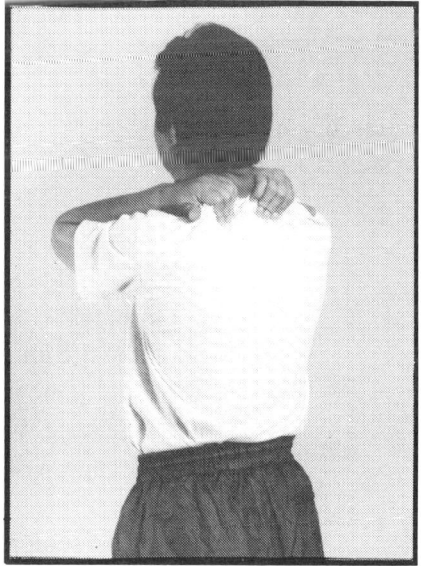

D

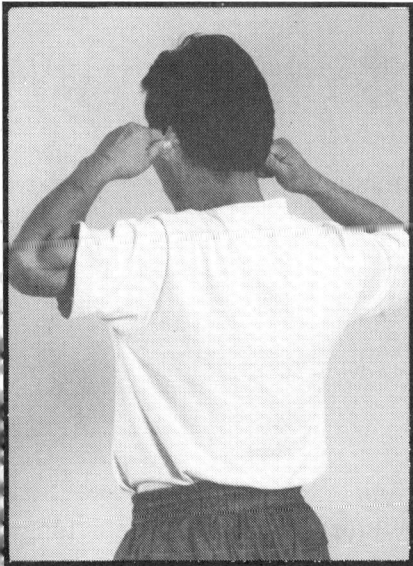

E

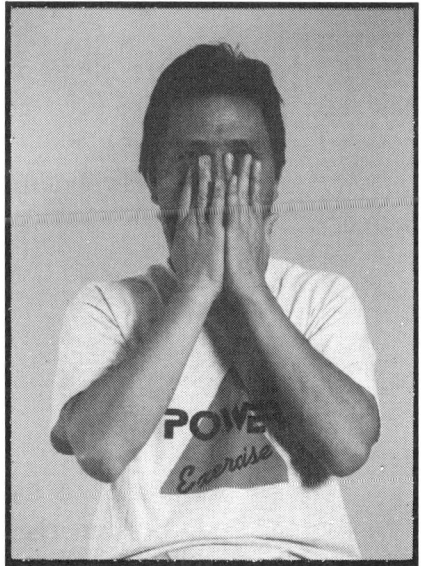

G

Benefits:

Moving the muscles of the eyes, nose, mouth, and face will:

* increase circulation and exercise those muscles, which are often ignored, and stimulate the organs that are connected through the nervous system:

> - chewing makes the jaw and teeth strong;
> - lip movements stimulate the lungs, stomach, pancreas, and kidneys;
> - eye massage and exercise will keep your eyes young, clear, and your vision sharp;
> - nose massage will help prevent colds;
> - ear massage will keep the hearing sharp.

* prevent skin discoloration, wrinkles, and keep you looking healthier and better.

Massaging with warm hands will:

* increase the circulation through your neck, face, and scalp.

* regulate your blood pressure, relieve tension, and help prevent neuralgia, insomnia, and even dandruff.

* stimulate your brain, reduce minor headaches, and improve memory.

6. Chest and Back Exercises

These exercises will loosen up your shoulder, chest, and back muscles, and open up your chest to allow more oxygen into your lungs. They are also good for the heart.

How to do it:

A. Maintain same stance as #5. (Bend your knees slightly, with your feet approximately shoulder width apart).

B. Inhale and grasp the air with your hands in front of your shoulders and slowly move your elbows back as far as possible, as if rowing a boat (count 1,2). It is important to keep the elbows the same level as the shoulders.

C. Exhale and extend your arms outward, palm up, and keep them straight as you pull them backward as far as possible (count 3,4).

D. Repeat B and C (count 5-8).

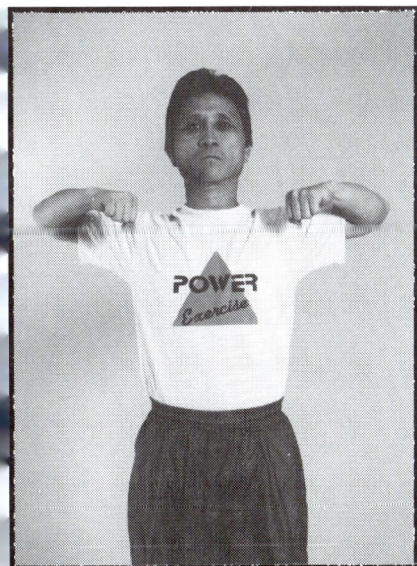

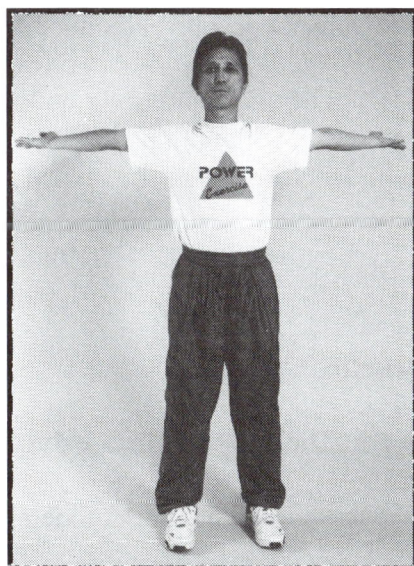

B   C

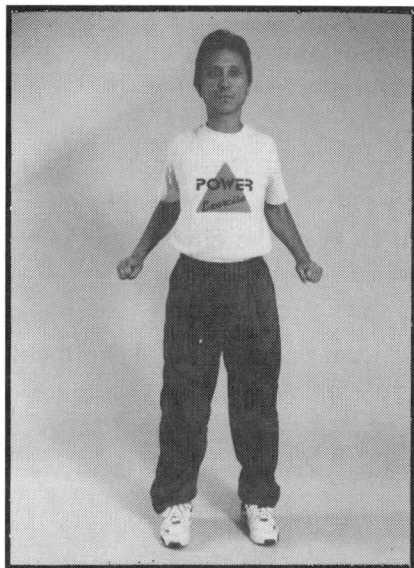

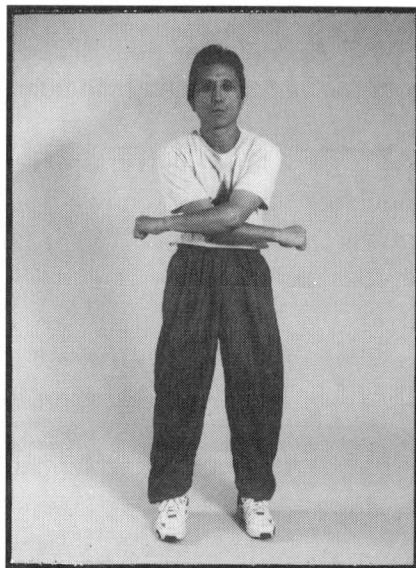

E   F

E. Drop your hands to waist level, inhale, and move them back as if rowing at waist level (count 1, 2).

F. Exhale and bring both fists all the way forward at waist level as if to punch with both hands, except that you cross your arms. Extend your shoulders forward as you punch, to stretch your back (count 3,4).

G. Repeat E and F (count 5-8).

Benefits:

The chest and back exercises will:

* loosen up the shoulders and elbow joints.

* expand and stretch the chest and back.

* open up the lungs to increase lung capacity.

* increase the oxygen content and circulation of the blood to make the heart work more efficiently, allowing it to relax more.

* prevent colds and fever.

Caution:

If you have weak shoulders or are subject to shoulder dislocation, do not stretch your hands too far either backward or forward.

7. Hip and Abdominal Exercises

The lower back is a point of nagging pain for many people. This exercise will loosen up the lower back and increase the circulation through that area.

How to do it:

A. Maintain same stance as #6. (Bend your knees slightly, with your feet approximately shoulder width apart). Inhale.

B. Put your hands on your hips. Exhale and shift your hips to the left (count 1-4). Inhale and return your hips to the center (count 5-8).

C. Exhale and shift to the right (count 1-4). Inhale and return your hips to the

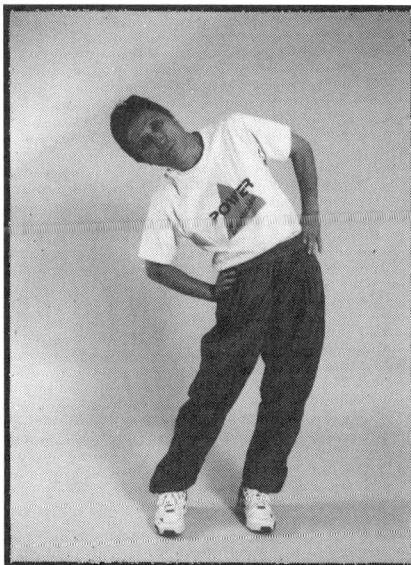

B

223

D. Exhale and bend your knees slightly and slowly tilt your pelvis forward by contracting your lower abdominal and buttocks muscles.

E. Inhale and tilt your pelvis backward by relaxing your lower abdomen and buttocks.

F. Repeat D and E three more times.

Benefits:

The lower abdominal exercises will:

* loosen up and strengthen lower back, hip joint, and lower abdomen.

* increase circulation and energy flow to lower back, hip, and groin area.

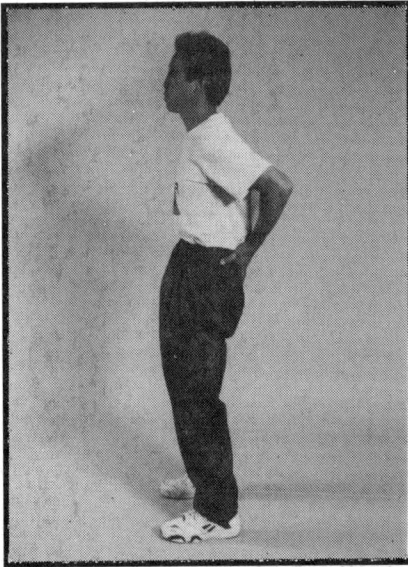

D

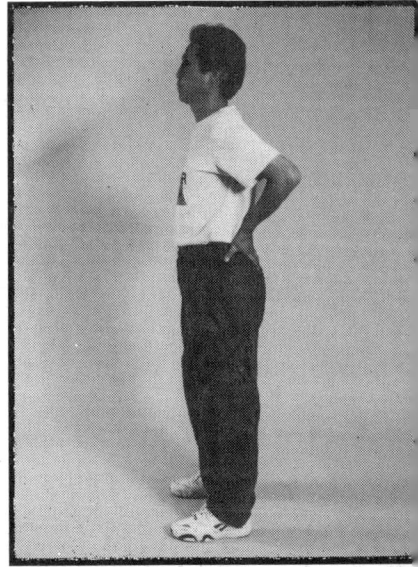

E

Caution:

Do not lean too far in any direction, but especially do not lean back. You are trying to loosen up, not strain yourself. If you have a bad back, bend only as far as comfortable.

8. Knee and Thigh Exercise

The knees are a common source of discomfort among even people with athletic backgrounds. As we grow older, we need to maintain the strength and flexibility of our legs.

How to do it:

A. Place your hands on your hips and step your left leg backward one shoulder width and bend your right knee. Inhale.

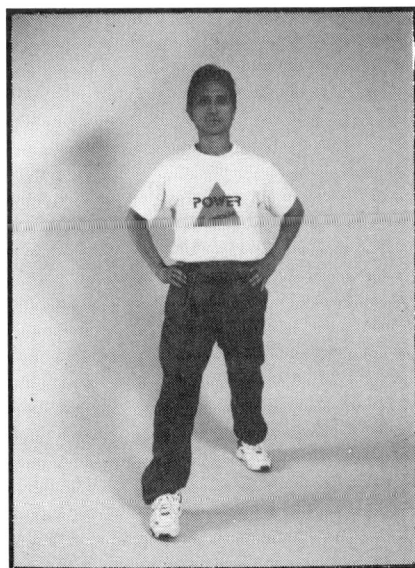

A, C

B. Exhale and bend your left knee and pick your left heel up off the floor as you tilt your pelvis forward as far as possible, as in #7, feeling a stretch throughout your left thigh muscle.

C. Inhale and raise your body by making your right knee nearly straight.

D. Repeat B & C three more times.

E. Inhale and raise your body. Switch stance by moving your left leg forward one shoulder width and your right leg back. Bend both knees and pick your right heel up off of the floor. Inhale.

F. Exhale and bend your right knee and pick your right heel up off the floor as you tilt your pelvis forward as far as possible, feeling a stretch throughout your right thigh muscle.

G. Inhale and raise your body by making your left knee nearly straight.

H. Repeat F and G three more times, stretching the right thigh.

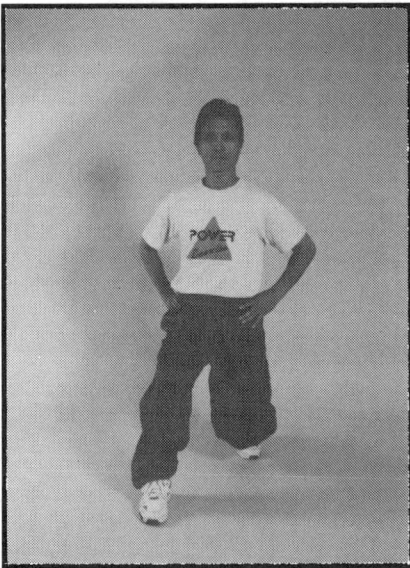

B, F

Benefits:

The knee and thigh exercise will:

* loosen up the knee and ankle joints.

* warm up and strengthen the thigh muscles.

* stretch the thigh muscles.

226

Caution:

People with bad or weak knees should not go down too far. No one should let the knee go forward of the ankle, or let the hip drop below the knee. You are trying to strengthen yourself, not strain yourself. Only go down as much as is comfortable for you.

Be careful not to turn your hips in B and F. You could risk knee strain by twisting your body.

9. Ankle and Shoulder Exercise

Up to this point we have been working with localized muscles -- muscles and joints all in the same area. Now we are going to start integrating body parts by working upper and lower body at the same time.

How to do it:

A. Bring both feet together, side by side.

B. Put your hands together in front of your chest as if praying.

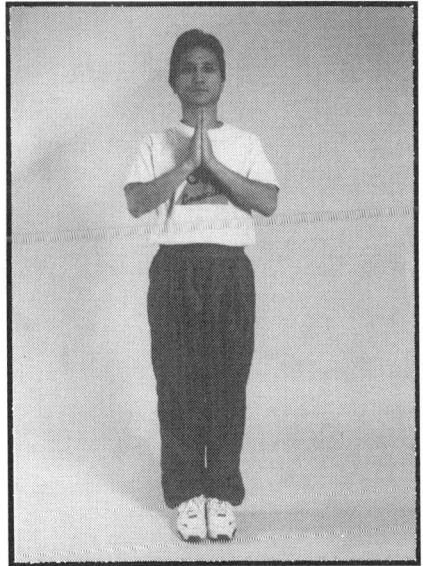

B

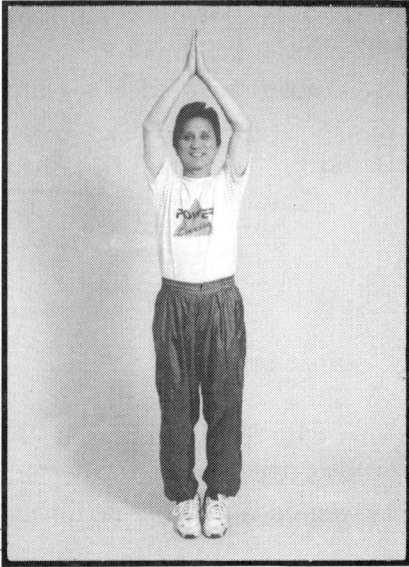

C

C. Inhale as you raise up on the balls of your feet at the same time you fully extend both hands directly over your head, and then exhale and return to position B.

D. Inhale as you raise up on the balls of your feet at the same time you fully extend both hands directly over your head, and then exhale as you open your hands outward and downward as two halves of a circle, while you lower your heels.

E. Repeat C and D.

F. Repeat B through E again.

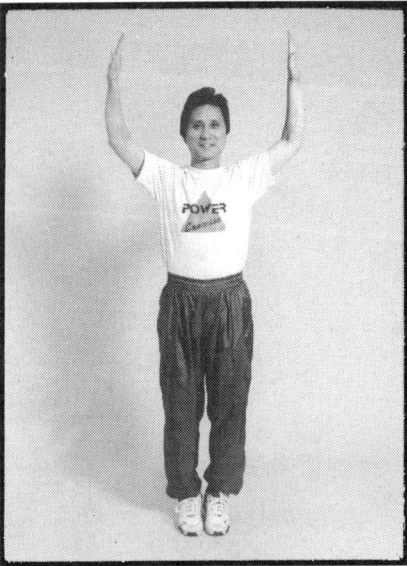

D (outward)

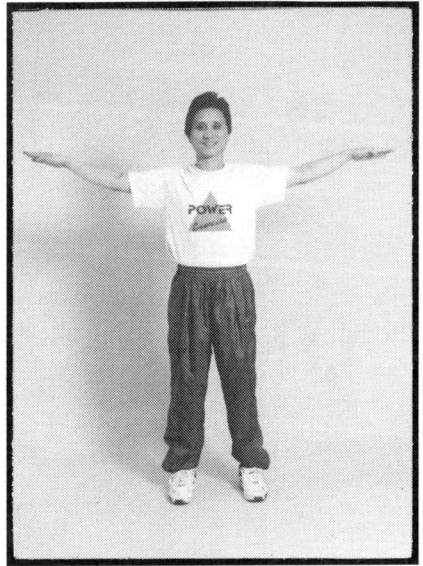

D (downward)

Benefits:

The ankle and shoulder exercise will:

* loosen up, build up, and strengthen the ankle joint.

* warm up the calf muscle.

* warm up the shoulder and back muscles.

* stimulate and increase the circulation to the entire body due to nerve connections between foot and the rest of the body.

* develop balance.

Caution:

People with weak or bad ankles should be very careful. Just raise up as far as comfortable.

10. Elbow and Hip Exercise

The back is a source of pain for many people in our modern society. We spend too much time sitting and standing with bad posture, and even when we lie down, our furniture does not always give us the proper support. This exercise will help loosen up the back and hips.

How to do it:

A. Assume front stance (step your right leg backward one shoulder width; bend both knees and pick your right heel up off of the floor.)

B. Inhale and lift both elbows up to the side above the shoulder. Point your fingers toward each other in front of your chest, palm down.

C. Bring your left elbow up to about a seventy-five degree angle, exhale and look over your left shoulder, twisting your body back to the left without moving your feet (count 1-7).

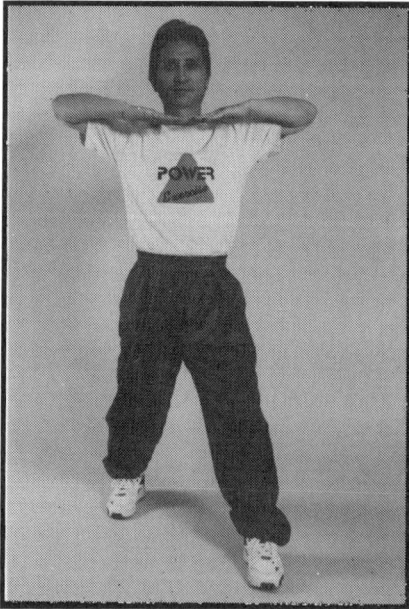

A, B

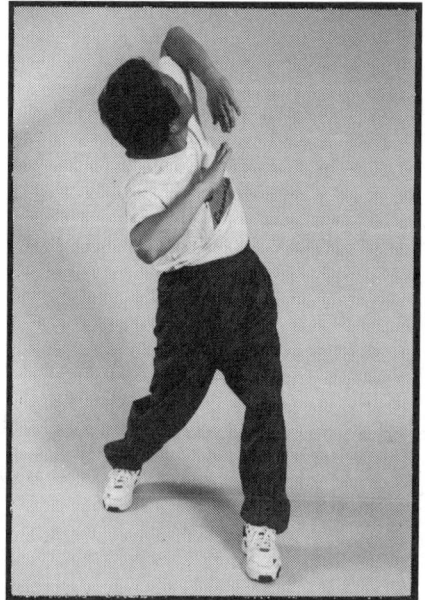

C

D. Inhale and return to center (on the 8th count), then switch feet by stepping your right leg forward one shoulder width, and your left leg backward.

E. Bring your right elbow up to about a seventy-five degree angle, exhale and look over your right shoulder, twisting your body back to the right without moving your feet (count 1-7.)

F. Inhale and return to center (on the 8th count).

Benefits:

The elbow and hip exercise will:

* warm up and strengthen the elbows and shoulders.

* strengthen and adjust the back.

* loosen up and strengthen the hips, lats, and thighs.

* improve digestion.

* release stress, tension, and headaches.

Caution:

If you have weak shoulders or are subject to shoulder dislocation, do not stretch your elbows too far either upward or backward.

11. Finger Chain Stretch

The *latissimus* (lat.) muscle is the largest muscle in the upper body. It is the main power muscle for most sports activities. This exercise will stretch your lat. muscle, as well as the arm, hands, and lower back. It also helps to re-adjust the spine.

How to Do it:

A. Return to ready stance (Bend your knees slightly, with your feet approximately shoulder width apart).

B. Interlock your fingers into a finger chain. Turn your palms upward, inhale, and extend your hands up over your head.

C. Exhale and lean to the left without bending forward (count 1-3), then inhale and return to upright (on the 4th count).

D. Exhale and lean to the right without bending forward (count 5-7), then inhale and return to upright (on the 8th count).

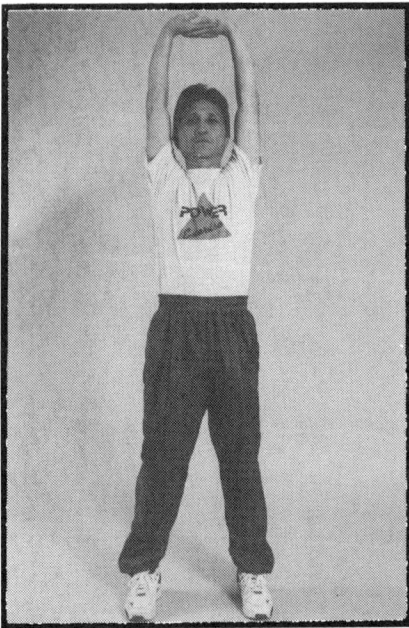

B

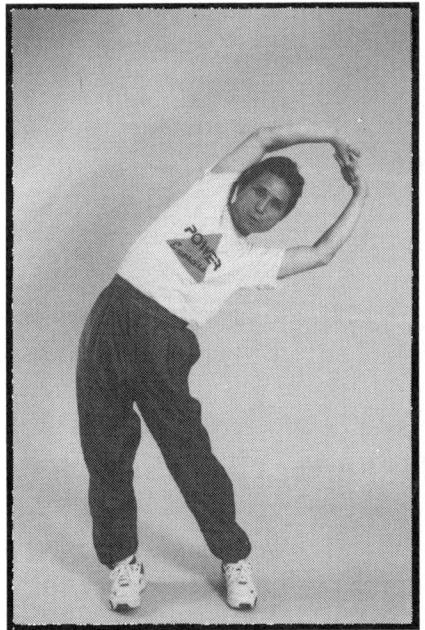

C

E. Release your fingers and bring your arms down, bend your knees a little deeper, and reach behind your back.

F. Inhale and interlock your fingers into a finger chain behind your back and twist your hands so that your palms face away from your body.

G. Exhale and bend forward until you head is at waist level but looking straight to the front (keep your back flat). Try to bring your hands to a vertical position (count 1-7).

H. Inhale and return to upright (on the 8th count). Release your fingers.

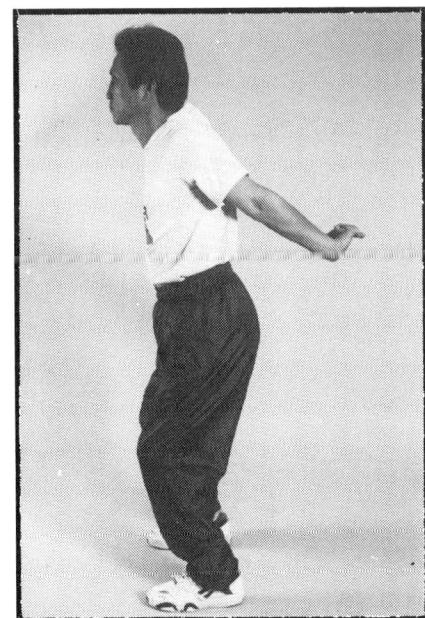

F

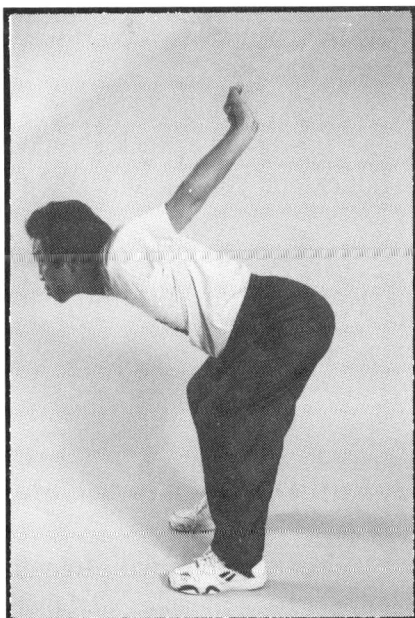

G

Benefits:

The finger chain stretch will:

* loosen the finger, wrist, and shoulder joints.

* loosen and stretch the side (lat. muscle).

* loosen the middle and lower back.

* adjust the spine.

* release stress and tension, and reduce headaches.

* stimulate the internal organs, improve digestion and release waste products.

Caution:

Do not lean too far in any direction -- you are trying to loosen up, not strain yourself. If you have a bad back, bend only as far as comfortable.

If you have weak shoulders or are subject to shoulder dislocation, do not extend your shoulders too far.

Be sure to keep your head up when leaning forward to avoid losing balance or straining the lower back.

12. Pull Down Exercise and Loosen Up

This exercise will strengthen the lat. muscle as well as the shoulder and upper back muscles, and then loosen them up.

How to do it:

A. Maintain same stance as #11. (Bend your knees slightly, with your feet approximately shoulder width apart).

B. Reach above your head as if grabbing a wide trapeze. Pull both hands straight down while keeping your shoulders as far back as possible. You should feel the muscles get tight across your upper back and shoulder.

C. Roll out of the pull down by moving your hands forward a few inches.

D. Repeat B and C seven more times.

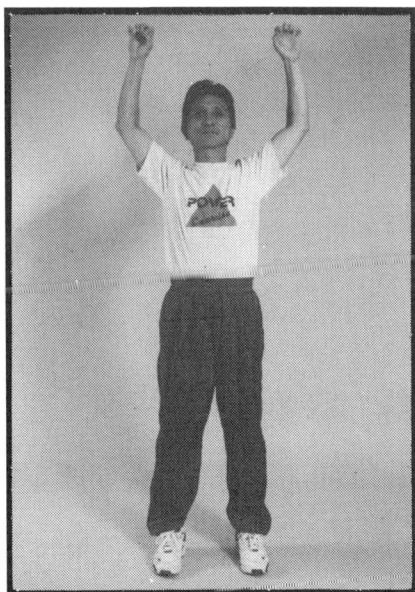

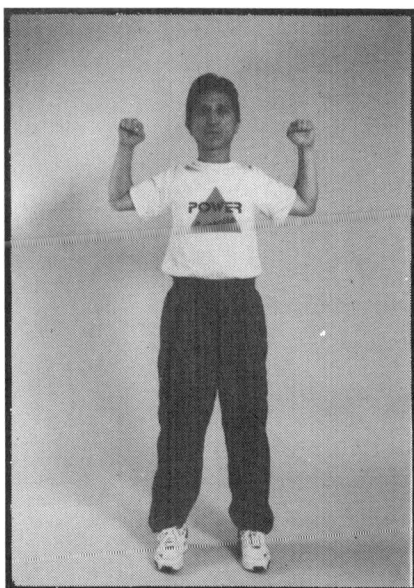

B (reach)   B (pull)

E. Loosen up your shoulder and upper back by grasping your left *triceps* (back of the arm) muscle in your right hand and pulling across your chest (count 1-4).

F. Loosen up your other shoulder by grasping your right triceps muscle with your left hand and pulling it across your chest (count 5-8).

G. Roll your shoulders four times to the front and four times to the back to loosen them up.

Benefits:

The pull down exercise, along with its loosening exercises will:

* loosen up the shoulder joint.

* loosen up the middle and lower back.

* strengthen the lat., shoulder, back, and arm muscles.

* release tension and stress; reduce headaches.

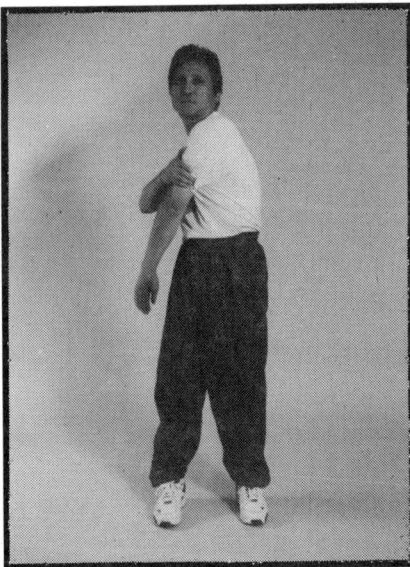

E

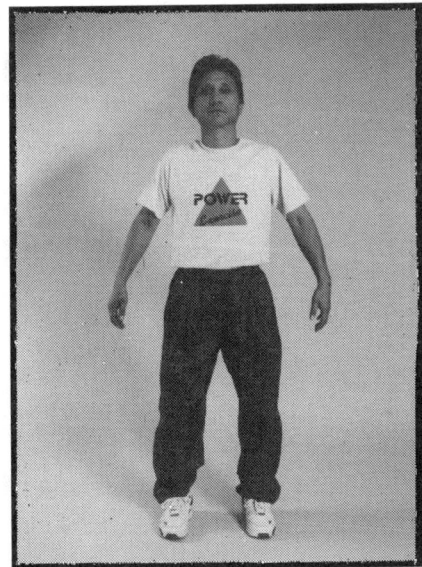

G

Caution:

People with bad or weak shoulders should not pull back too far, it is possible to pull a weak shoulder out of socket in this exercise.

13. Abdomen and Back Exercise

This exercise is another combination upper body and lower body exercise. The combined movement while breathing will help remove waste products from the body and improve digestion.

How to do it:

A. Maintain same stance as #12. (Bend your knees slightly, with your feet approximately shoulder width apart.)

B. Extend your hands and arms straight out to each side. Inhale.

C. Fix your eyes on your left hand. Exhale for as long as possible as you slowly bend forward and touch your right hand above your left knee, while your left hand points directly to the ceiling.

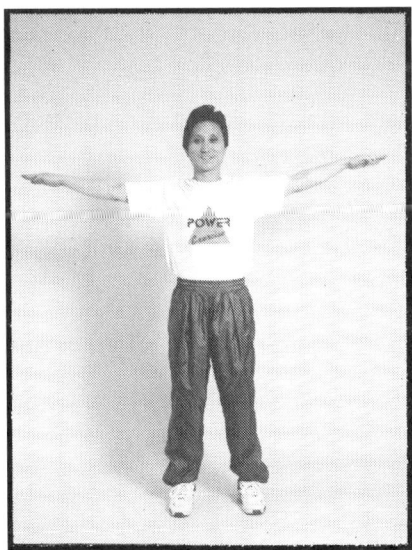

B, D, F

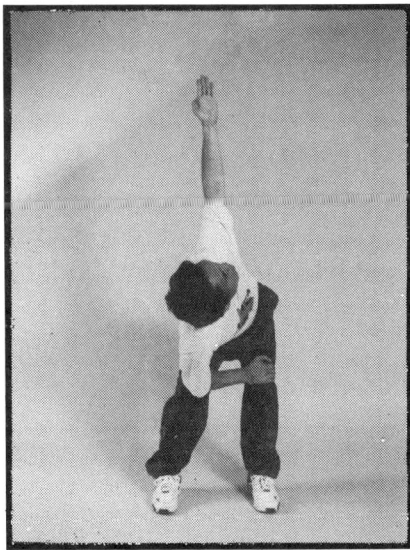

C

D. Inhale as you straighten up.

E. Fix your eyes on your right hand. Exhale for as long as possible as you slowly bend forward and touch your left hand above your right knee, while your right hand points directly to the ceiling.

F. Inhale as you straighten up.

G. Exhale for as long as possible as you slowly bend forward and place both palms above both knees, while keeping your head up.

H. Inhale as you arch your back down and extend your abdomen.

I. Exhale and arch your back upward as you pull in your stomach, and slowly raise your head and shoulders approaching an upright position.

J. Inhale as you place both hands on your lower back and stretch upward (but do not lean backward).

K. Exhale and relax.

Benefits:

The abdomen and back exercise will:

* loosen up and strengthen the lower back, abdomen, hamstrings, and shoulders.

* cleanse the body by expelling waste products (CO_2) and replacing them with fresh nutrients (O_2).

* aid digestion by compressing and expanding the abdomen and digestive organs.

* release tension and stress.

* prevent diarrhea and constipation.

* prevent and heal asthma.

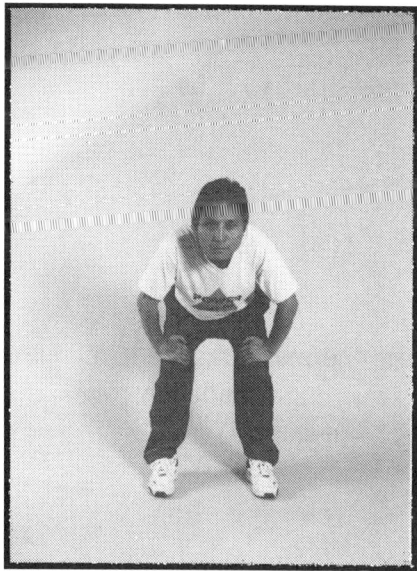

G

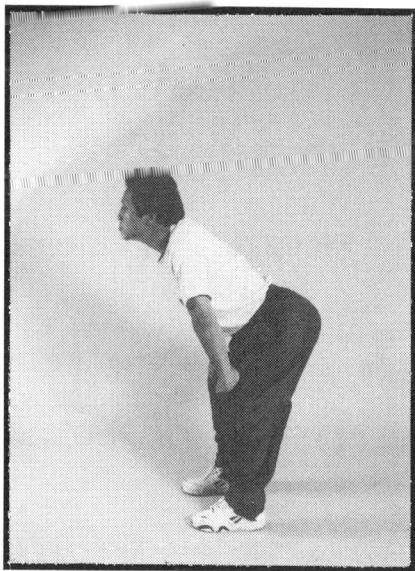

H

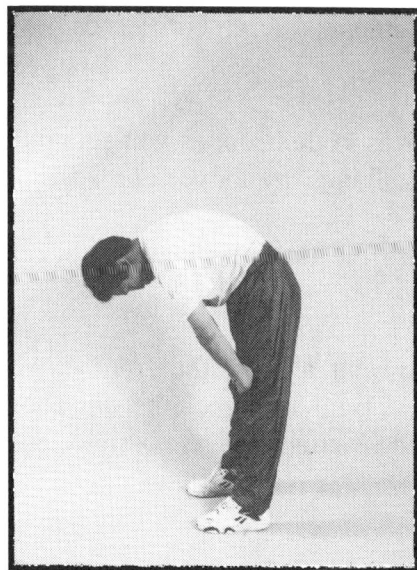

I

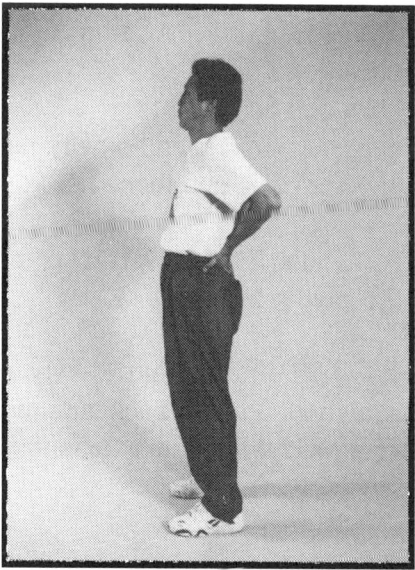

J

239

Caution:

Keep your head up whenever you bend forward to protect your lower back.

Do not lean backward in J, as you may strain your back.

14. Shoulder and Lower Back Exercises

The front stance is a basic stance in the martial arts. It increases leg and lower back strength and develops a strong foundation for martial art techniques. This exercise is done in the front stance.

How to do it:

A. Step your right foot backward approximately two shoulder widths, while maintaining your feet one shoulder width apart. Bend the front (left) knee, while keeping the back (right) knee straight.

B. Lean forward as far as comfortable, and reach both hands down toward the floor.

C. Inhale and slowly raise both arms to the front as you straighten up your back, and then raise your arms up all the way above your head .

D. Exhale and lower both arms to the floor by bending forward (keep your head up).

E. Inhale and slowly raise your right arm to the front as you straighten up your back, and then raise your right arm up all the way above your head while you extend the left arm backwards as far as possible.

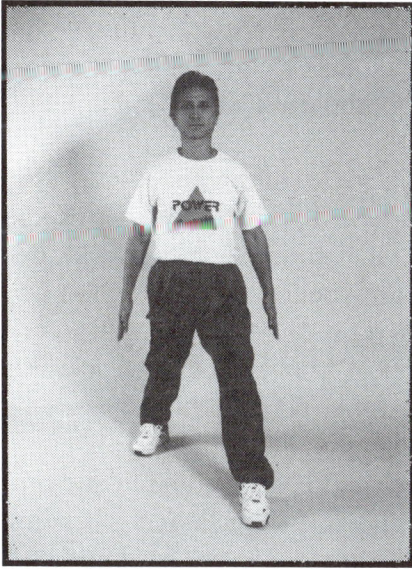

A

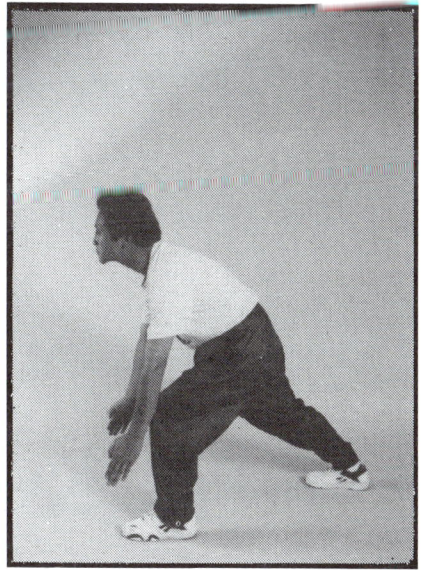

B,D,F,H

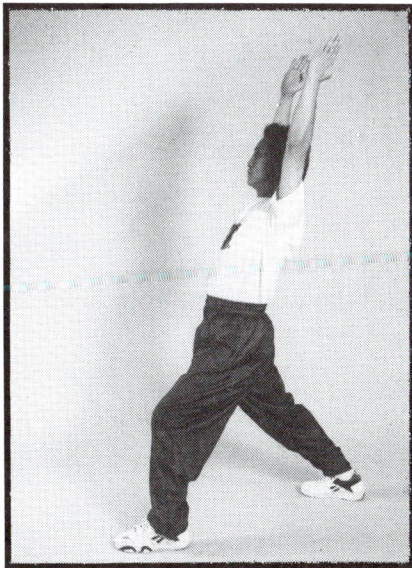

C

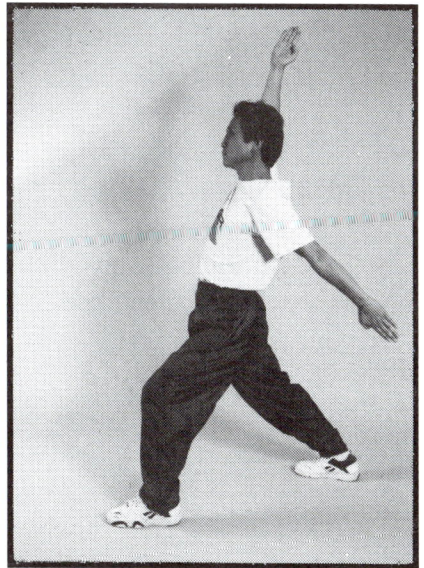

E

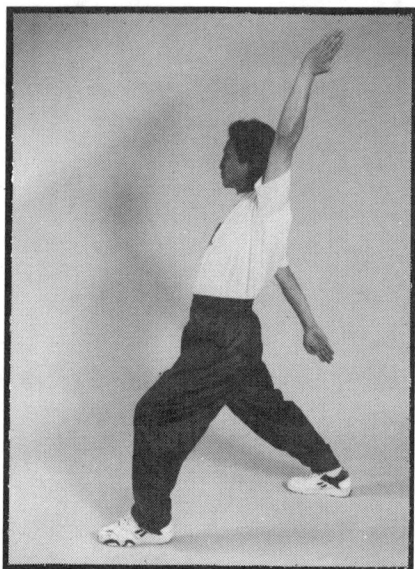

F. Exhale and lower your right arm to the floor by bending forward (keep your head up).

G. Inhale and slowly raise your left arm to the front as you straighten up your back, and then raise your left arm up all the way above your head while you extend your right arm back-wards as for as possible.

H. Exhale and lower your left arm to the floor by bending forward (keep your head up).

G

I. Change stance by stepping your left foot back and your right foot forward approximately two shoulder widths, while maintaining your feet one shoulder width apart. Bend the front (right) knee, while keeping the back (left) knee straight.

J. Lean forward as far as comfortable, and reach both hands down toward the floor.

K. Inhale and slowly raise both arms to the front as you straighten up your back, and then raise your arms up all the way above your head and lean your head back.

L. Exhale and lower both arms to the floor by bending forward (keep head up).

M. Inhale and slowly raise your left arm to the front as you straighten up your back, and then raise your left arm up all the way above your head while you extend your right arm as far backwards as possible.

242

N. Exhale and lower your left arm to the floor by bending forward (keep head up).

O. Inhale and slowly raise your right arm to the front as you straighten up your back and then raise your right arm up all the way above your head while you extend your left arm as far backwards as possible.

P. Exhale and lower your right arm to the floor by bending forward (keep head up).

Q. Return to comfortable stance.

Benefits:

The shoulder and lower back exercises will:

* loosen up and strengthen the lower back, middle back, shoulder, neck, and all spinal muscles.

* open up the lungs and increase the blood circulation. It will get rid of toxins and waste products while increasing nutrients in the blood.

* stretch the hip flexor muscles, strengthen the quadriceps (thigh) muscles, and loosen up the knee joint.

* release stress and tension.

* increase the blood circulation throughout the entire body.

Caution:

Those with bad knees should be very careful not to bend the front knee too much. Even people with good knees should not bend the front knee more than ninety degrees.

15. Hamstring and Back Stretch

The hamstrings are the muscles that run up the back of your leg, between your buttocks and the back of the knee. When the hamstrings are inflexible, you have poor mobility and poor circulation in your legs.

This exercise will also help relieve lower back pain and massage your internal organs.

How to do it:

A. Stand with your weight on your right leg. Step your left foot forward about one foot in front of your right.

B. Place the palms of both hands on your respective thighs, close to the hip, while tilting your left foot up so that only the heel touches the floor.

C. Inhale deeply into your abdomen and extend your stomach as you lift your right hip up as high as possible to stretch the left hamstring (count 1-8).

D. Bring your left foot close to your right foot, exhale and arch your back as high as possible, while sucking your stomach up against your backbone and slowly raising your head and shoulders upward, approaching an upright position (count 1-8).

E. Switch feet by standing with your weight on your left leg. Step your right foot forward about one foot in front of your left.

F. Place the palms of both hands on your respective thighs, close to the hip, while tilting your right foot up so that only the heel touches the floor.

G. Inhale deeply into your abdomen and extend your stomach as you lift your left hip up as high as possible to stretch the right hamstring (count 1-8).

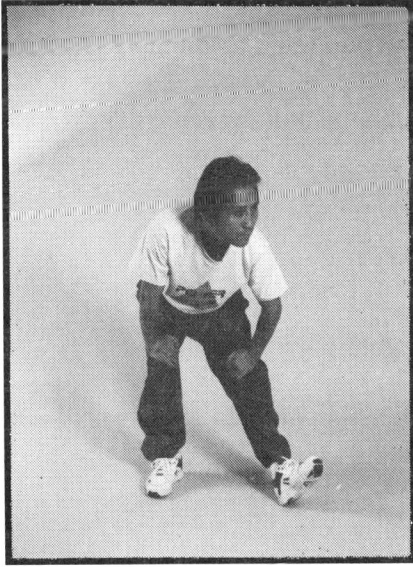 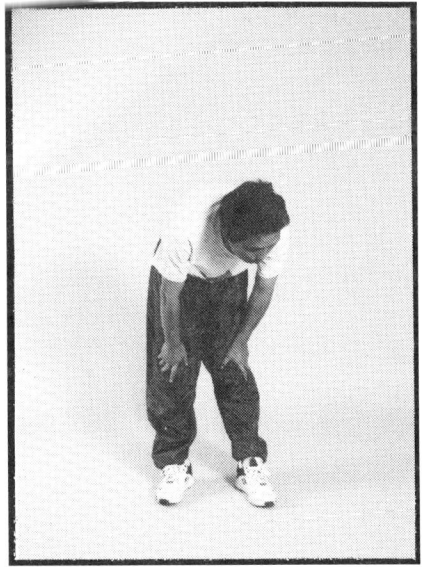

| A, B, C, | D |

H. Bring your right foot close to your left foot, exhale and arch your back as high as possible, while sucking your stomach up against your backbone and slowly raising your head and shoulders upward, approaching an upright position (count 1-8).

I. Inhale and relax.

Benefits:

The hamstring and back stretch will:

* loosen and stretch the hamstrings (back of the leg).

* loosen and stretch the calf muscle.

* freshen thigh and shin muscles and improve blood circulation throughout the leg.

* develop body balance.

* loosen up the lower and middle back. The reverse arch will separate the vertebrae and allow fresh circulation into the spinal column.

* sucking the stomach up to the backbone will massage the internal organs of the abdomen.

Caution:

Do not press on the knee joint with your hands.

Keep your head tilted back to reduce strain on your lower back.

16. Balance Stretch

The balance stretch will help you develop your sense of balance while it stretches the hip and lower back area.

How to do it:

A. Return to ready stance (bend your knees slightly, with your feet approximately shoulder width apart).

B. Inhale and lift your left knee as high as possible and clasp your hands together so that they hold the back of the left thigh near the knee.

C. Exhale and use your hands to pull your left thigh against your abdomen (count 1-8).

D. Release your leg and return to ready stance.

E. Inhale and lift your right knee as high as possible and clasp your hands together so that they hold the back of the right thigh near the knee.

F. Exhale and use your hands to pull your right thigh against your abdomen (count 1-8).

G. Release your leg and return to ready stance.

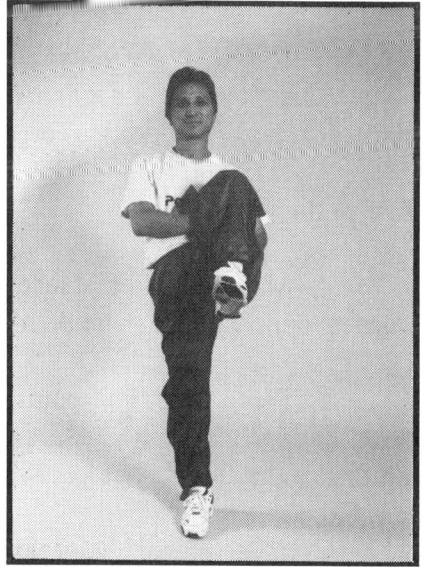

Benefits:

C

The balance stretch will:

* loosen and stretch the lower back, buttocks, and hips.

* strengthen the entire leg.

* develop balance.

* loosen up ankles.

Caution:

For better balance, slightly bend the knee of the support leg. If you have a bad knee, be careful when trying to balance on that leg (you don't want to put your knee out or fall). Also do not clasp your hands on the shin of your bent leg because that may also strain the knee.

If you do not have good balance, be prepared to unclasp your hands quickly to release your leg and regain balance.

17. Internal Organ Massage

This exercise is a good for the digestion because it massages the internal (especially digestive) organs.

How to do it:

A. Maintain same stance as #16. (Bend your knees slightly, with your feet approximately shoulder width apart).

B. Place your left palm over your lower energy center (thumb above the belly button and index finger just below it) with the fingers pointing to the side. Place your right hand over your left hand.

C. Inhale through your nose into your lower abdomen.

D. Exhale slowly through the mouth and roll your hand up and down about one 1 inch, first applying pressure with the thumb and pushing down, and next applying pressure with the pinkie and pushing up.

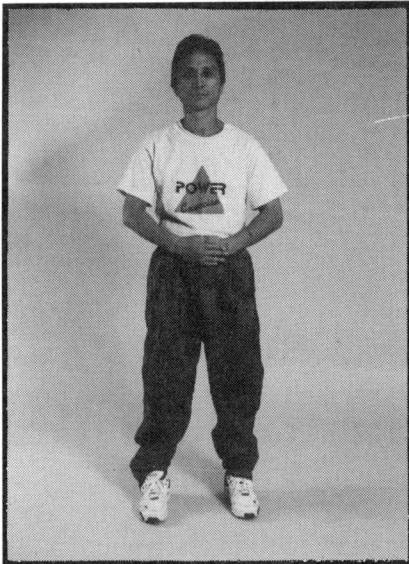

B

E. Change hands so that the left hand is over the right.

F. Repeat steps C and D.

Benefits:

The internal organ massage will:

* stimulate internal organs, specifically: the liver, stomach, pancreas, large and small intestines, kidneys, and bladder.

248

* stimulate the internal organs to secrete the proper chemicals. The rolling motion also helps to move the contents around for proper chemical balance.

* prevent and heal stomach ache.

* prevent and heal diarrhea and constipation.

* encourage good digestion.

* aid in the discovery of internal problems, so they can be treated immediately.

* Shake all the stale gas out of your stomach and other digestive organs.

Caution:

You may burp or "break wind" as the gasses in your organs are shaken loose and expelled. Do not worry even the slightest; this is completely normal, and a desirable effect of this exercise.

18. Skin Massage

Part of this massage will be done with a cupped hand. The cupped hand contains a small amount of air, which, when used to massage, is gentler and more evenly distributed than massaging with flesh on flesh. This whole body massage increases circulation and relaxes muscle tension.

How to do it:

A. Maintain same stance as #17. (Bend your knees slightly, with your feet approximately shoulder width apart).

B. Cup your hands as if you were trying to hold a few ounces of water. The air in this little "cup" will be what massages you in the first part of this exercise.

C. Pat yourself with the left cupped hand up and down the center of the chest and abdomen, then use both hands and move to every part of the chest and abdomen.

D. Return to using only the left hand, and pat the right side of your torso, from arm pit to hip.

E. Using only the right hand, pat the left side of your torso, from arm pit to hip.

F. Move the left hand to the back of the neck and pat yourself along the back of the neck and shoulder, down the outside of the right arm, and up the inside of the same arm.

G. Move the right hand to the back of the neck and pat yourself along the back of the neck and shoulder, down the outside of the right arm, and up the inside of the same arm.

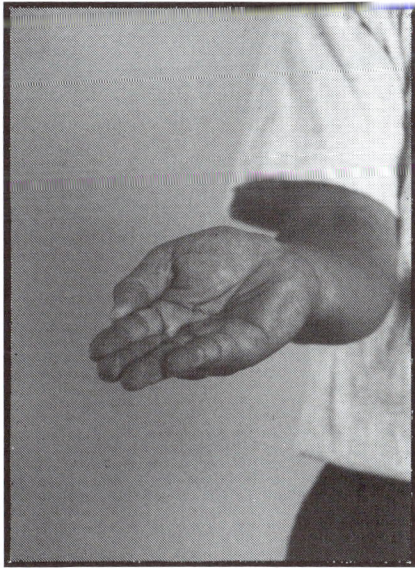

B

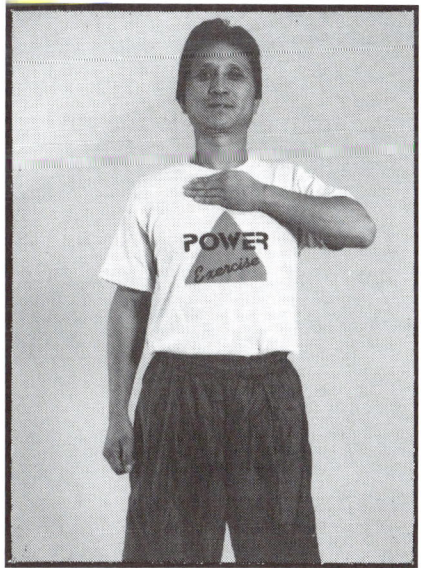

C

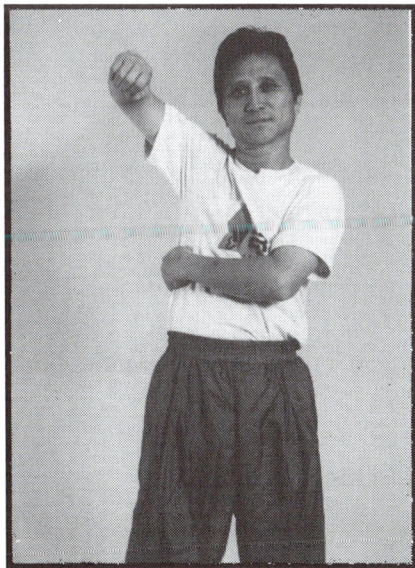

D

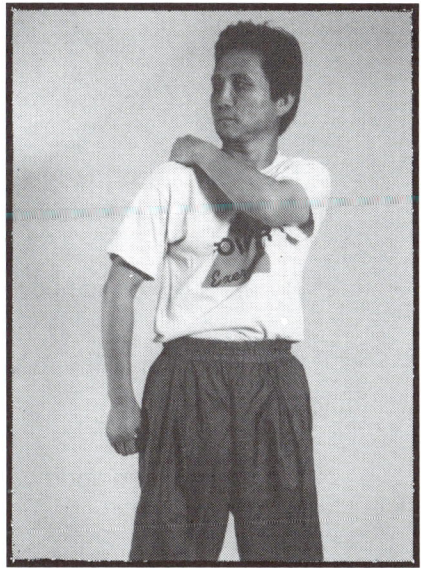

F

H. Using both hands at the same time, begin patting yourself along the middle back, down the buttocks and back of the legs, to the front of the feet and back up the front of the legs.

I. Move both hands to the outside of the legs and work your way down from the hip to the ankle, then come back up the inside of the leg to the groin.

J. Separate your fingers as if grabbing a soft ball and use your finger tips to pat your neck, face, side and top of head.

K. Wash your face and hair with air.

Benefits:

* The patting stimulates the blood to come to the surface, to increase the circulation.

* The patting also stimulates all the internal organs, especially the heart, lungs, and brain.

* The patting helps to relax the muscle and reduce tension.

* By massaging the abdomen, you stimulate the flow of digestive juices and the movement of food to improve digestion.

* By massaging the neck and head, you can reduce headaches.

* By massaging the whole body, you complete the whole body standing warm-up.

* You strengthen and make your muscles shapely.

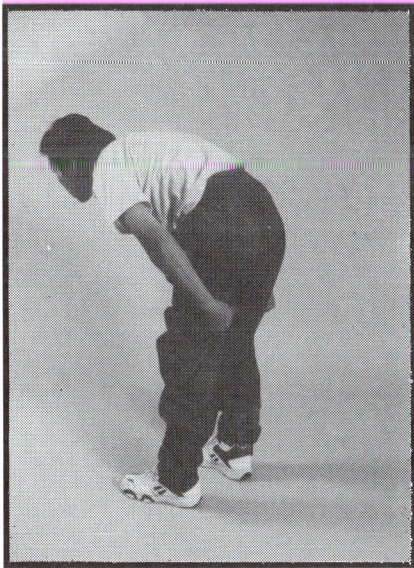

H

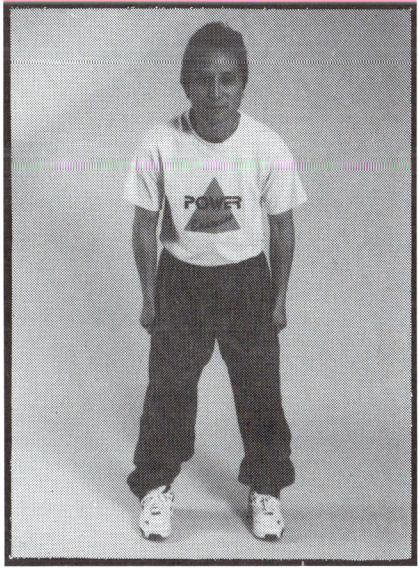

I

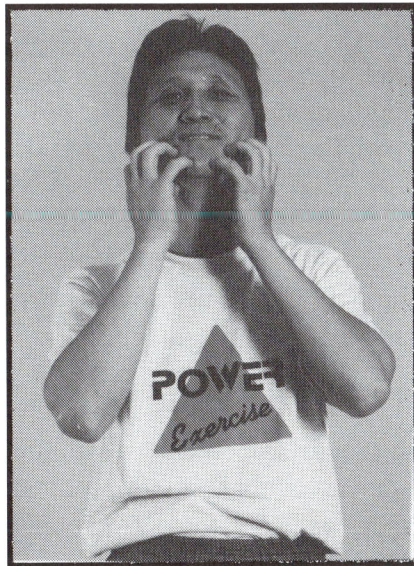

J

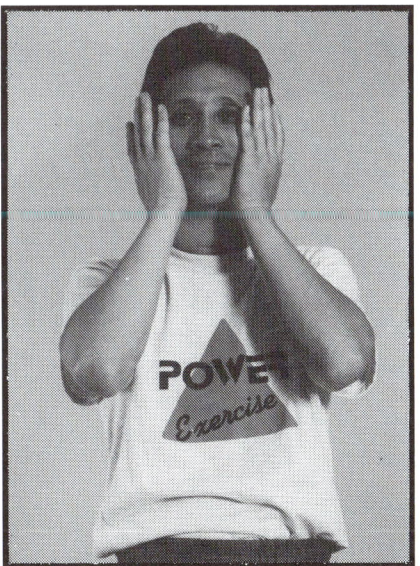

K

Caution:

You must pat the body with the correct force: if you do not pat hard enough, you will not bring the blood to the surface; if you pat too hard you could bruise yourself or otherwise make this exercise uncomfortable. Be sure to massage every part of your body.

If you are somewhere where the sound of the patting will disturb others, just squeeze the muscles in a massaging motion instead of patting.

19. Body Bouncing

This exercise, after stretching and massaging the muscles in a proper warm-up, will help you relax and integrate flexible muscles into graceful movements.

How to do it:

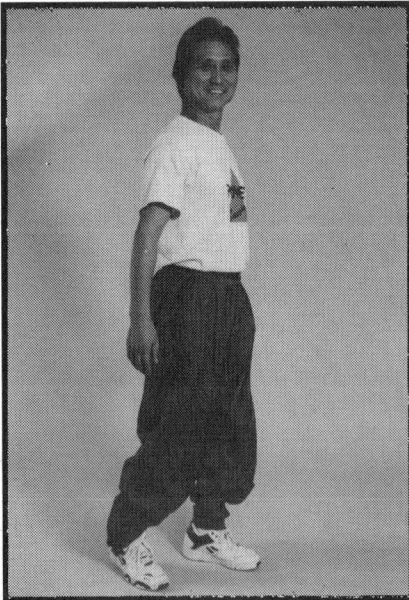

A. Maintain same stance as #18. (Bend your knees slightly, with your feet approximately shoulder width apart.)

B. Rise up on the balls of your feet, and bounce by jumping up and down very slightly (less than one inch).

C. Relax your entire body so that every part flows with the bounce. Inhale for 2 counts, and exhale for 2 counts throughout the exercise.

D. Turn your torso to the left gradually, so that your torso has turned ninety degrees in 4 counts.

E. Turn your torso to the right gradually, so that your torso has turned ninety degrees in 4 counts. Continue to turn right for 4 more counts.

F. Turn your torso to the left again for 4 counts, so that you finish facing front.

E. Continue to bounce facing the front for 8 counts.

F. Return to ready stance (knees slightly bent with feet approximately shoulder width apart.)

Benefits:

The body bouncing exercise will:

* warm up the entire body through increased circulation and increased flexibility.

* massage the internal organs through bouncing and vibrating them.
* release tension and stress.

Caution:

Keep your weight on the balls of your feet, never letting the heels strike the ground and jar your body.

If you have bad knees or a bad back, be careful never to leave the ground. Bounce by bending the knees but keeping the feet in contact with the floor.

If you are only going to do the standing exercises, do the deep breathing exercise described as #1 in this section one more time at this point as #20. As a closing exercise, it was designed to restore more oxygen to your system. For this reason, breathe deeply but a little bit faster than you did at the beginning of the exercises.

Finish with standing Concentration Meditation, Reflective Meditation, or Power Meditation (pp. 166-188).

If you are going to continue doing seated or other Power Exercises, do the breathing and meditation at the end of your complete Power Exercise session.

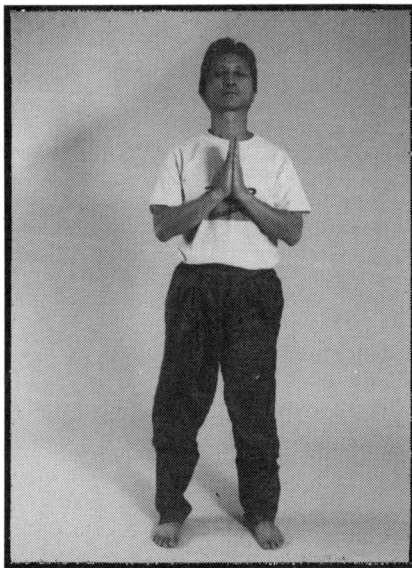

SEATED POWER EXERCISES

The seated exercises as a whole can more properly be named "stretching" than "warm-up" exercises, because they concentrate more on stretching muscles and loosening joints than on increasing the heart rate and body temperature. Whenever you perform stretching exercises, be certain to

A. Be gentle to the muscle,

B. Go slowly as not to strain the muscle,

C. Adapt the directions to your body: stretch as far as is possible for you, but do not over-pull and end up straining yourself.

D. Keep the head back whenever you bend forward, to avoid lower back strain.

Seated Exercises

1. Foot Massage

2. Single Leg Stretch

3. Butterfly

4 Open Leg Stretch

5. Double Leg Stretch

6. Seated Adjust the Spine

7. Rhythm Breathing

8. Finger Chain Breathing

1. Foot Massage

According to the science of reflexology, different areas of the foot are connected to every part of the body. By massaging the feet, we can stimulate any organ, joint, or muscle. Therefore, by massaging the whole foot, we can stimulate the whole body.

How to do it:

A. Sit on the floor with your right leg extended directly in front of you.

B. Cross your left leg over your right so that the knee is fully bent and the ankle extends over the right thigh.

C. Grasp the left foot in both hands.

D. Massage the foot completely: each toe, ball, arch, heel and ankle (count 1 - 8).

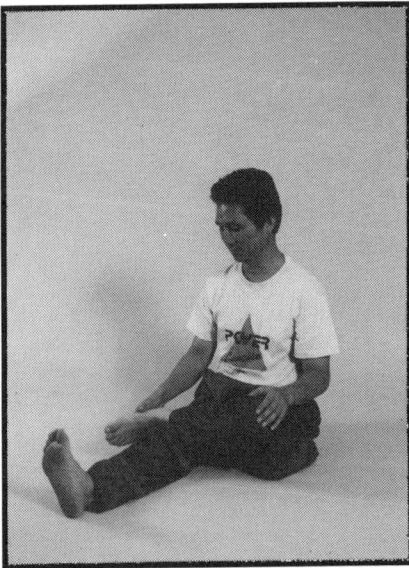

A, B

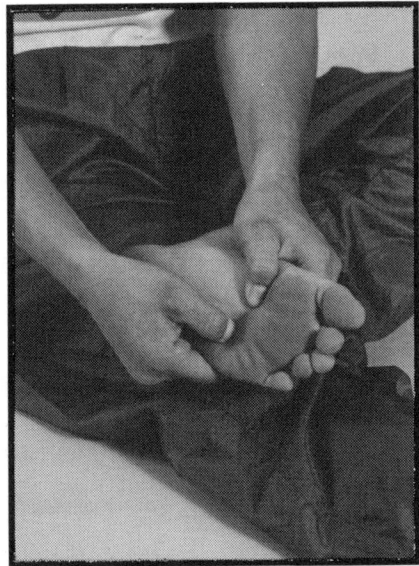

C, D

E. Switch feet by extending your left foot directly in front of you.

F. Cross your right leg over your left so that the knee is fully bent and the ankle extends over the left thigh.

G. Grasp the right foot in both hands.

H. Massage the foot completely: each toe, ball, arch, heel and ankle (count 1 - 8).

Benefits:

The foot massage will:

* loosen the ankles and feet.

* stimulate the entire body to increase circulation.

* reduce headaches.

Caution:

It is not necessary to put the ankle over the leg. If you have a bad knee, just place your bent leg and foot on the floor by your groin.

If you find any areas on your foot that are sensitive to the touch, it may indicate there is a problem in the organ that corresponds to that area of the foot. Consult a reflexology chart, or consult a certified reflexologist or other health care professional.

2. Single Leg Stretch

This posture will stretch the hamstring (back of the thigh), lower back, hip, and knee. This is a basic stretch to loosen up many connected areas of the body.

How to do it:

A. Sit on the floor with your left leg extended directly in front of you.

B. Bend your right leg at the knee and place the sole of the right foot against the inside of the left thigh. Move the right knee back to open as wide an angle as possible between your two thighs.

C. Extend both your arms straight out from the shoulder to the side as you inhale.

D. Exhale slowly for as long as possible and bend your body forward, reaching both hands toward the foot, attempting to put your chin on your shin, with your head up.

E. Inhale and sit upright.

F. Switch feet by extending your right foot directly in front of you. Bend your left leg at the knee and place the sole of the left foot against the inside of the right thigh, again opening as wide an angle as possible between the two thighs.

G. Extend both your arms straight out from the shoulder to the sides as you inhale.

H. Exhale slowly for as long as possible and bend your body forward, reaching both hands toward the foot, attempting to put your chin on your shin, with your head up.

I. Inhale and sit upright.

A,B,C

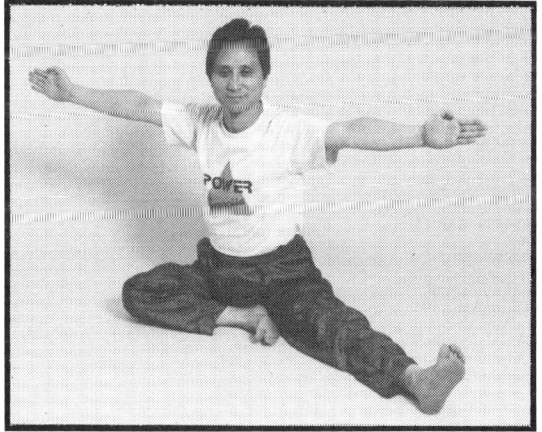

D

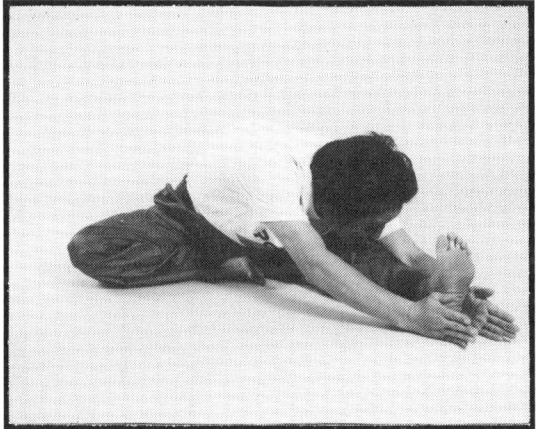

Benefits:

The single leg stretch will:

* loosen and stretch the hamstring, lower back, hip and knee.

* release and remove waste products from your body.

Caution:

Always remember to bend the head back whenever you bend the body forward to reduce the possibility of lower back strain. If you are prone to hip dislocation, be very careful.

3. Butterfly

The butterfly stretch will loosen your hip and groin muscles, as well as the lower back muscles. It is a good exercise to restore sexual drive.

How to do it:

A. Sit on the floor. Pull both feet in to the groin, and place them sole to sole. Hold your feet in your hands, palms against the insteps.

B. Use your hip muscles to pull your knees gently toward the floor, then release them, in a motion that resembles a butterfly flapping its wings (16 repetitions).

C. Inhale. Exhale for as long as possible and slowly bend forward, trying to lower your chin to the floor in front of your feet with your head back.

D. Inhale and sit upright.

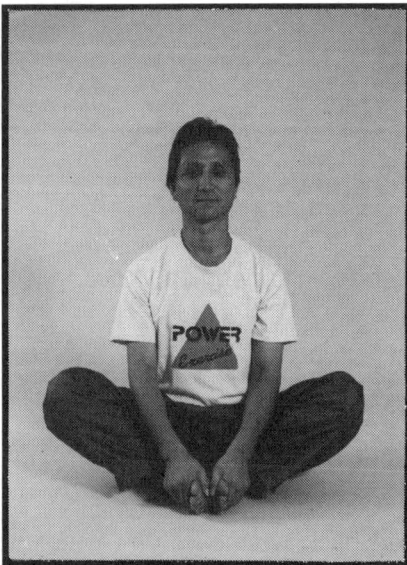

A

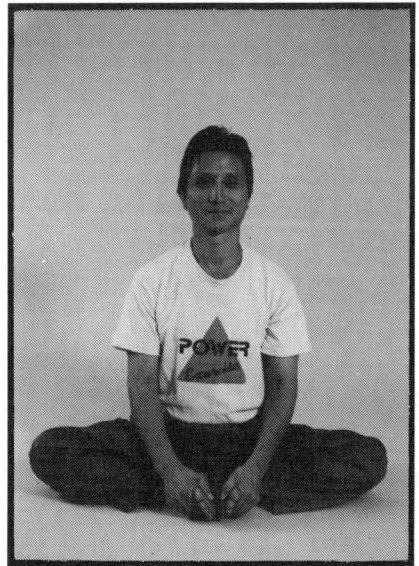

B

Benefits:

The butterfly stretch will:

* loosen and stretch groin muscles and hip joints.

* increase circulation and energy flow to the lower energy center, restoring inhibited sexual drive.

* loosen and stretch lower back.

* expel waste products from internal organs.

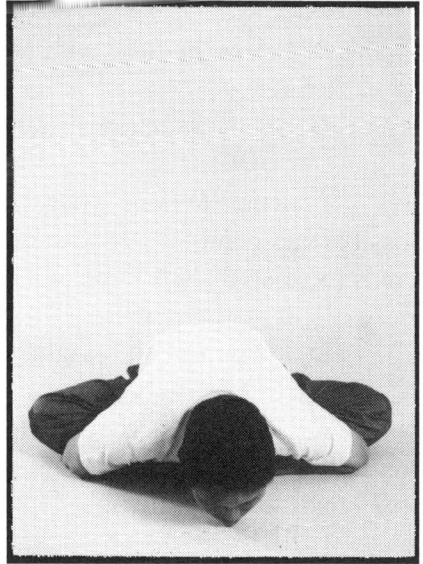

C

Caution:

If you are prone to hip displacement, be very careful.

4. Open Leg Stretch

The open leg stretch will stretch many hip, leg, and back muscles at the same time. There are three different ways to do it, and each one changes the target muscles slightly.

How to do it:

A. Sit on the floor with both legs extended as far apart as possible.

B. Extend both arms straight out from the shoulders and inhale.

C. Turn to face your left foot. Exhale slowly for as long as possible and gently lower your chest to your left thigh, while reaching both hands to grasp the left foot and tilting the head back.

D. Inhale and sit upright, extending both arms.

E. Turn to face your right foot. Exhale slowly for as long as possible and gently lower your chest to your right thigh, while reaching both hands to grasp the right foot and tilting the head back.

F. Inhale and sit upright, extending both hands.

G. Exhale slowly for as long as possible and gently lean to the left, trying to touch your left ear to your left knee. Reach your left hand to your left foot, thumb down, palm facing the sole. Reach your right hand straight over your head and point it toward the ceiling.

H. Inhale and sit upright, extending both arms.

I. Exhale slowly for as long as possible and gently lean to the right, trying to touch your right ear to your right knee. Reach your right hand to your right foot, thumb down, palm facing the sole. Reach your left hand straight over your head and point it toward the ceiling.

J. Inhale and sit upright, extending both arms.

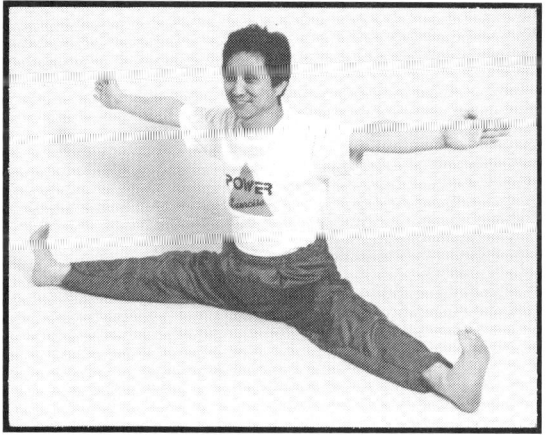

A, B, D, F,
H, J, L

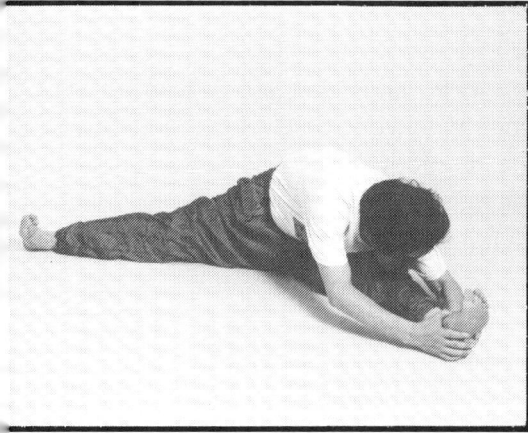

C

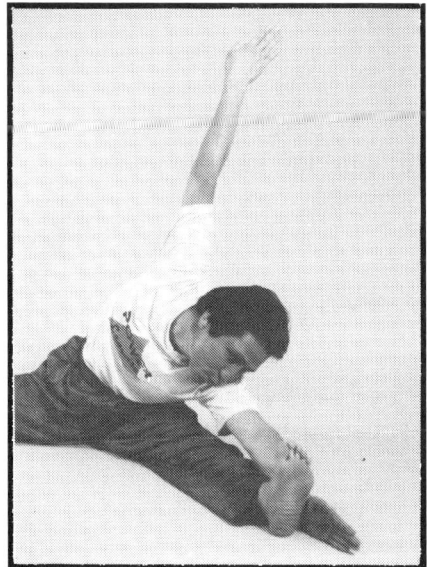

G

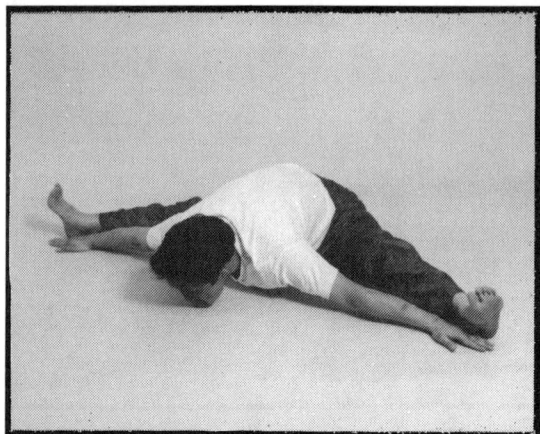

K

K. Exhale slowly for as long as possible and gently lean forward, trying to touch your chin to the floor with your head back. Reach each hand for the ankle or sole of its respective foot.

L. Inhale and sit upright, extending both arms.

Benefits:

Open leg stretching will:

* loosen and stretch the hamstrings, sides (lat.), lower back, and groin muscles, and hip joints.

* release tension and stress by stretching the spinal muscles.

* stimulate the lower energy center and increase sexual energy.

* stimulate the lower digestive and elimination tract to prevent constipation and bladder control problems.

* adjust the spine.

Caution:

If you have a bad back, be very careful of over-extending it, especially in G and I.

5. Double Leg Stretch

The double leg stretch stretches both hamstrings at the same time. It is a little more advanced than the single leg stretch.

How to do it:

A. Sit on the floor with both legs extended directly in front of you. Place both hands palm to palm in front of the chest, as if praying, and then extend your hands over your head as you inhale.

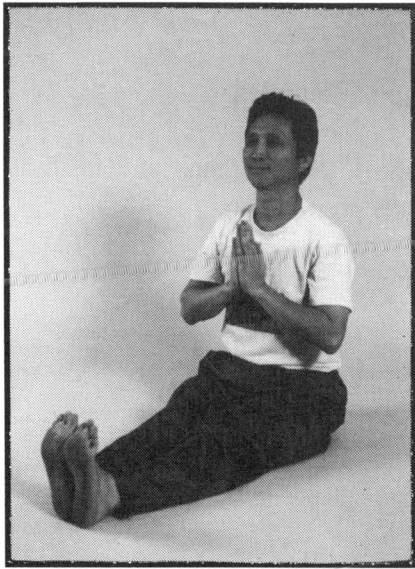

A (front), C

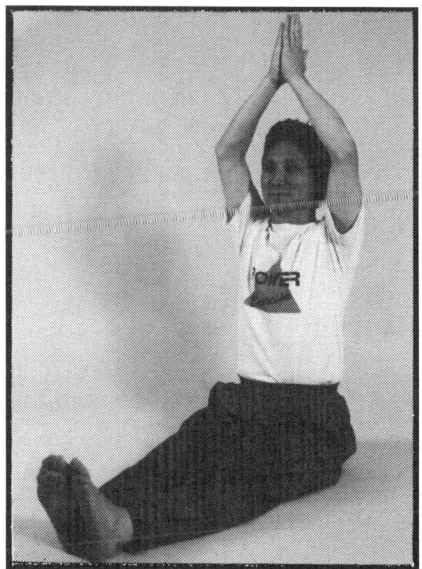

A (up)

267

B. Exhale slowly for as long as possible as you separate your arms and lower them to the side, then gently bend forward as far as possible, reaching your hands to grasp your ankles or feet. Try to touch your chest to your thighs and keep your head back.

C. Inhale and sit up.

D. Repeat A through C.

Benefits:

The double leg stretch will:

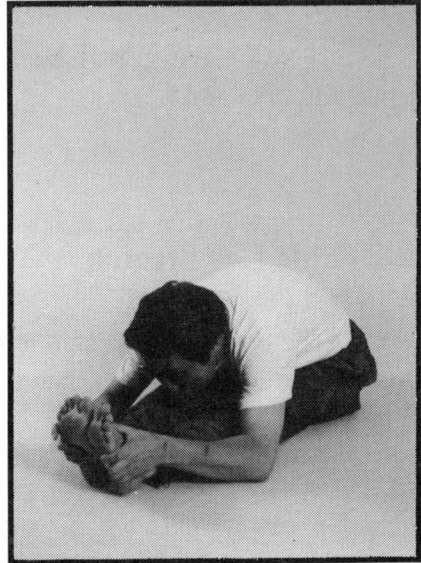

B

* increase blood circulation throughout the whole body.

* loosen up and stretch the hamstrings, lower back, arms, and shoulders.

* release tension by stretching the spinal muscles.

* aid digestion by strengthening the internal organs and pushing out carbon dioxide, stale gas, and other waste products.

Caution:

Tilt your head back to avoid straining the lower back.

Do not strain yourself by pulling too fast or too hard. Stretch as far as you can comfortably.

6. Seated Adjust the Spine

This exercise is excellent for loosening up the lower back and reducing back pain.

How to do it:

A. Sit on the floor with your left leg extended directly in front of you.

B. Cross your right leg over your left so that the knee is up and the right foot is flat on the floor to the left of the left thigh.

C. Reach your left elbow across your right knee and use the elbow to move the knee to the left as far as possible, while maintaining a straight body. Inhale.

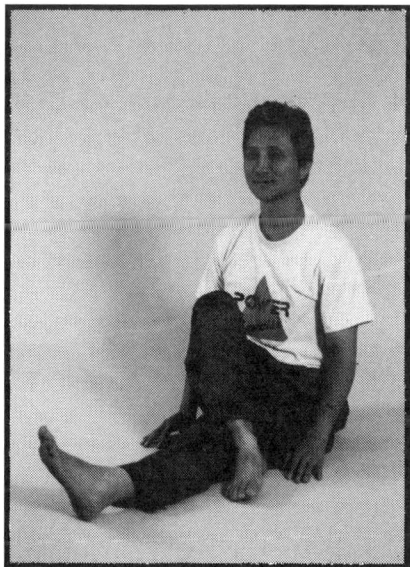
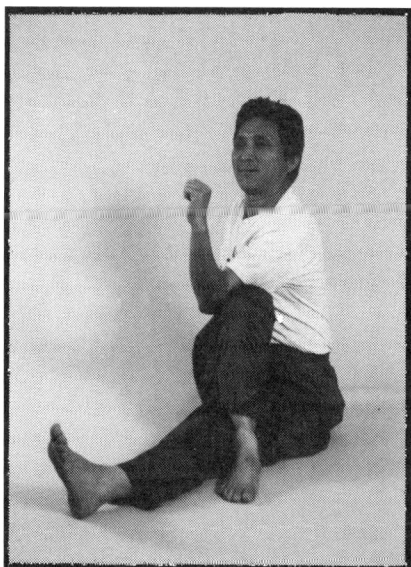

A, B   C

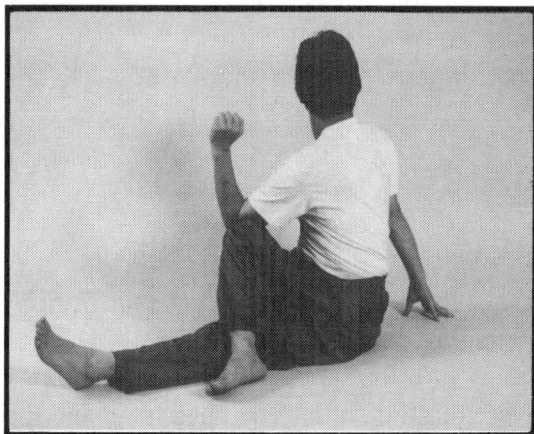

D. Place the right hand on the floor directly behind you with the fingers spread wide. Exhale, and turn your head as far as possible to look behind you to the right, slowly twisting your torso.

E. Inhale and return to center.

D

F. Switch feet by extending your right leg directly in front of you.

G. Cross your left leg over your right so that the knee is up and the left foot is flat on the floor to the right of the right thigh.

H. Reach your right elbow across your left knee and use the elbow to move the knee to the right as far as possible, while maintaining a straight body. Inhale.

I. Place the left hand on the floor directly behind you with the fingers spread wide. Exhale, and turn your head as far as possible to look behind you to the left, slowly twisting your torso.

J. Inhale and return to center.

Benefits:

The seated adjust the spine will:

* loosen and stretch the spinal muscles, lower back, and hip joints.

* allow vertebrae that are slightly "out of place" to re-align themselves when the muscles relax.

* allow hips that are slightly out of place to go back where they belong.

* strengthen kidney, liver, and spleen, and regulate bladder problems.

* prevent and heal headache, back ache, stomach ache, and other digestion problems.

* increase blood circulation greatly.

Caution:

People prone to hip or shoulder displacement should not apply too much pressure to either joint.

People with back problems should not twist too far.

7. Rhythm Power Breathing

This exercise is especially good for the digestion. The rocking motion will adjust the digestive organs and digestive juices to release excess gas. It will also adjust your spine.

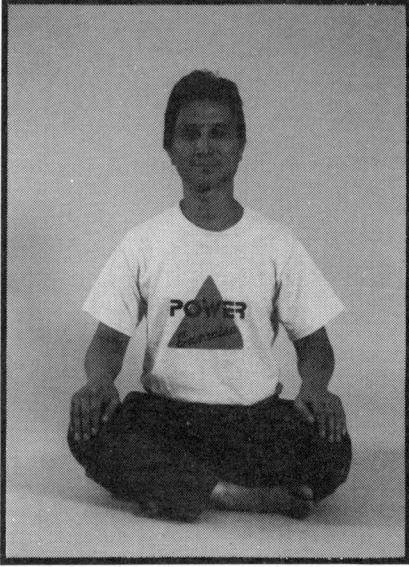

A, B, C

How to do it:

A. Sit comfortably on the floor with your legs crossed.

B. Place your hands comfortably with the palms against abdomen or on the knee.

C. Slowly inhale into the lower abdomen through the nose.

D. Exhale and tighten your lower abdomen as you gently rock your body from side to side, while keeping the head still.

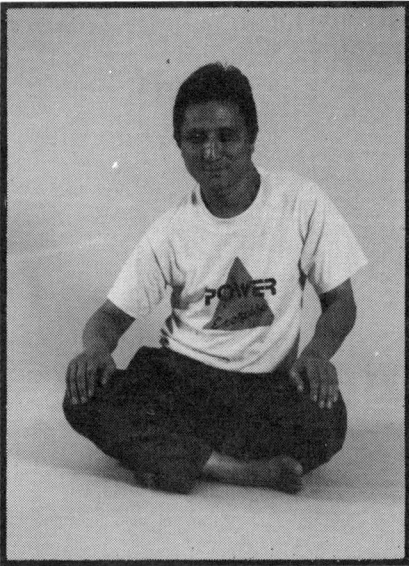

D (left)

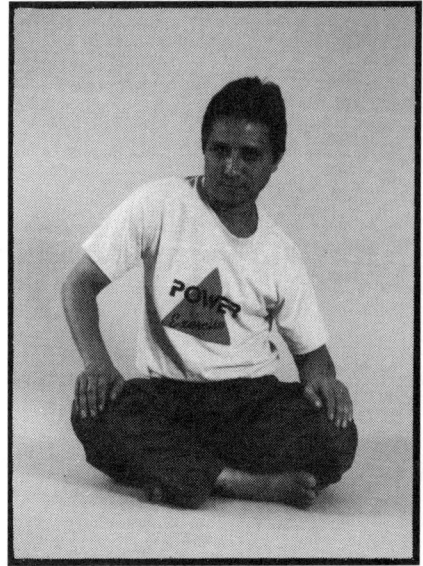

D (right)

E. Repeat A through D.

Benefits.

Rhythm power breathing will:

* loosen the spinal muscles, adjust the vertebrae, and strengthen the lower back.

* massage the internal organs.

* release trapped gas in the digestive tract.

* prevent stomach aches, constipation, and diarrhea.

* release stress and tension.

Caution:

If you have bad knees, you need not cross your legs uncomfortably. If you have a bad back, do not rock very much.

Be prepared to burp as the digestive gasses are released. Do not do this exercise immediately after eating.

8. Finger Chain Breathing

This exercise can loosen up the hands, arms, and shoulders at the same time it releases the tension in your back.

How to do it:

A. Sit comfortably on the floor with your legs crossed, as in # 7.

273

B. Place your palms together and interlock your fingers into a finger chain. Inhale and extend your hands up over your head with your palms up.

C. Release your fingers and bring your extended arms down each side as you exhale.

D. When your hands reach waist level, bring your hands forward and together again.

E. Repeat B through D three more times.

Benefits:

Finger chain breathing will:

* loosen the fingers, shoulders, and the entire back.

* release tension and stress.

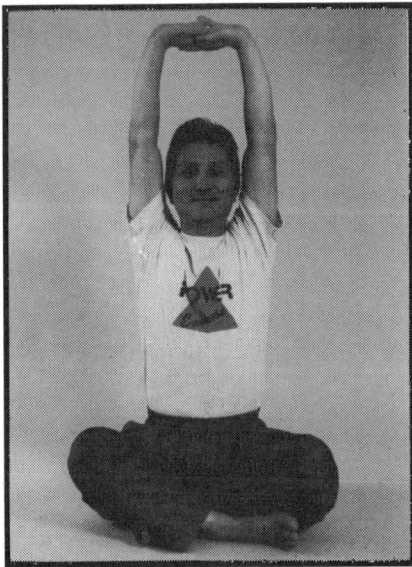

B

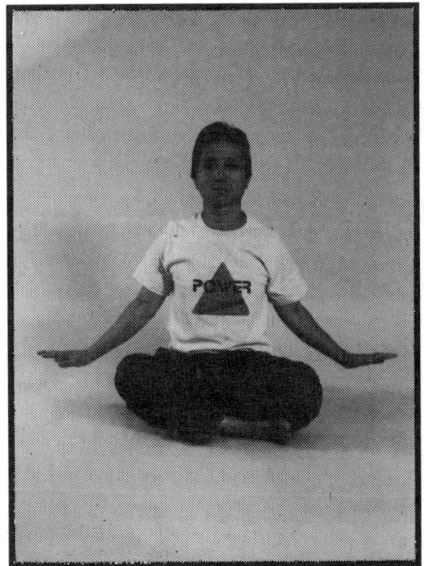

C

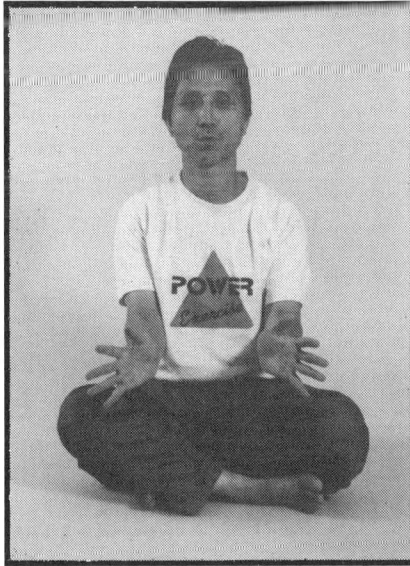

D

Caution:

If you have bad knees, you need not cross your legs uncomfortably. If you have a bad back, do not bend forward too far.

If you are going to finish your Power Exercises here, begin Concentration, Reflective, or Power Meditation (see pp. 166-188). If you are going to continue, meditate at the end of your complete Power Exercise session.

LYING DOWN POWER EXERCISES

Lying Down Power Exercises are a little more challenging than the standing or seated exercises, but they are very worthwhile. Do them the best you can until you can slowly build up the strength and flexibility necessary. You will have a lot of fun and a sense of accomplishment.

Lying Down Exercises

1. Push-up Stretch

2. Side Push-up

3. Hip-up

4. Sit-ups

5. Single Leg Pull

6. Inverted Butterfly Pull

7. Adjust the Spine

8. Full Body Stretch

1. Push-up Stretch

This version of the push-up will not only strengthen your arms and chest, but adjust your spine as well.

How to do it:

A. Lie on the floor on your stomach. Extend your legs with your toes pointed and your ankles together. Bend your elbows and place your palms on the floor next to your shoulders, with your fingers pointing straight ahead.

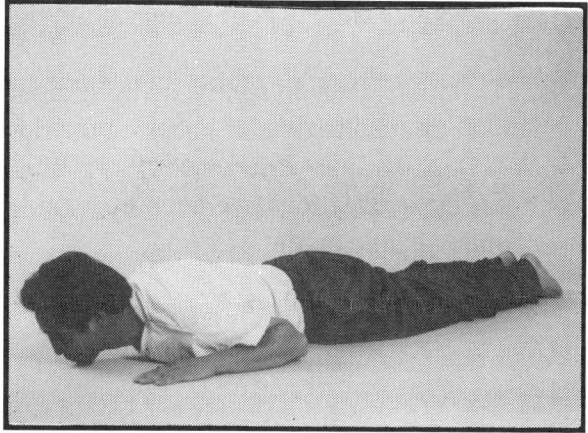

A, F

B. Inhale and slowly straighten your arms to lift your shoulders up off of the floor, so that you can look at the ceiling, while leaving your hips down.

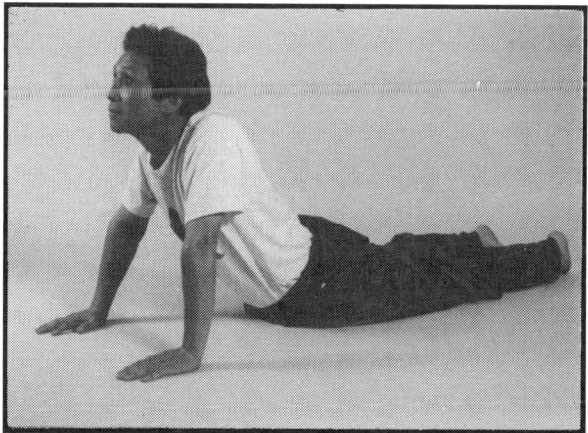

B

277

C. Lift up your hips to the same height as your shoulders.

D. Exhale and lean back so that your buttocks rest on your heels and your arms are fully extended.

E. Inhale and lift your hips up and forward, into the same resting position as C.

F. Exhale and lay your stomach on the floor again as in A.

G. Inhale, then do a push-up by straightening your arms as you exhale (ladies may leave their knees on the floor).

H. Do at least four to nine more push-ups, inhaling on the way down, and exhaling on the way up.

I. Lay your stomach on the floor again as in A.

C, E

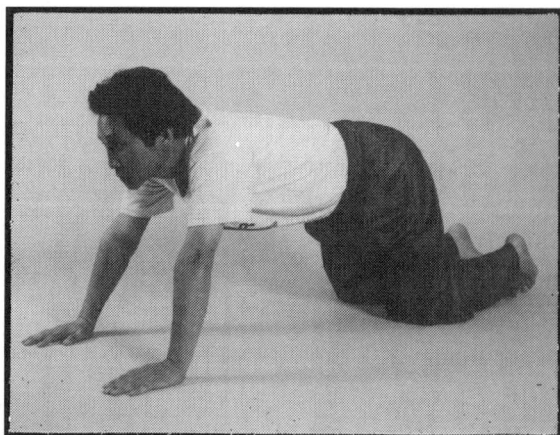

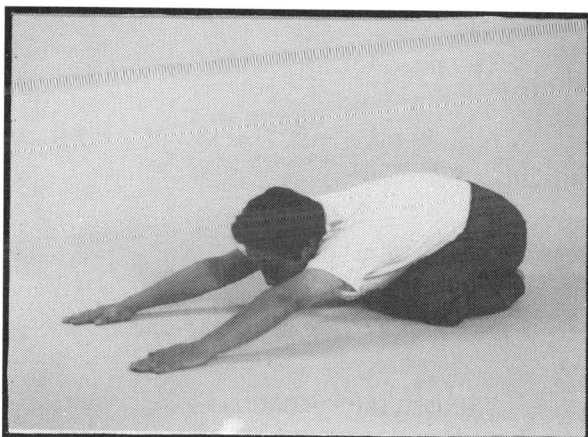

D

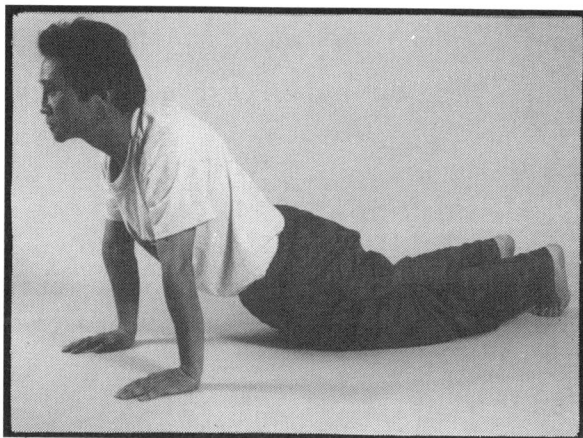

G (lady)

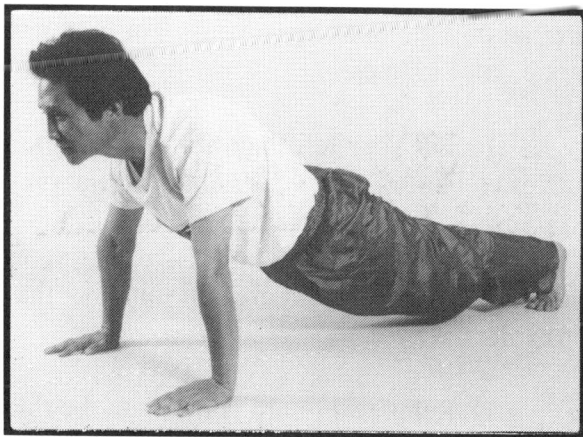

G (man)

279

Benefits:

The push-up stretch will:

* loosen the back (backwards and forward), and stretch lower back muscles.

* adjust the spine.

* strengthen the arms and chest.

* loosen the knee joints.

Caution:

Those with bad knees should not sit all the way back on their heels.

2. Side Push-up

This exercise will help improve your balance while it strengthens your arms, abdomen, sides, buttocks, and lower back.

How to do it:

A. Roll over on your left side, so that your left hip, knee, and ankle are flat on the floor. Place your right foot on top of your left foot, ankle to ankle, knee to knee.

B. Put your left hand flat on the floor in a straight line with your ankles and knees. Put your right hand flat on your right hip. Inhale.

C. Lift your body up so that it is straight, and only your hand and the side of your left foot are still touching the floor. Exhale for as long as possible.

D. Relax and return your hip to the floor, and sit down.

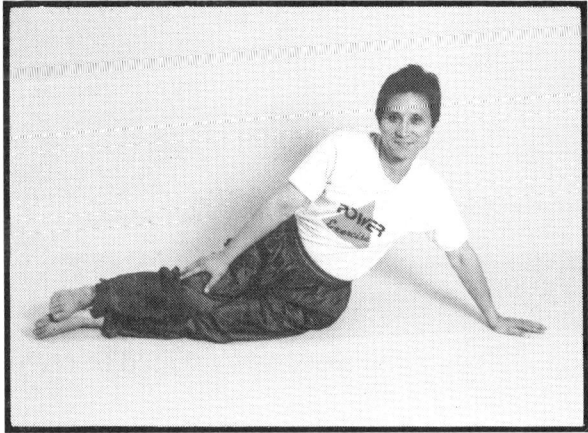

A, B

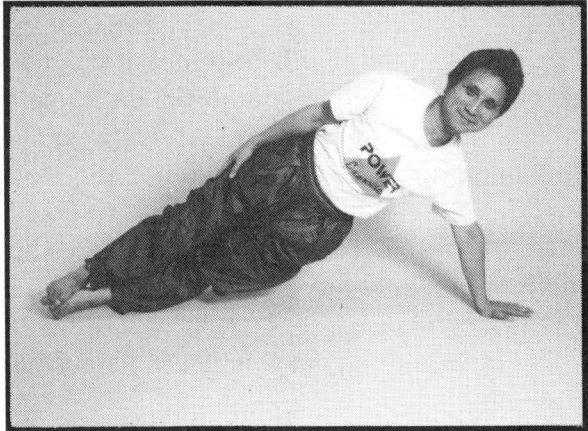

C

E. Roll over on your right side, so that your right hip, knee, and ankle are flat on the floor. Place your left foot on top of your right foot, ankle to ankle, knee to knee.

F. Put your right hand flat on the floor in a straight line with your ankles and knees. Put your left hand flat on your left hip. Inhale.

G. Lift your body up so that it is straight, and only your hand and the side of your right foot are still touching the floor. Exhale for as long as possible.

H. Relax and return your hip to the floor, and sit down.

Benefits:

The side push-up will:

* strengthen your arms.

* improve your body balance

Caution:

Those with weak backs should be careful not strain their backs.

3. Hip-up

This exercise will help loosen up and strengthen your lower back and buttocks, as well as your lower abdominal muscles.

How to do it:

A. Lie on your back with your knees bent and your soles flat on the floor.

B. Inhale and put your hands flat on the floor.

C. Exhale and lift your hips up off the floor by tightening the buttocks and lower abdomen (but keep your back flat on the floor).

D. Inhale and relax so that your hips rest on the floor.

E. Repeat C and D three more times.

Benefits:

The hip-up will:

* loosen up and strengthen the buttocks, lower abdomen, and lower back.

* increase the circulation and energy flow to the hip area.

Caution:

Keep the back flat on the floor from the waist up (belt line), throughout the exercise. Lifting the back off the floor risks straining the back without any significant muscle advantage.

A, B, D

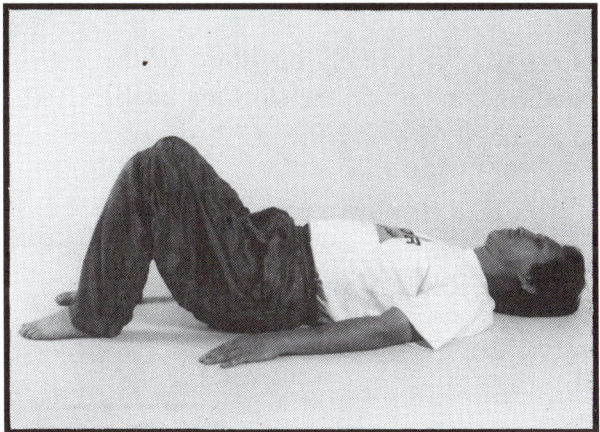

C

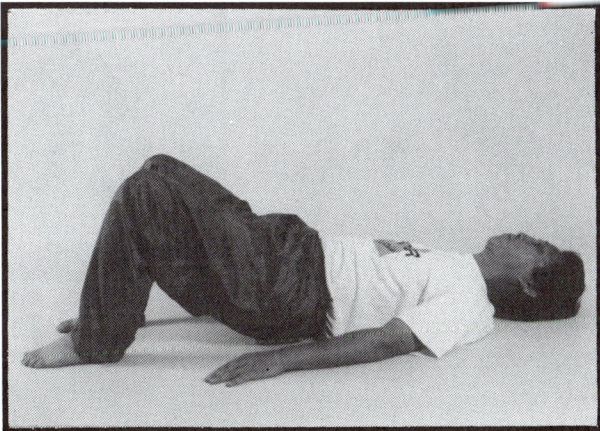

4. Sit-ups

Many people do sit-ups to strengthen the abdomen and lower back, but they do not realize that sit-ups also release nervous tension, aid digestion, and help prevent insomnia.

How to do it:

A. Lie on your back with your knees bent and your soles flat on the floor.

B. Reach your hands up as if to grab two handles about knee height directly above your abdomen. Inhale.

C. Sit up only one-third of the way by pulling on the imaginary handles, contracting the stomach muscles, exhaling, and touching the chin to the chest.

D. Relax by returning to position B.

E. Repeat C and D seven more times.

A, B, D

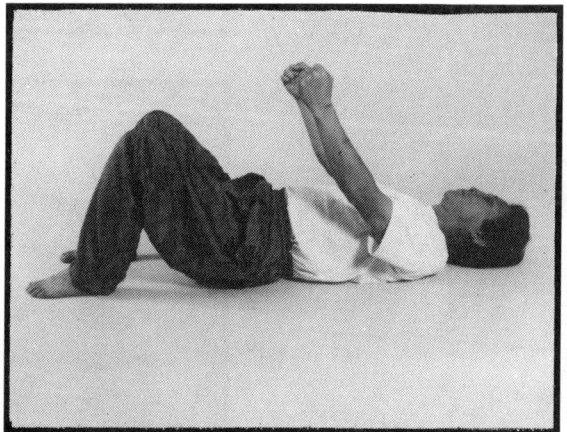

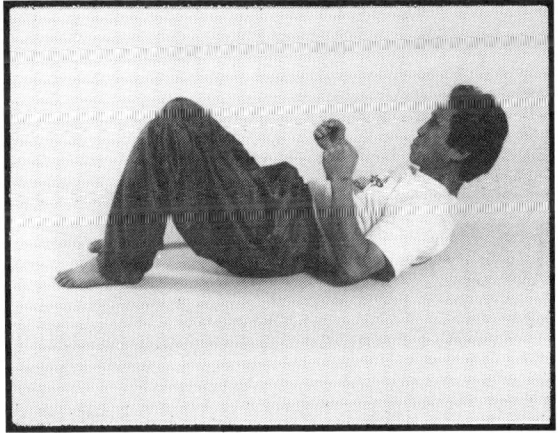

C

Benefits:

Sit-ups will:

* strengthen the abdomen and lower back muscles.

* adjust the spine.

* release nervous tension and stress, and help prevent insomnia.

* aid indigestion and help prevent burping.

* aid in bladder control.

* release stale gasses from the system.

Caution:

This exercise is very safe as described. Do not do sit-ups with the knees straight, as you may strain the lower back. Likewise, only come up one-third of the way to avoid straining the back.

5. Single Leg Pull

This is a good static stretch to loosen up the hamstring, hip, and lower back. It is a good stretch to increase flexibility for high kicking.

How to do it:

A. Lie on the floor on your back. Inhale.

B. Lift the left leg with the knee bent and grab the back of the thigh with both hands close to the knee.

C. Exhale and pull the leg so that your thigh touches your abdomen (count 1-4).

D. Release the thigh and grab the ankle with both hands as you straighten your knee. Inhale.

E. Exhale and pull the leg up toward your shoulder, as high as is comfortably possible (count 1-8).

F. Release your leg and gently return it to the floor. Inhale.

G. Lift the right leg with the knee relaxed and grab the back of the thigh with both hands close to the knee.

H. Exhale and pull the leg so that your thigh touches your abdomen (count 1-4).

I. Release the thigh and grab the ankle with both hands as you straighten your knee. Inhale.

J. Exhale and pull the leg up toward your shoulder, as high as is comfortably possible (count 1-8).

K. Release your leg and gently return it to the floor.

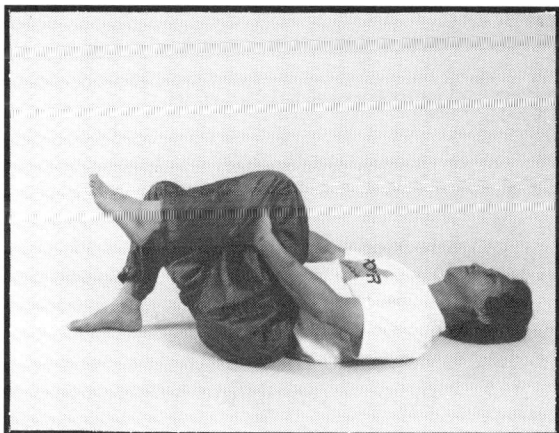

A, B

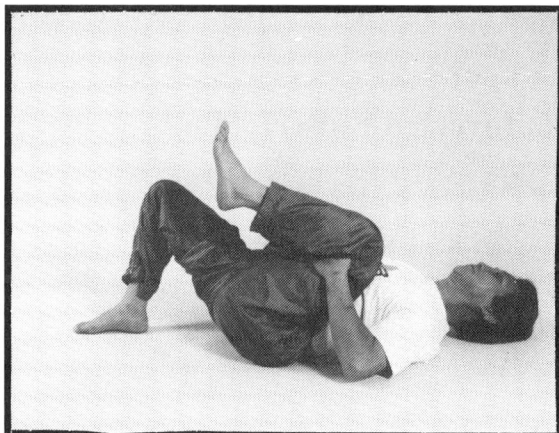

C

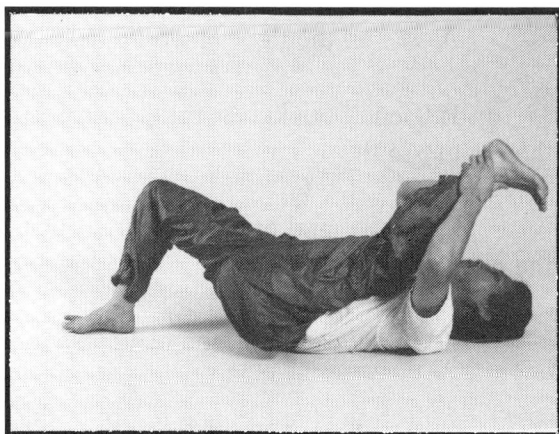

E

287

Benefits:

The single leg pull will:

* loosen and stretch the hamstring and lower back muscles.

* loosen and stretch the hip and lower back joints.

* stimulate the nervous system.

* increase circulation by using gravity to drain blood out of the legs and increase the blood supply to the brain.

* build good body balance by building a strong lower body.

6. Inverted Butterfly Pull

This exercise will loosen up your hip joints, which will and increase the circulation and energy flow to the hip area and extend them downward into the legs.

How to do it:

A. Lie on the floor on your back.

B. Bend both knees, bring your feet together, sole to sole, and bring them close to the groin.

C. Inhale and grab the feet so that each hand grasps the instep in the palm.

D. Exhale and pull the feet close to the belly button (count 1-8).

E. Release the feet and return to the lying position as you inhale.

B, C

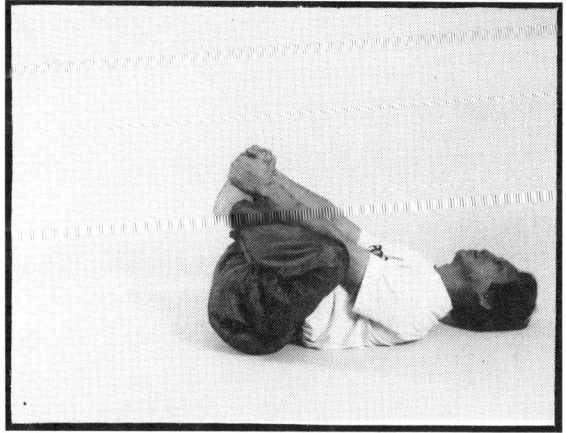

D

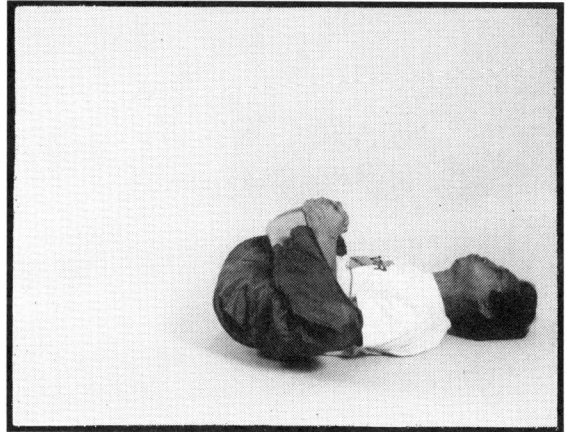

Benefits:

The inverted butterfly will:

* loosen the hip, knee, and lower back.

* loosen the groin muscles.

* stimulate the internal organs, specifically the digestive tract and the bladder.

7. Adjust the spine

This exercise will loosen up and re-align the spine, as well as help regulate the digestive tract.

How to do it:

A. Lie on your back in the shape of a cross, with your legs straight and your arms straight out from your shoulders.

B. Inhale and bend your left knee.

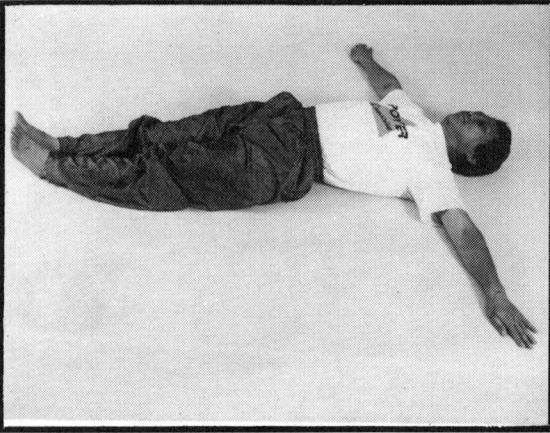

A

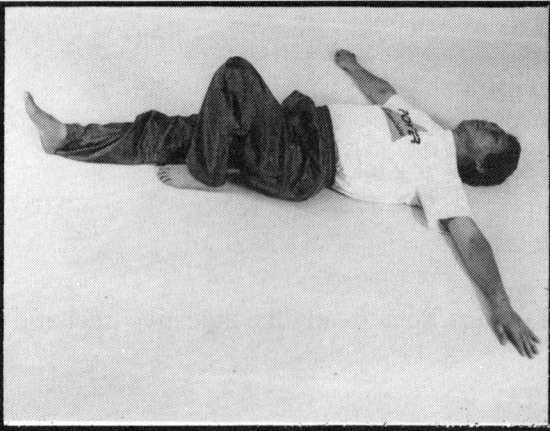

B

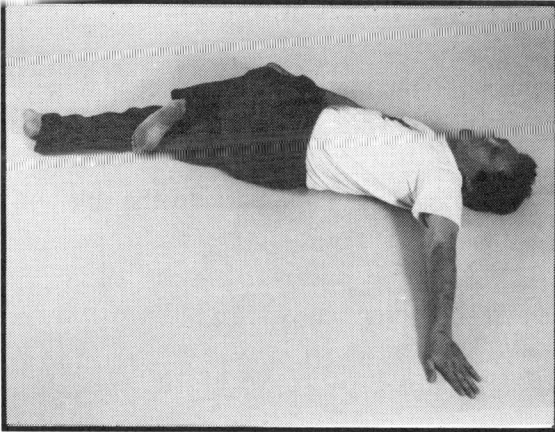

C

C. Exhale and bring your left knee across your right, placing your right hand on your left knee in order to help it reach toward the floor on the right side of your body. Do not let your left shoulder or arm come up off the floor.

D. Inhale and bring your knee back to the upright position as you put your right hand back on the floor.

E. Exhale and straighten out your left knee.

F. Inhale and bend your right knee.

G. Exhale and bring your right knee across your left leg and try to touch it to the floor on the left side of your body.

H. Place your left hand on your right knee and help your knee reach toward the floor. Do not let your right shoulder come up off the floor.

I. Inhale and bring your knee back to the upright position as you put your left hand back on the floor.

J. Exhale and straighten out your right knee.

Benefits:

The adjust the spine exercise will:

* adjust your back bone: loosen and re-align lower back and neck muscles, and then strengthen them in the correct position.

* adjust your internal organs into their proper position, stimulating the liver and kidneys, and controlling constipation and diarrhea.

8. Full Body Stretch

This exercise will loosen up your whole body in preparation for stretching and other exercises. If you are doing only lying down exercises, do this as the first exercise. If you began with standing, seated, or any other exercise, use the full body stretch as the LAST exercise before you stand up.

How to do it:

A. Lie on the floor with your back straight.

B. Interlock your fingers into a finger chain. Turn your palms away from your body and extend your hands over your head.

C. Inhale and stretch yourself as much as possible by reaching the hands over the head and flexing (bending) your ankles.

B

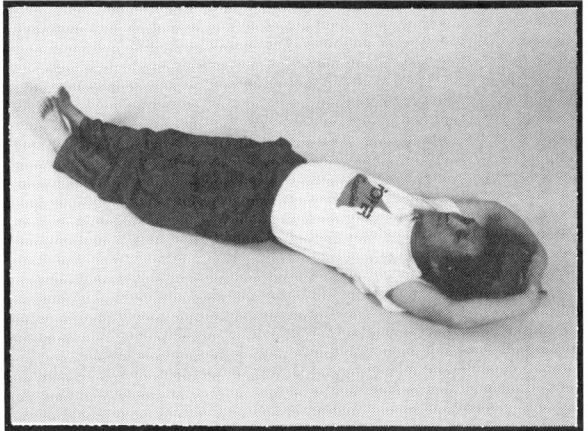

C

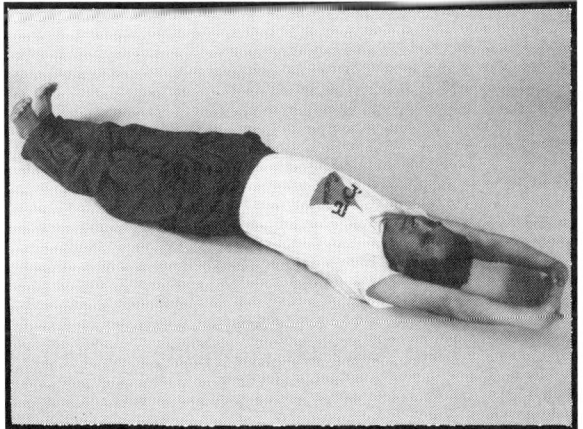

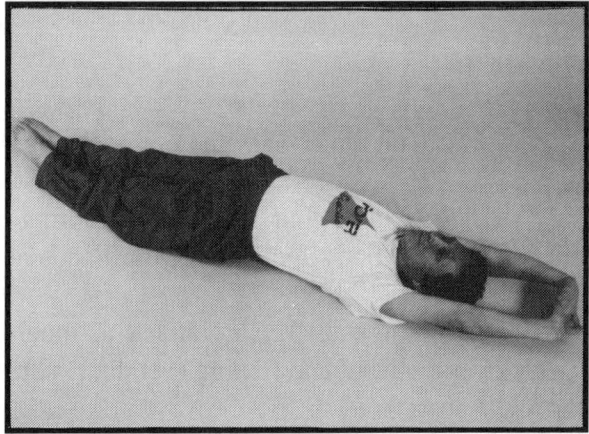

E

D. Exhale, release your fingers, return your arms to your sides, and relax your whole body.

E. Repeat steps A through D, this time extending (straightening) the ankles C.

Benefits:

The full body stretch will:

* loosen and stretch entire body, especially the torso in preparation for further exercise.

* release stress and tension.

* refresh and make comfortable the entire body by stimulating nerves through tensing and relaxing.

* help you sleep better.

* help you wake up when your body doesn't want to wake up.

Caution:

Those with shoulders prone to dislocation should be careful when extending the arms.

At the completion of your Power Exercises it is important to refresh yourself and clear your mind. If this is the end to your exercise session, sit up and perform Concentration, Reflective, or Power Meditation (pp. 166-188).

If you are using Power Exercises as a warm-up to a more strenuous aerobic exercise, stand up and do the body bouncing (#19) and deep breathing (#20) exercises described at the end of the standing Power Exercises (pp. 254-256) before you begin your strenuous exercise.

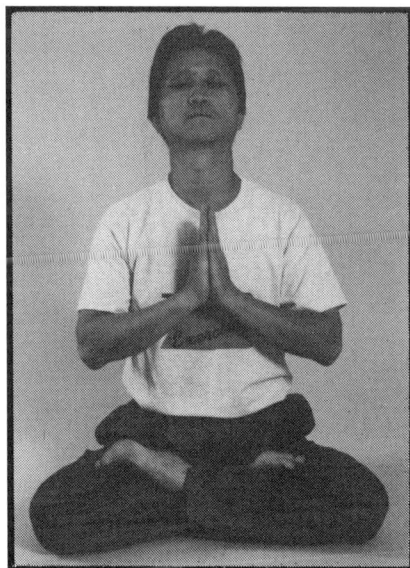

POWER EXERCISES WITH A PARTNER

Exercising with a partner is not only more fun, it can accelerate your results. Sharing any meaningful experience will create a new friendship or deepen an existing friendship. When you have someone to train with, you challenge and motivate each other to improve. In muscle work, whether it is stretching or strengthening, the strength of a training partner will allow you to push farther with a greater margin of safety.

Power Exercises with a Partner

1. Partner Sit-ups
2. Partner Open Leg Stretch
3. Single Leg Stretch
4. Standing Back to Back Stretch
5. Front Leg Stretch
6. Side Leg Stretch
7. Shoulder and Chest Stretch
8. Massage

1. Partner Sit-ups

Regular sit-ups strengthen the abdomen and hip flexor muscles, as well as loosen up the back and hips. Partner sit-ups allow those who are not yet strong enough to do many sit-ups a chance to utilize their partner's strength to help them do more. Partner sit-ups also strengthen the lower back muscles.

How to do it:

A. Sit on the floor facing your partner. Cross your knees over each other (partner X bend knees with feet shoulder width apart; partner Y assume same position and place partner X's knees and upper shins against the back of partner Y's knees) and place your feet one on each side of your partner's hips.

B. Grasp each other by the wrists (Partner X both palms up, partner Y both palms down).

C. Partner X inhale and slowly lean back to touch the floor, while partner Y exhales and leans forward.

A, B

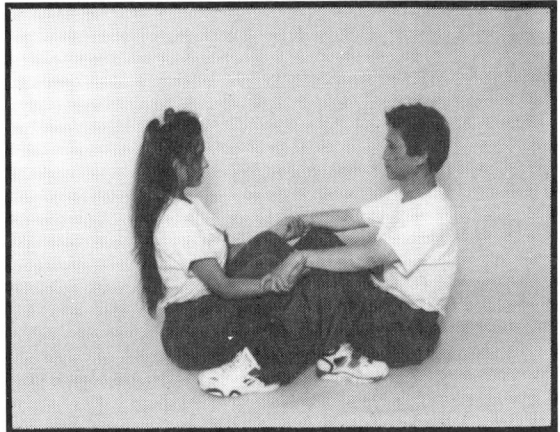

C

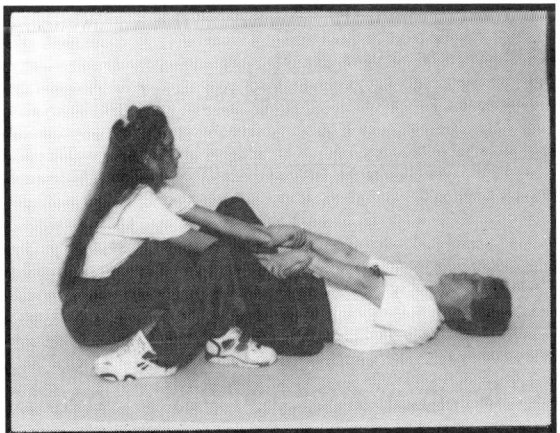

297

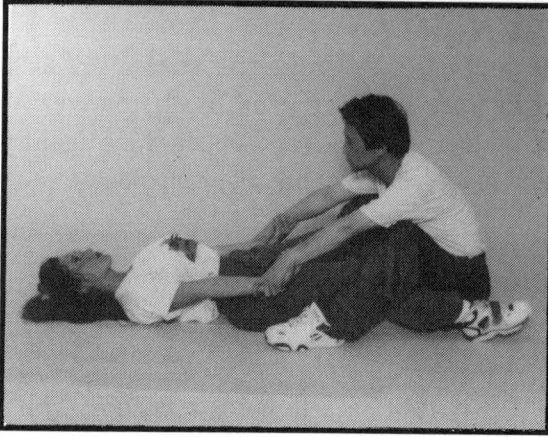

D

D. Partner Y inhale and slowly lean back to touch the floor, while partner X exhales and leans forward.

E. Repeat steps C and D from five to ten times.

Benefits:

Partner sit-ups will

* strengthen lower abdomen, hip flexor, and lower back (*erector spinae*) muscles.

* loosen up hip, lower back, and shoulder muscles.

* massage internal organs.

* relieve stress and tension by removing waste products.

Caution:

The partner who leans back must lean back slowly the first time until he can gauge the flexibility of the other partner.

2. Partner Open Leg Stretch

This exercise will help you stretch your hips, legs, and lower back.

How to do it:

A. Sit on the floor facing each other. If both partners are the same size, place your feet sole to sole. If both partners are not the same size, the shorter or less flexible partner should place the soles of his feet against the inside ankles of the taller/more flexible partner. Both open your legs as far as possible.

B. Both partners inhale and interlock your fingers (place hands palm to palm and move hands slightly left or right so that one's fingers fit between the other's, and grasp.) Inhale.

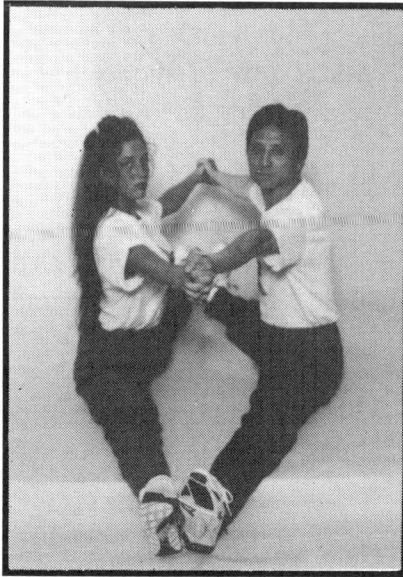

A, B

C. Partner X exhale and lean to the left, laying your left side on your left thigh, extending both your hands toward your left foot, reaching the right arm over the head. Partner Y is mirror reflection of partner X, maintaining interlocked fingers.

D. Inhale and return to position B.

E. Partner X exhale and lean to the right, laying your right side on your right thigh, extending both your hands toward your right foot, reaching the left arm over the head. Partner Y is mirror reflection of partner X, maintaining interlocked fingers.

F. Inhale and return to position B.

G. Partner X exhale and lean to the left, laying your left side on your left thigh, extending your left hand toward your left foot and your right hand directly overhead. Partner Y is mirror reflection of partner X, maintaining interlocked fingers.

H. Inhale and return to position B.

I. Partner X exhale and lean to the right, laying your right side on your right thigh, extending your right hand toward your right foot and your left hand directly overhead toward the ceiling. Partner Y is mirror reflection of partner X, maintaining interlocked fingers.

J. Inhale and return to position B.

K. Partner X inhale and lean back as far as possible, within his own and his partner's limitations. Partner Y exhale and lean forward as far as possible.

L. Partner Y inhale and lean back as far as possible, within his own and his partner's limitations. Partner X exhale and lean forward as far as possible.

M. Inhale and return to center position.

300

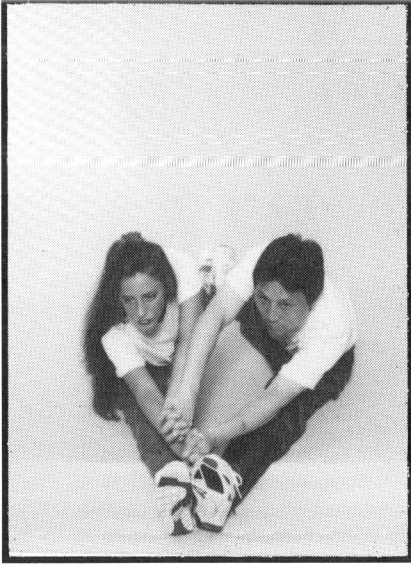

C

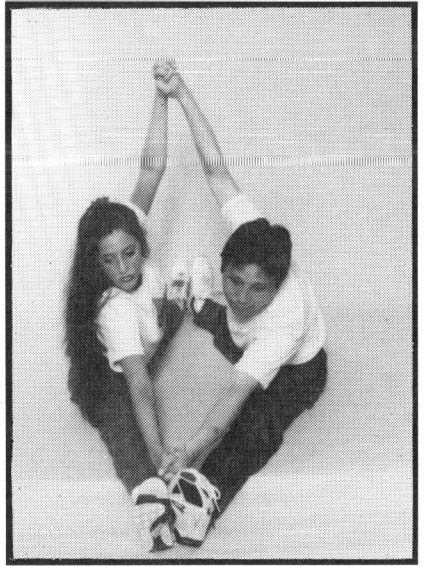

G

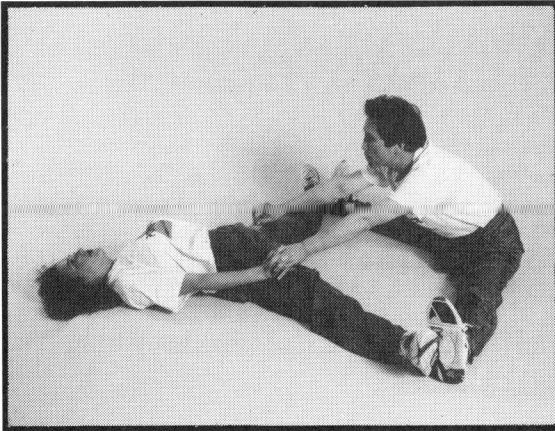

L

Benefits:

Partner open leg stretch will:

* loosen the groin, complete back (including lat.), and shoulder muscles.

* loosen the hip and shoulder joint, and adjust the spine.

* improve the digestion by stimulating and massaging the internal organs.

* release tension and stress.

Caution:

Do not use too much pressure to spread the legs too far. Do not press on the ankles of a person with bad knees. Instead, move the soles of the feet to the inside of the thigh, just above the knee, and spread their legs as far as possible.

3. Single Leg Stretch

This is an intense stretch of the hamstring that can increase flexibility for high kicking.

How to do it:

A. Partner Y lie on your back on the floor, inhale, and lift your right knee straight up toward the ceiling.

B. Partner X step your right foot on Partner Y's lower inside left pant leg. (If your partner is not wearing long pants, you may use your toes to hold his foot down, but do not stand on his leg.

C. Partner X bend Partner Y's right leg and gently push his thigh against his chest as he exhales.

D. Partner X gently pull partner Y's thigh away from his chest as he inhales and straighten his right leg, putting your right hand behind his ankle while keeping your left hand over his knee.

A, B, C

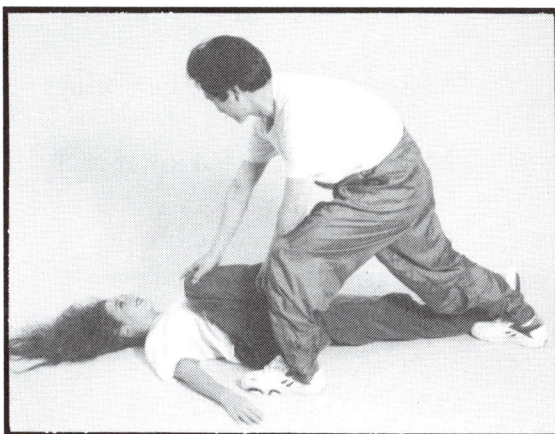

D

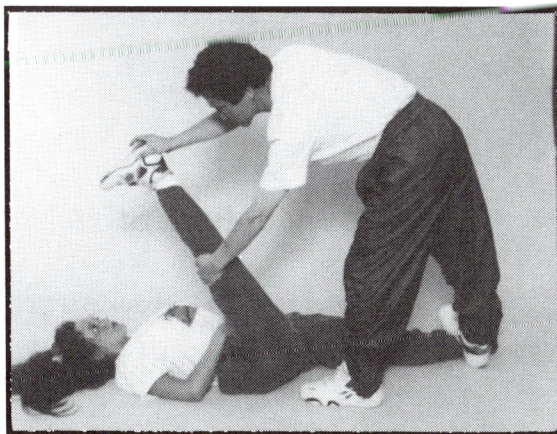

E. Partner X move Partner Y's straightened leg as close to his chest as possible, trying to direct his foot over his right shoulder and slightly to the outside.

F. Partner X release Partner Y's leg and allow it to return to the floor as he inhales.

G. Repeat steps A through F for partner Y's left leg.

H. Repeat steps A through G for partner X's right and left legs.

Benefits:

The single leg stretch will:

* intensely stretch the hamstrings.

* loosen the hips and lower back.

* wash the blood out of legs and improve the circulation to the whole body, especially the head.

Caution:

Do not push too hard or too far. Do not over-extend the knee while trying to keep it straight.

4. Standing Back to Back Stretch

The standing back to back stretch will continue to loosen your back, sides, and shoulders.

How to do it:

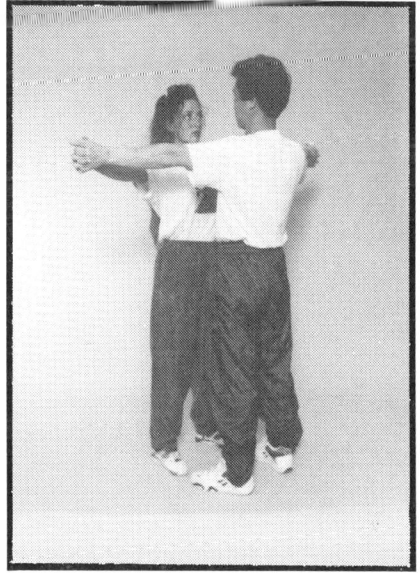

A

A. Stand facing each other. Both partners inhale and interlock your fingers as in open leg stretching (place hands palm to palm and move hands slightly left or right so that one's fingers fit between the other's, and grasp.)

B. Remain interlocked, and move both hands to one side. Continue to twirl around until you end up back to back.

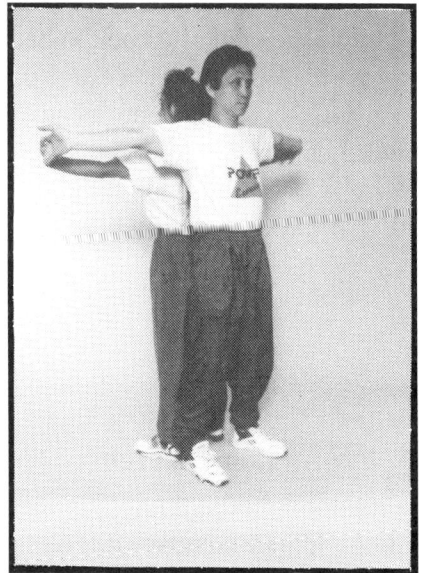

B

305

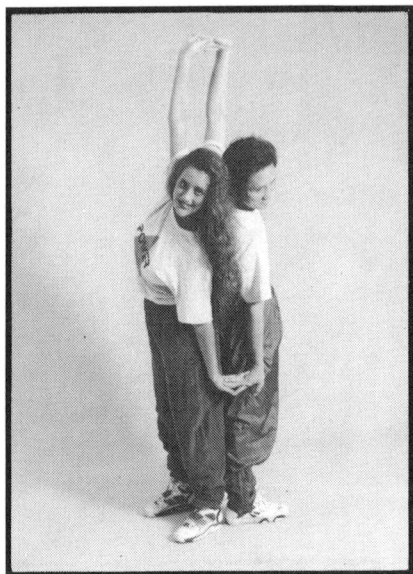

C. Extend interlocked hands straight out from the shoulders and lean to partner X's right side.

D. Lean to partner Y's right side.

E. Return to upright.

F. Release your fingers and relax.

C

Benefits:

The standing back to back stretch will:

* loosen the entire back (including *lat.*) and shoulders, and adjust the spine.

* relieve stomach ache and improve digestion.

5. Front Leg Stretch

This exercise allows you to develop balance while gaining flexibility, which will help develop higher and stronger kicks for the martial arts or dancing.

How to do it·

A. Partner Y stand in left front stance (feet shoulder width apart, front leg bent and back leg straight.)

B. Partner X inhale and lift your right leg and place your Achilles tendon on partner Y's shoulder, and grab his shoulders for balance and support.

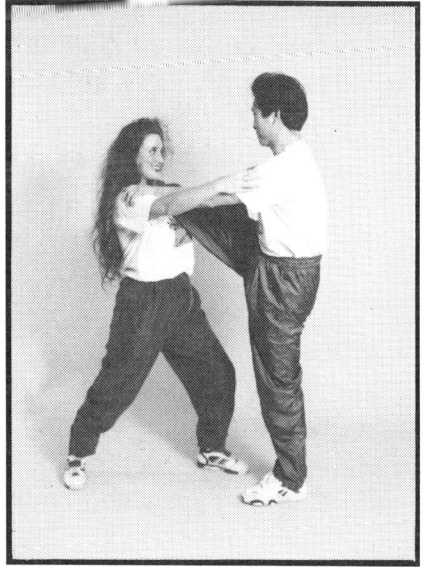

A, B

C. Partner X exhale slowly as partner Y places his right hand over your knee to keep it from bending; partner Y slowly stand up higher and higher to stretch partner X's right hamstring.

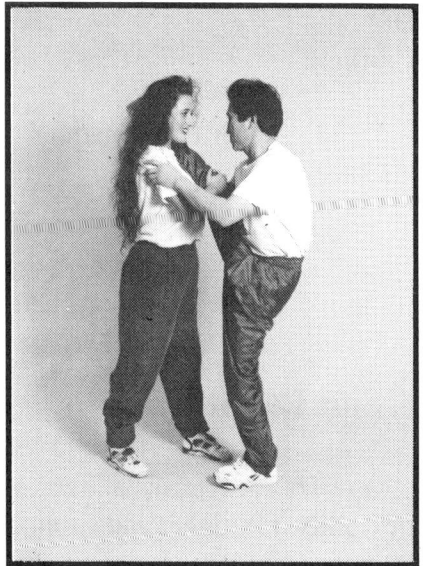

C

307

D. Partner Y lower himself until partner X can lower his leg safely.

E. Repeat steps A through D changing stance and legs so that you stretch partner X's left hamstring.

F. Exchange roles and repeat steps A through E stretching partner Y's legs.

Benefits:

The front leg stretch will:

* intensely stretch your hamstrings for high kicking.

* develop your balance and strengthen your legs.

* increase blood circulation throughout body.

Caution:

Do not lift your partner's leg too high or put too much pressure on his knee.

6. Side Leg Stretch

This exercise allows you to develop balance while gaining flexibility, for higher and stronger kicks to the side (rather than to the front as in the front leg stretch).

How to do it:

A. Partner Y stand in left front stance, as in #5 (feet shoulder width apart, front leg bent and back leg straight.)

B. Partner X inhale and lift your right leg and place the inside of your right ankle on partner Y's shoulder, wrapping your foot around the back of his neck, and grabbing his hands for balance and support.

C. Partner X exhale as partner Y slowly stands up higher and higher to stretch your groin muscles.

D. Partner Y lower himself until partner X can lower his leg safely.

E. Repeat steps A through D changing stance and legs so that you stretch partner X's left leg.

F. Exchange roles and repeat steps A through E stretching partner Y's legs.

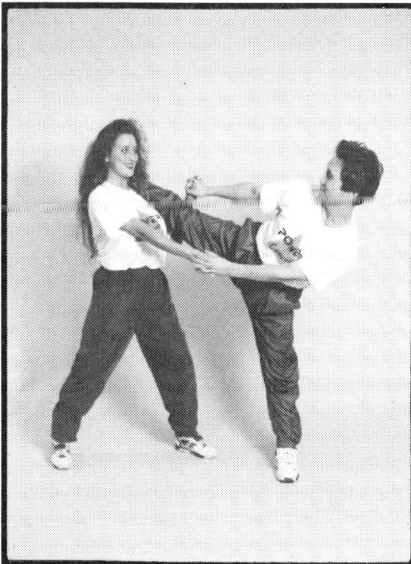

A, B

Benefits:

The side leg stretch will:

* intensely stretch your groin muscles for high side kicking.

* develop your balance and strengthen your legs.

* increase the blood circulation in your lower body.

Caution:

Do not lift your partner's leg too high or put too much pressure on his knee.

7. Shoulder and Chest Stretch

This exercise will help you stretch your shoulder and chest muscles.

How to do it:

A. Partner Y turn away from Partner X. Partner X face partner Y's back.

B. Partner X grab partner Y's wrists and gently pull his arms behind his back, with his palms facing each other. Try to cross the arms over each other.

C. Open the arms a little and stretch again, this time switching the top and bottom arm.

D. Gently release partner Y's arms and wrists.

E. Both partners turn around and repeat B through D with Partner Y stretching Partner X's shoulders and chest.

Benefits:

The shoulder and chest stretch will:

* loosen and stretch your shoulders and chest muscles much more intensely than you could by yourself.

* release emotional stress and tension stored in the chest area.

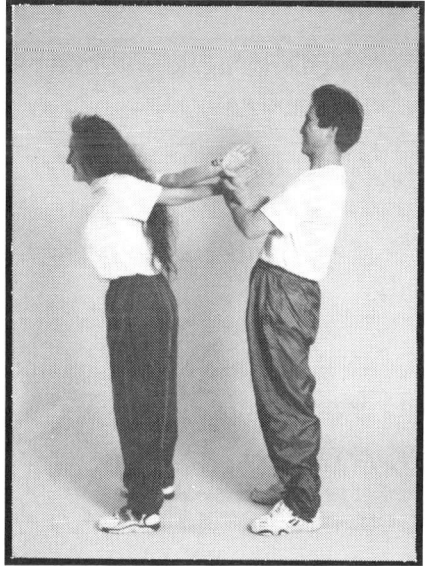

A, B

Caution:

Those prone to shoulder dislocation and other shoulder problems should be very careful.

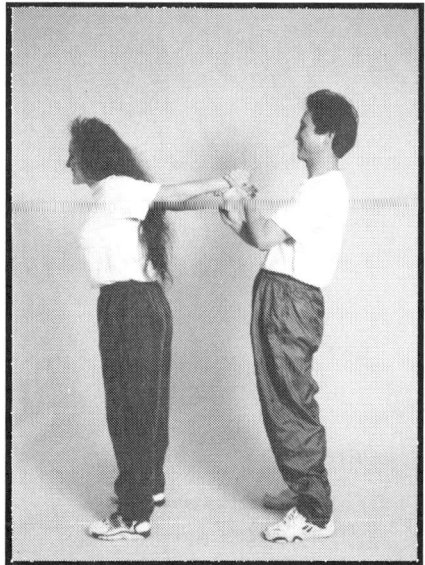

C

8. Massage

This massage will bring the blood to the surface, and you will feel refreshed and enlivened.

How to do it:

A. Partner Y turn away from partner X. Partner X face partner Y's back.

B. Partner X massage the muscles of partner Y's neck, shoulders, and back with the fingers, as if kneading bread.

C. Partner X cup your hands and pat partner Y's shoulders, neck, back, sides, legs, and arms.

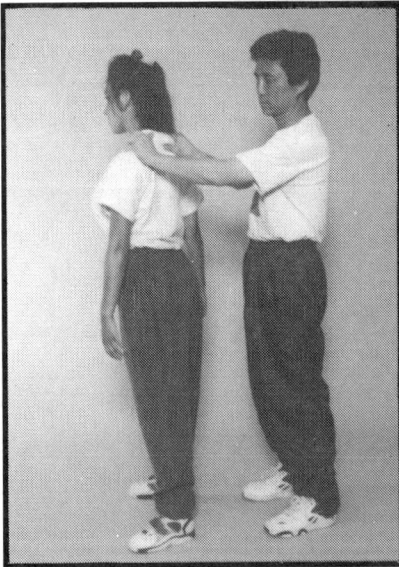

B (knead)

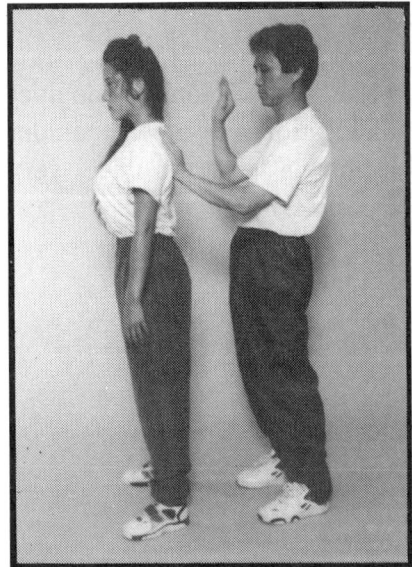

C (pat)

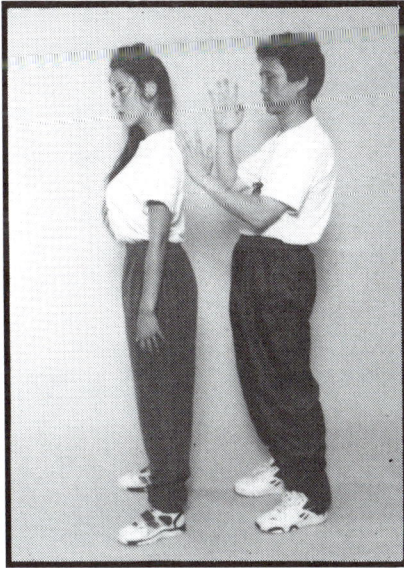

D (chop)

D. Partner X open spaces between the fingers of each hand and use the fingers to "chop" the muscles of partner Y's neck, shoulders, and back, striking lightly with the pinkies, not with the edge of the hand.

E. Both turn around so that partner Y can massage partner X.

Benefits:

This massage will:

* increase circulation to the surface of the body.

Caution:

Be gentle whenever massaging. Pat your partner, do not pound on him.

At the end of the Power Exercise session with your partner, motivate each other to feel good: smile, laugh, admire each other and tell each other good things.

If you are going to finish your Power Exercises here, do the deep breathing exercise (#1) in the standing Power Exercises (pp. 207-210) and perform standing Concentration, Reflective, or Power Meditation (pp. 166-188). If you are going to continue to exercise, meditate at the end of your complete workout.

Aerobic Self-Defense

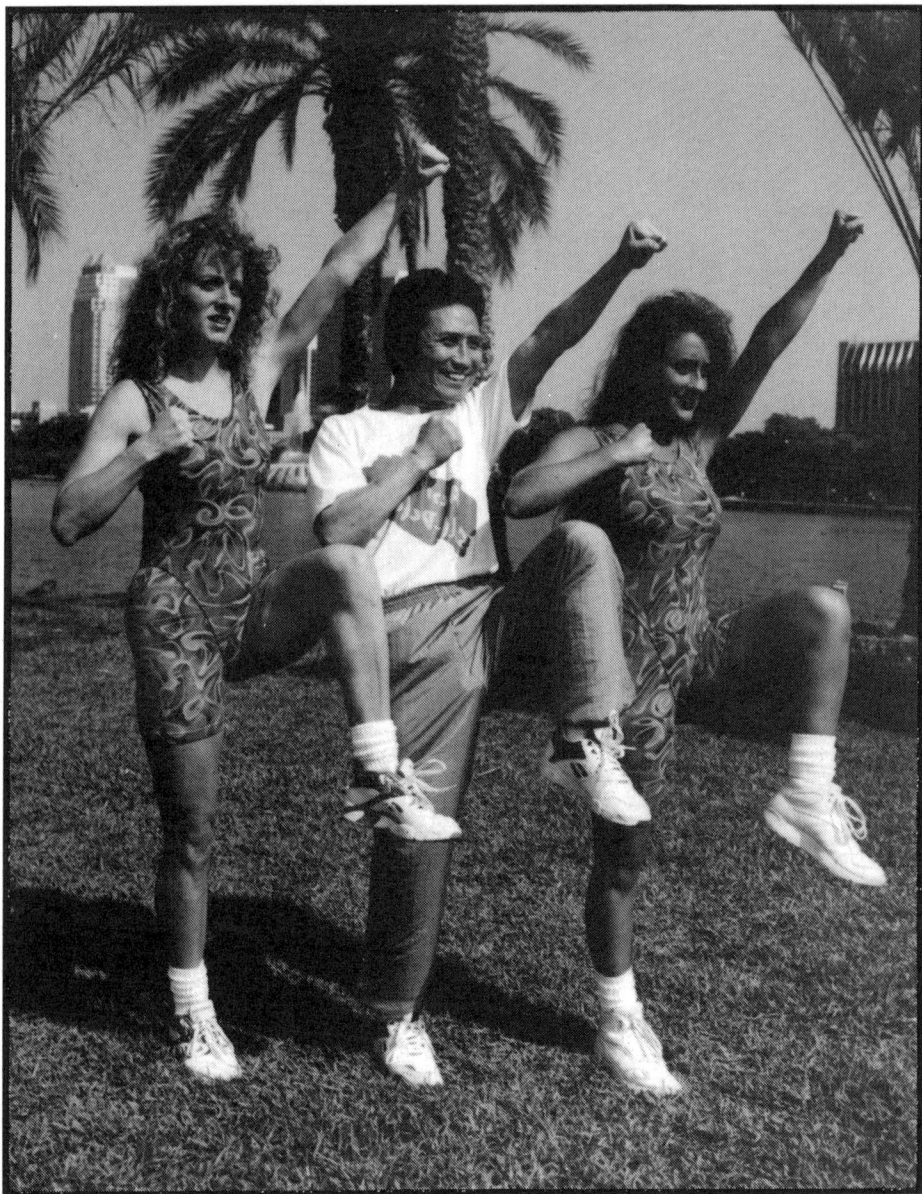

"The best self-defense is positive thinking, which is self- confidence."

What is Aerobic Self-Defense?

Aerobic self-defense is a combination of an aerobic workout and practical self-defense training. The purpose is to learn self-defense and get In shape at the same time, while building self-esteem and peace of mind.

What is an aerobic workout?

There are two kinds of exercise: aerobic and anaerobic. Loosely translated, these words mean "with air" and "without air." An anaerobic exercise is very strenuous, and your muscle cannot do it very long before it runs out of air. For example, push ups are anaerobic: you can do ten, twenty, maybe fifty or more, but then your muscle will reach the point where it does not have enough oxygen to power its movement. It reaches fatigue, and cannot do another push-up. After a brief rest the oxygen can be restored, and you can do more push-ups.

Aerobic exercises are ones that can be performed at a pace in which the body can replace the oxygen used in this movement. Jogging or dancing are examples of aerobic exercise: you can jog or dance for thirty minutes or even an hour or more without your muscle reaching fatigue. The more aerobic exercise you do, the better your body will be able to replace the oxygen, and the better you will be "in shape". For example, the first time you jog, you may only be able to go a half mile or so before you feel you have to stop. Within a week you should be able to go a mile, and soon two miles, etc. This is the training effect. Your body becomes better able to replace the oxygen, and you can continue to work aerobically for longer periods.

Through research, exercise physiologists have come up with a formula to determine whether or not you are getting the "training effect." It is not 100% accurate, but is useful for the average person. It is based on heart rate over time. If you can maintain your target heart rate for twenty minutes (some authorities say thirteen minutes is sufficient, but twenty minutes is a more widely accepted norm), you will increase your ability to use oxygen and burn fat. The target heart rate can be found by taking 60%

to 80% of your maximum heart rate, which is 220 minus your age. To make this more clear, here is a sample formula for a 30 year old man or woman:

220
-30   age
190   maximum heart rate for 30 year old.

190 (max. heart rate)   190 (max. heart rate)
x.60 (60%)   x.80 (80%)
114   152

A 30 year old man or woman should keep his/her heart rate between 114 and 152 beats per minute for twenty minutes to improve oxygen utilization and burn fat -- to get in better condition.

You can measure your heart rate by finding your pulse with your first two fingers (don't use the thumb because it has a pulse of its own) either on the wrist or on the side of the neck. Once you find your pulse, you want to know how many times your heart beats in a minute. You can

A. count heartbeats for a whole minute.

B. count heartbeats for 10 seconds and multiply by 6.

C. count heartbeats for 6 seconds and multiply by 10.

Option C is the easiest; option A is the most accurate. For training effect purposes you don't need complete accuracy, and you probably want convenience, so I recommend C.

To find your own training heart rate just substitute your age for the 30 in the above equations, and do the math.

What is self-defense?

Self-defense is the ability to defend or protect yourself from a negative, evil, or violent attacker.

What is the best self-defense?

Self-confidence. You do not have to become a technical expert to defend yourself. If you want to defend yourself, you can defend yourself beginning today. If you really do not want to defend yourself, no amount of training will enable you to do it.

Many people do not realize that prevention is better than cure when it comes to self-defense, too. What I mean is that the best self-defense is never to get into trouble . . . then you never have to get out of trouble.

The true best self-defense is:

1. Do not ask for trouble:

　　　- do not go to "bad" places where trouble is likely to occur.
　　　- do not associate with people who are negative or bad.

2. When trouble comes to you, if you have a choice, try to walk away or talk your way out of it.

3. Smile. A smile is one of the best weapons for self defense. Remember: nobody likes to see an ugly face. A smile brings an open mind and breaks a cold mind.

When do you really have to defend and protect yourself?

Only fight an attacker if he threatens your life, your family, or presents an evil to your town or nation.

Let's talk about an individual situation: it should only be necessary to use the physical aspect of self-defense if someone threatens your life or your family. How? You have to use your strong points against your opponent's weak points. Everybody has strong points -- arms, legs, brains -- and everybody has weak points -- groin, neck, brains. Even if you punch someone in the shoulder (a strong point) a million times, you will not kill him. You may destroy the shoulder muscle. You may even break the bone, but it will take too long to defend yourself this way. Sometime before you got the first ten punches off, he will have gotten you back.

However, if you use the same strong point in your fist and punch to his throat (a weak point), in one second you can walk away from the attacker. The same would be true if you were to kick with the ball of the foot (strong point) into the groin (weak point) of the attacker. Try this little exercise: bend the second knuckle of each finger on your strong hand to make a bear paw (see page 338 for a picture). Now tap those knuckles against the bottom part of your throat (between the collar bone and the Adam's apple). Can you feel how vulnerable that place is? It is a weak point for everybody, no matter how big or strong. Just remember to use your strong point (these knuckles) against your opponent's weak point (the throat), and you will be able to defend yourself, but only if you believe you can.

Your whole body and mind are weapons for self-defense, but the body and mind must work together. Without believing in yourself, which is self-confidence, even basic physical self-defense techniques will not work. If your mind gets out of control with fear or depression, your own mind becomes a weapon against you. You must control your own fear and depression with self-confidence.

How can you build the self-confidence to defend and protect yourself?

In order to build the self-confidence to protect yourself physically, you have to understand life self-defense. Life self-defense involves many aspects:

1. Health Self-Defense

You have to protect your health from so many new, modern sicknesses and diseases, which is health self-defense. If you do not, you will become weak, sick, and die. Health self-defense is building your immune system to act like security guards for your body. When you build your health from the inside out, it is much more permanent. Even when germs or viruses attack you, your immune system will kick and punch them out of your body. You will keep a healthy and strong body so you can maintain self-confidence and be able to defend yourself from violent attack if it becomes necessary.

2. Relationship Self-Defense

You have to protect your relationships from the things that threaten them like jealousy, and negative or nasty attitudes. Relationships like husband/wife, boyfriend/girlfriend, boss/employee, teacher/student, parent/child, brother/sister, friend/friend, and co-worker/co-worker are important for happiness, so you must learn relationship self-defense or social self-defense. If you do not, you will lose your relationships, have emotional trouble, and be alone.

In order to learn relationship self-defense or social self-defense, you must learn to compete only with yourself. If you compete with others, you will cause more trouble than you solve. Second, you must learn the value of sacrifice. You must know the right time to yield to someone else, and the right time to stand firm. Knowing how and when to sacrifice will help you create strong relationships.

3. Financial Self-Defense

You have to protect your business or your job from lots of competition, bad economic times, and being fired, which is financial self-defense. If you do not defend yourself financially, you can lose your business, job, or money, and have no way to pay for your food, shelter, car, or anything else. You will become a street bum.

I think now you can understand that violent self-defense is just part of true self-defense. No matter what the circumstance, you must control yourself by showing self-confidence. If you cannot control yourself (lack of self-confidence), you cannot control others, and you will never defend yourself.

Another thing to consider in life self-defense is that if you face many enemies, it is very difficult to win. If you could limit the number of enemies you face to one, you would have a much better chance of winning. When you learn to compete with yourself and no one else, you can limit your enemies to only one. That way you can become a true winner in your life. When you compete with others, you become a loser.

319

What do I mean by competing with others? A person who blames others for things that are his own fault competes with others, because he is trying to be better than they are. When he tries to be better than someone else he becomes jealous, hesitates, has a negative or violent mind, and talks bad about other people. He focuses on them and not on himself. Someone who competes with himself only focuses on himself and his own performance. When he tries to become better today than he was yesterday, he becomes positive, cooperative, responsible, and self-disciplined.

Let's look at an example: thirteen to sixteen year old girls have the highest suicide rate in the U.S.A. today. I believe this is true because they compete with others. If they have a friend who has more beautiful clothes, a popular boyfriend, clearer skin, or a new car, they do not feel happy for themselves or their friend. Instead, they concentrate on the negative (what they don't have themselves) and get depressed. They compete with their friends on a superficial level that has nothing to do with their real value. If these girls would just discipline themselves to concentrate on the good things they do have and to compete only with themselves, they could be much happier.

In order not to compete with others, we must realize that every human being has strong points and weak points. If we think about our weak points, we will become depressed. If we think about our strong points, we start to become proud of ourselves. That pride makes us love, trust, and respect ourselves, and lets us believe in ourselves.

The 21st Century will be a very competitive world. It will be like a war for survival. In order not just to survive but to become successful, you will need to build up a great deal of self-confidence. Self-confidence begins by believing in yourself. When you believe in yourself, you are not afraid to compete with yourself to become a winner in life. Then you can defend and protect yourself, release all your fear and depression, and enjoy your life. You can become an expert in life self-defense, and truly happy.

Aerobic Self-Defense Outline

Warm-up:

    7 minutes of standing Power Exercises

Aerobics:

Exercise	Attack (Response)
March	2 sets 8 count

1. Make a Fist

Ready Stance		Grab (Claw Face)
Front		Headlock (Claw Groin)
	Low palm up	alt L&R 8 counts
	High palm down	alt L&R 8 cts.
Side		
	Low palm up	alt L&R 8 cts.
	High palm down	alt L&R 8 cts.

    Repeat

2. Outside Wrist Escape   Same Side Wrist Grab
                                      (Escape)

Ready Stance		
Side		Punch (Outside Block)
	Low	alt L&R 8 cts.
	High	alt L&R 8 cts.
Front		
	Low	alt L&R 8 cts.
	High	alt L&R 8 cts.

    Repeat

3. Clap   Front Bear Hug (Clap Ears)

      Ready Stance
      Close, Far
            Diagonal   alt L&R 2 x 8 cts.
            Straight   alt L&R 2 x 8 cts.

   Repeat

4. Inside Wrist Escape   Opposite Wrist Grab (Escape)
      Ready Stance   Two Hand Wrist Grab (Escape)
      Side
            Low   alt L&R 8 cts.
            High   alt L&R 8 cts.
      Front
            Low   alt L&R 8 cts.
            High   alt L&R 8 cts.

   Repeat

5. Bear Paw   Grab Shoulder (Bear Paw)
      Ready Stance
            Diagonal   alt L&R 2 x 8 cts.
            Front   alt L&R 2 x 8 cts.

   Repeat

6. High Block   Overhead Club (Block)
      Ready Stance
            Side   alt L&R 2 x 8 cts.
            Front   alt L&R 2 x 8 cts.

   Repeat

7. Punch   Grab from Side (Punch)
    Ready Stance
        Side   alt L&R 2 x 8 cts.
        Front   alt L&R 2 x 8 cts.

    Repeat

8. Inside Block   Lapel Grab (Escape)
    Ready Stance   Punch (Block)
        Side   alt L&R 2 x 8 cts.
        Front   alt L&R 2 x 8 cts.

    Repeat

9. Elbow to Chin   Two Hand Wrist Grab (Escape)
    Ready Stance
        Front   alt L&R 4 x 8 cts.

10. Knee Kick   Front Bear Hug (Knee Groin)
    Ready Stance   (Grab Head and Smash Face)
        Groin (1 hand slap)   alt L&R 2 x 8 cts.
        Face (2 hand slap)   alt L&R 2 x 8 cts.

    Repeat

11. Finger Up and Turn   Double Lapel Grab (Escape)
    Ready Stance
        up, step across   alt L&R 4 x 8 cts.

March (HEART RATE CHECK)   2 x 8 cts.

12. Front Kick   Choke from Front (Kick)
    Ready Stance
        Low   alt L&R 2 x 8 cts.
        Middle   alt L&R 2 x 8 cts.

Repeat (middle may become high)

13. Palm Up Strike   Hair Grab (Escape)
    Ready Stance
        Diagonal   alt L&R 2 x 8 cts.
        Front   alt L&R 2 x 8 cts.

Repeat

14. Side Kick   Purse Snatch (Shin Kick)
    Ready Stance   Shoulder Grab (Middle Kick)
        Low   alt L&R 2 x 8 cts.
        Middle   alt L&R 2 x 8 cts.

Repeat

15. Elbow Up and Back Turn   Back Shoulder Grab (Escape)
    Ready Stance
        Back Step   alt L&R 4 x 8 cts.

16. Back Kick   Back Shoulder Grab (Kick)
    Ready Stance
        Low   alt L&R 2 x 8 cts.
        Middle   alt L&R 2 x 8 cts.

Repeat

17. Double Arm Wrist Escape   Two Hand Wrist Grab (Escape)
       Ready Stance
            Front (out and in)   alt O&I 4 x 8 cts.

18. Pushing Kick   Shoulder Grab (Kick)
       Ready Stance
            Middle   alt L&R 4 x 8 cts.

19. Claw Groin, Elbow   Arm Choke (Strike)
       Ready Stance
            Claw Groin,
            High Elbow Strike   alt L&R 4 x 8 cts.

March   2 x 8 cts.

20. Multiple Kick   Gang Attack (Kick)
       Ready Stance
            F, F, S, S, B, B, S, S
            Low   alt L&R 2 x 8 cts.
            Middle   alt L&R 2 x 8 cts.

   Repeat

March   2 x 8 cts.

21. Multiple Punch   Two Man Attack (Punch)
       Ready Stance
            L, M, MH, H
            Diag. L   alt L&R 1 x 8 cts.
            Diag. R   alt L&R 1 x 8 cts.
            Front   alt L&R 1 x 8 cts.
         Repeat
         Front
            Double Time   alt L&R 2 x 8 cts.

March   2 x 8 cts.

| 22. Two Knife-Hand Strike | Double Lapel (Escape/Strike) |
| Ready Stance | 4 x 8 cts. |

23. Claw Groin and Double Arm Up	Bear Hug Behind (Strike/Escape)
Attention Stance	
Sidestep	alt L&R 2 x 8 cts.
Sidestep and	
Elbows up	alt L&R 4 x 8 cts.

24. Elbow Strike	Continue from # 23
Ready Stance	
Mid & High	alt L&R 4 x 8 cts.

25. Low Block	Front Kick (Block)
Ready Stance	
Side Step	alt L&R 2 X 8 cts.
Sidestep and	
Down Block	alt L&R 2 x 8 cts.
Front	alt L&R 2 x 8 cts.

26. Stomp	Bear Hug Behind (Stomp)
Ready Stance	
Heel	alt L&R 1 x 8 cts.
Blade	alt L&R 1 x 8 cts.

Repeat

| March | 2 x 8 cts. |

| 27. Side Step and Shake | 2 x 8 cts. |

| 28. Deep Breathing | up, low |

WARM-UP:

Seven minutes of standing Power Exercises (see pp. 206-256).

AEROBICS:

March

The march is a way for you to get your body moving in rhythm with the music.

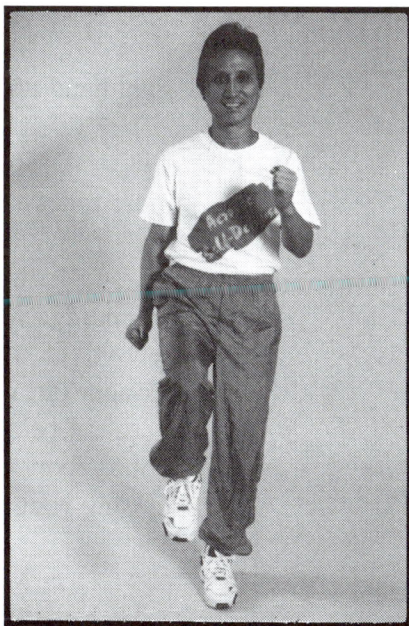

March

327

1. Make a Fist

The grasping action may be used to make your hand into a fist. The fist is the most basic weapon in self-defense. First of all, it protects the fingers from being broken. Second, it creates a hard and well supported striking surface. Third, and most important for health self-defense, is that each of the fingers is connected to one of the five major hollow organs. When we move the fingers, we stimulate the organs to make them healthier.

Grasping can be used as a self-defense move when you claw the face of an attacker, or claw the groin.

How to do it:

A. Stand with your legs shoulder width apart and your knees bent (ready stance).

B. Make a fist with your left hand by extending your left arm in front of your body with the palm up and pulling your elbow straight back while closing your hand into a fist.

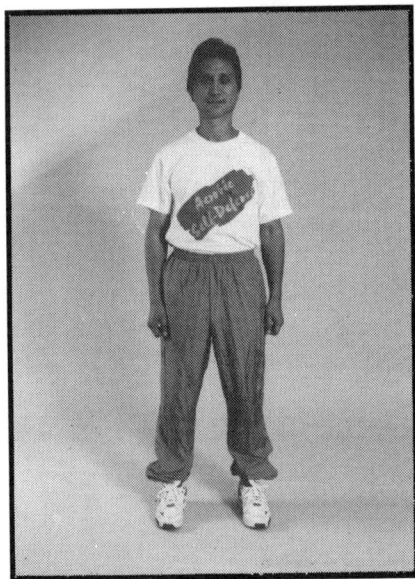

A

C. Make a fist with your right hand with the same action.

D. Repeat B and C three more times.

E. Make a fist high by extending your left arm at a forty-five degree angle up, straight out in front of your face with the palm down, and pulling your elbow straight back while closing your hand into a fist.

F. Make a fist high with your right hand with the same action.

328

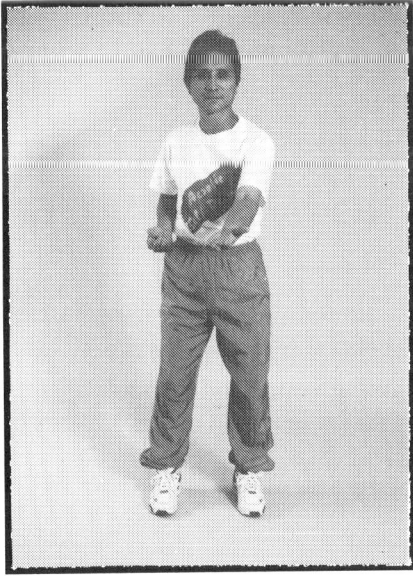

B

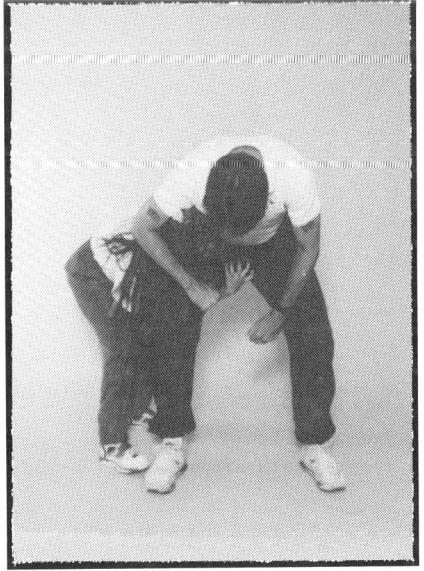

B application

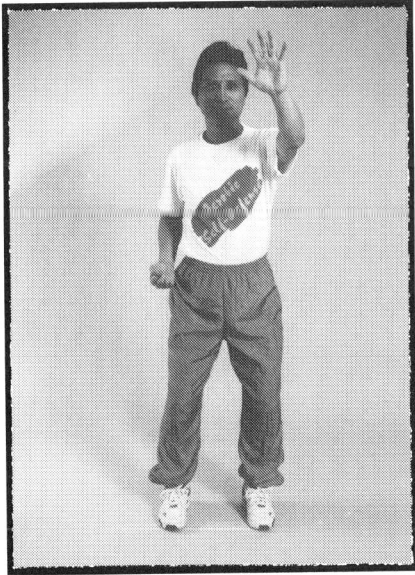

E

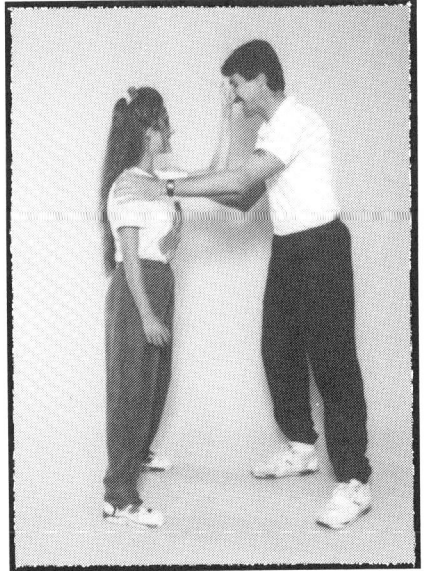

E application

G. Repeat E and F three more times.

H. Make a fist to the side by extending your left arm to the side of your body at rib height with the palm up and pulling your hand to your shoulder while closing your hand into a fist.

I. Make a fist to the other side.

J. Repeat H and I three more times.

K. Make a fist high to the side by extending your left arm at a forty-five degree angle up and directly to the side with the palm down, and pulling your hand to your shoulder while closing your hand into a fist.

L. Make a fist high to the other side.

M. Repeat K and L three more times.

N. Repeat B through M once again.

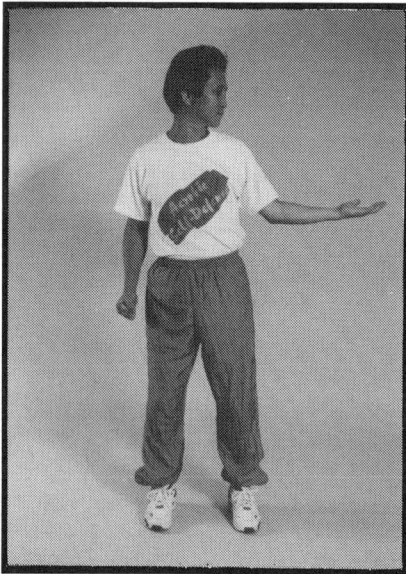

H

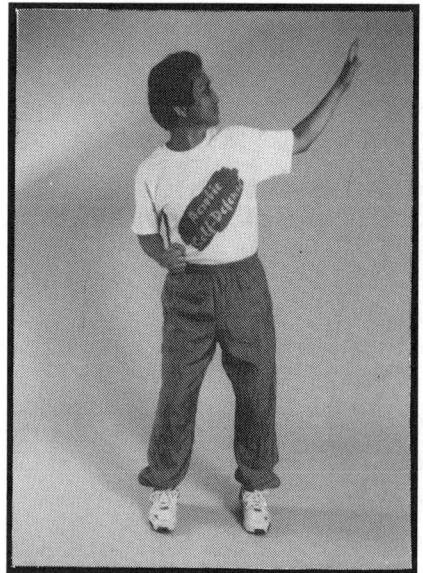

K

2. Outside Wrist Escape

The simplest escape is from the simplest grab: a hand grab to the wrist. The structure of the human hand gives it considerably more strength in the four fingers than in the thumb. If you try to escape by pulling your wrist straight back, you will not get away from a stronger attacker. If you turn your wrist into his four fingers, he will probably have the strength to hold on. If you turn your wrist against his thumb, your wrist is going to be stronger than his thumb, and you will escape.

This escape works when an attacker grabs you with the hand on the same side (his right grabs your left as he faces you.) The same motion when done above the shoulder would be an outside block, which could be used to block a punch.

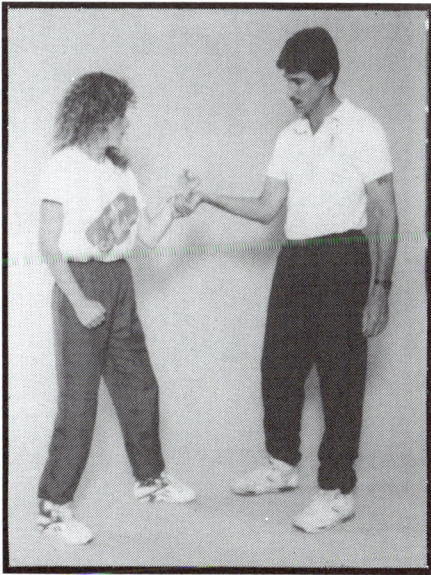

Escape (B)

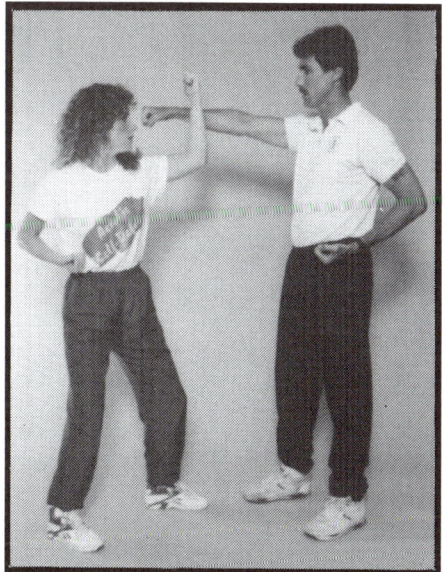

Block (E)

How to do it:

A. Maintain ready stance (stand with your legs shoulder width apart and your knees bent). Make a fist with both hands.

B. Perform a left outside wrist escape to the side by turning ninety degrees to the left and extending your left hand in front of your left hip. Circle your left hand upward and outward in a counter-clockwise semi-circle.

C. Perform a right outside wrist escape by turning one hundred and eighty degrees to the right and extend your right hand in front of your right hip. Circle your right hand upward and outward in a clockwise semi-circle.

D. Repeat B and C three more times.

E. Perform a high outside wrist escape to the side (arm at shoulder level) four times to each side.

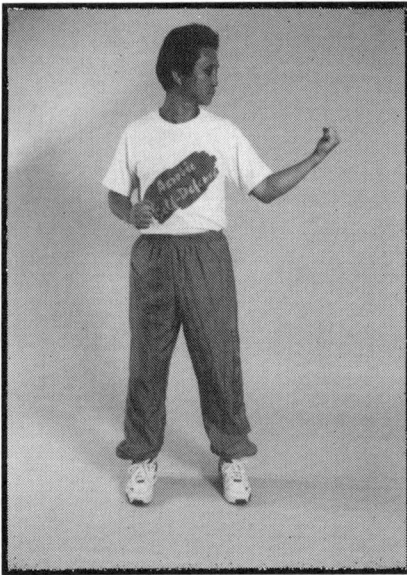

B

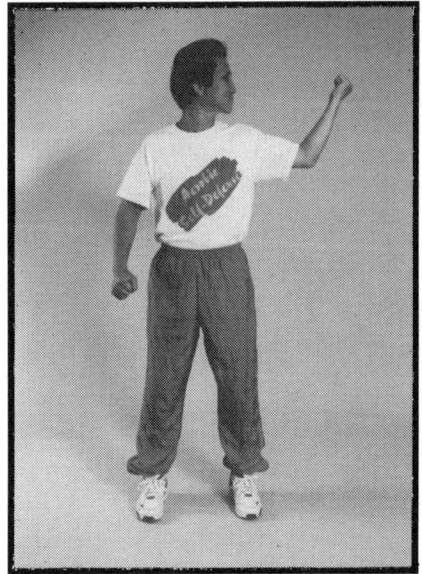

E

F. Perform an outside wrist escape to the front (extending hand at hip level) four times with each hand.

G. Perform a high outside wrist escape to the front four times with each hand.

I. Repeat B through G once again.

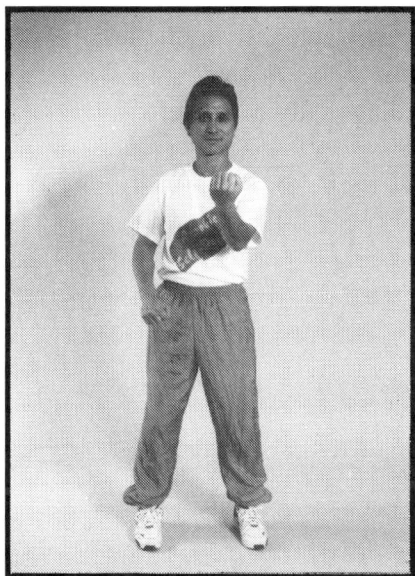

F

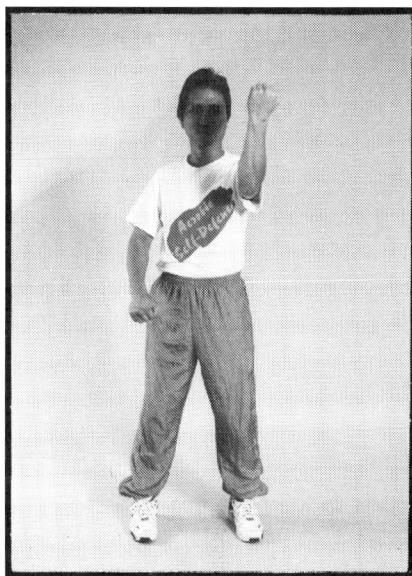

G

3. Clap

Most people clap during aerobics for fun. Few realize it has a self-defense application. If you cup your hands slightly so that they can hold a little more air, and clap your hands against the ears of an attacker, the hands will force air into his ear canal with enough pressure to burst his ear drums. This will not only affect his hearing, it will hurt him badly enough to encourage him to let you go, and affect his center of balance so that he will not be chasing you.

How to do it:

A. Maintain ready stance (stand with your legs shoulder width apart and your knees bent).

B. Clap your hands close to your chest, diagonally to the left.

C. Clap your hands fully extended, diagonally to the left.

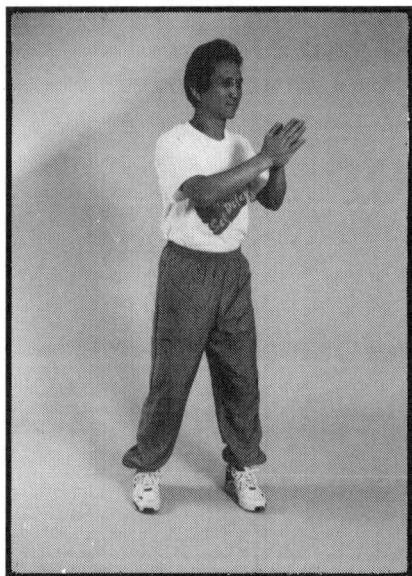

B

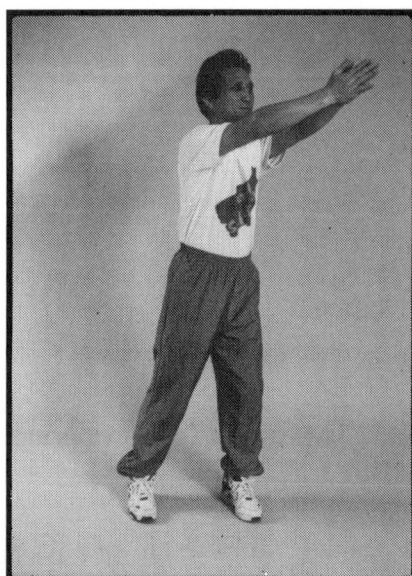

C

D. Clap your hands close to your chest, diagonally to the right

E. Clap your hands fully extended, diagonally to the right.

F. Repeat B through E three more times.

G. Clap your hands close to your chest, directly in front of you.

H. Clap your hands fully extended, directly in front of you.

I. Repeat G and H three more times.

J. Repeat B through I once again.

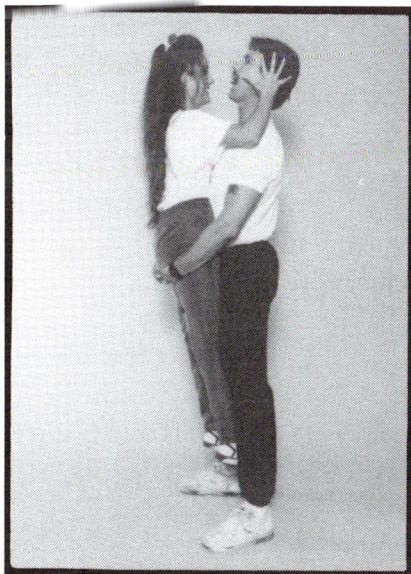

Application

4. Inside Wrist Escape

When the attacker grabs you with the opposite, or cross hand (his left grabs your left as he faces you), his thumb is on the other side, so you must turn your hand the opposite way that you did in #2 in order to escape against the thumb. Once you understand this simple principle, escape is just a matter of locating the thumb, and escaping in that direction.

How to do it:

A. Maintain ready stance (stand with your legs shoulder width apart and your knees bent). Make a fist with both hands.

B. Perform a low inside wrist escape to the side by turning ninety degrees to the left, extending your left hand in front of your left hip, and making a small circle by moving your left hand upward and inward in a clockwise semi-circle.

C. Perform a low inside wrist escape to the other side.

D. Repeat B and C three more times.

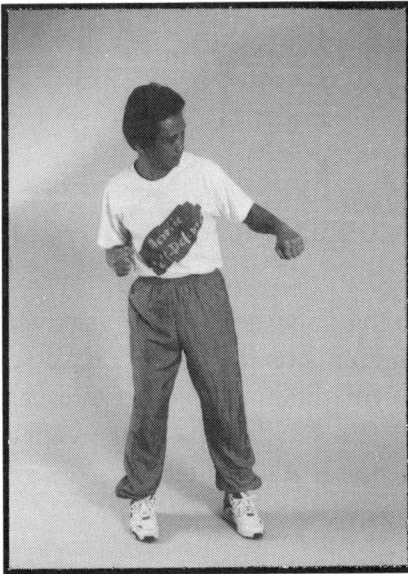

B

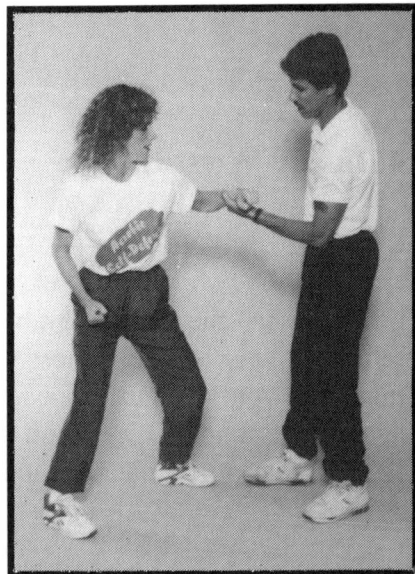

B application

E. Perform a high inside wrist escape to the side (arm at shoulder level, making a big circle) four times to each side.

F. Perform a low inside wrist escape to the front four times with each hand.

G. Perform a high inside wrist escape to the front four times with each hand.

H. Repeat B through G once again.

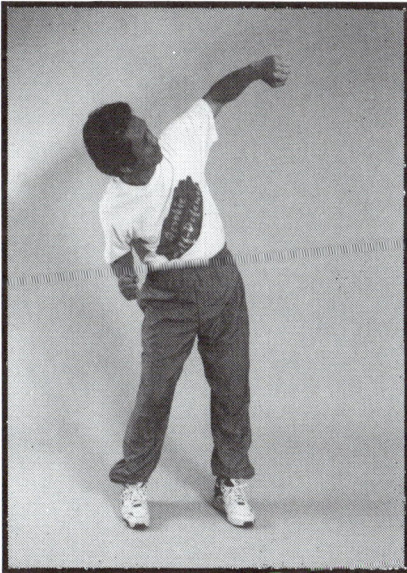

E

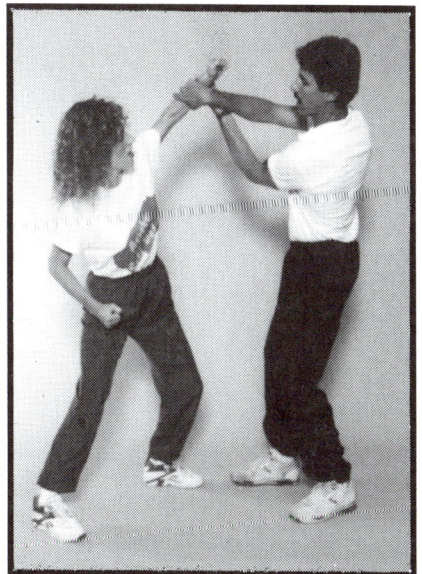

E application

5. Bear Paw

Sometimes it is difficult for a weak individual, especially a woman, to hurt someone with a punch. The bear paw is a special adaptation of the fist designed to increase the power of impact without increasing the force exerted. In other words, a bear paw concentrates the power of a punch into a smaller area. It will do more damage.

How to do it:

A. Maintain ready stance (feet shoulder width apart and knees bent).

B. Make your fists into bear paws by straightening the third knuckles (at the base of the fingers) on each hand.

C. Turn ninety degrees to the right and punch by extending the left bear paw.

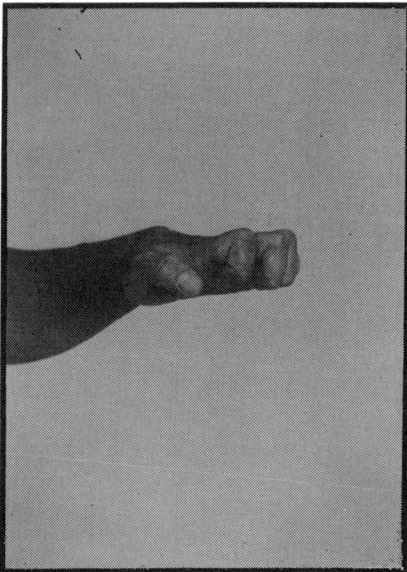

B

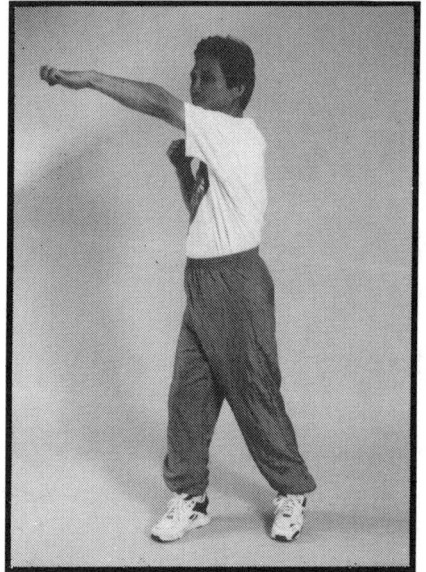

C

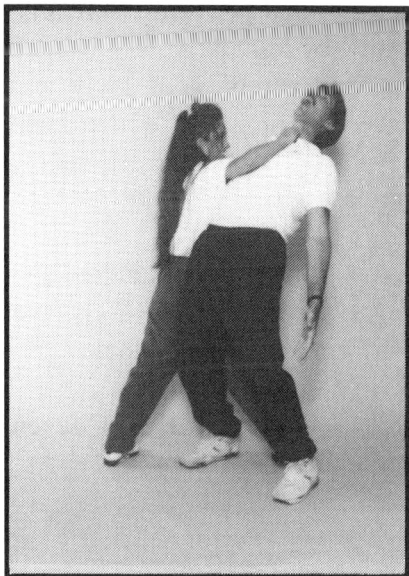

Application

D. Turn one hundred and eighty degrees to the left and punch by extending the right bear paw.

E. Repeat C and D seven more times.

F. Punch to the front by extending the left bear paw and pulling it back in.

G. Punch to the front by extending the right bear paw and pulling it back in.

H. Repeat F and G seven more times.

I. Repeat B through H once again.

6. High Block

The high block is designed to protect you from an attack to the head or face. It can be used to block a punch or a strike with a weapon like a club.

How to do it:

A. Maintain ready stance (stand with your legs shoulder width apart and your knees bent). Get into guarding position (make a fist with both hands, place your hands in front of your shoulders, and your elbows covering your ribs).

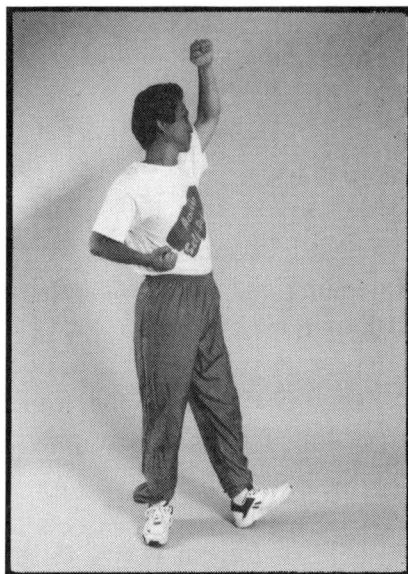

B. Turn ninety degrees to the left and perform a left high block by moving your left hand up in front of your body and face, stopping just above head level at a forty-five degree angle.

C. Turn one hundred and eighty degrees to the right and perform a right high block.

D. Repeat B and C seven more times.

E. Perform a left high block to the front.

B

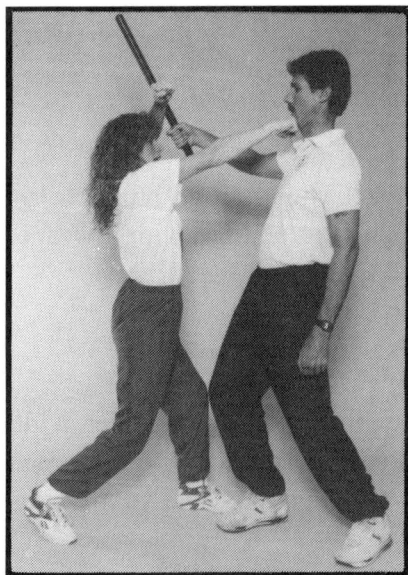

B application

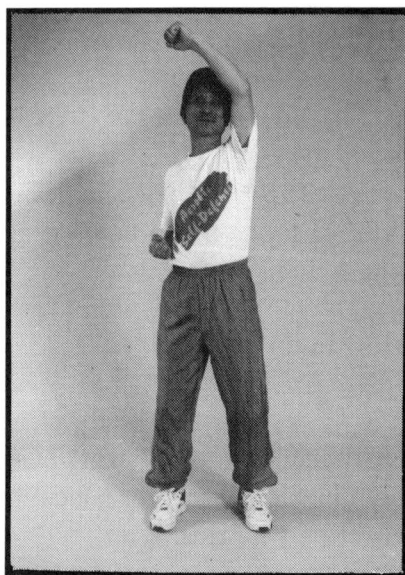

E

F. Perform a right high block to the front.

G. Repeat E and F seven more times.

H. Repeat B through G once again.

7. Punch

The punch is the simplest attack for Americans (and Europeans) to incorporate because we are accustomed to doing things with our hands. When you make a proper fist, the hand can become a deadly weapon for self-defense. The punch is the safest, simplest, and most direct means of self-defense without using a weapon.

How to do it:

A. Maintain ready stance (stand with your legs shoulder width apart and your knees bent). Get into guarding position (make a fist with both hands, place your hands in front of your shoulders and your elbows covering your ribs).

B. Turn ninety degrees to the right and punch by extending the left fist straight out from the shoulder, then pulling it back to the shoulder.

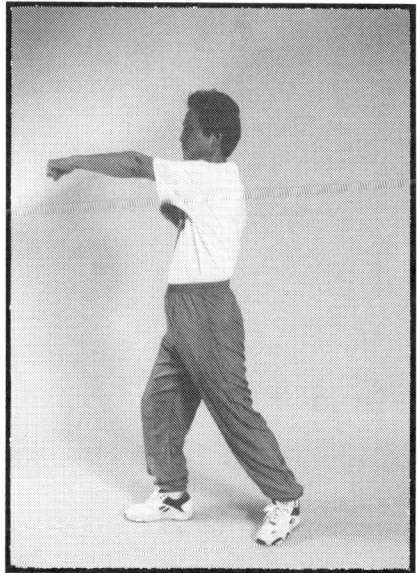

B

C. Turn one hundred and eighty degrees to the left and punch with the right hand.

D. Repeat B and C seven more times.

E. Assume a walking stance in guarding position (move your right foot back at a forty-five degree angle and about one shoulder width from your left foot, as if you were walking.)

F. Punch to the front with the left hand and then the right, four times with each hand.

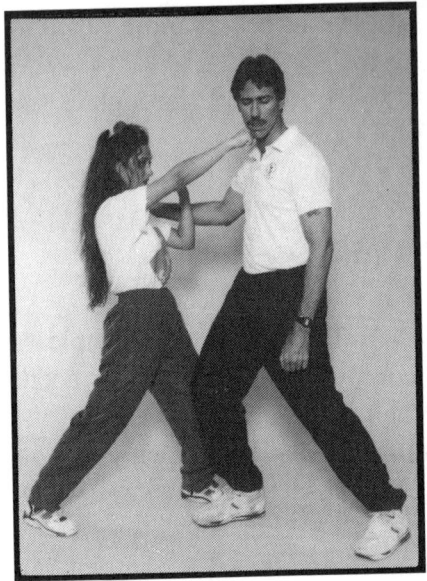

Application

G. Switch stance by moving the right foot forward almost one shoulder width, and the left foot back the same distance.

H. Punch to the front with the right hand and then the left, four times with each hand.

I. Repeat B through H once again.

8. Inside Block

The inside block is designed to protect you from an attack to the vital areas of the body. It can be used to block a punch, a kick, or a grab to the torso.

How to do it:

A. Maintain ready stance in guarding position (stand with your legs shoulder width apart and your knees bent. Make a fist with both hands, place your hands in front of your shoulders and your elbows covering your ribs).

B. Twist your body ninety degrees to the right and perform an inside block with the left hand by bringing your left fist across the front of the body and stopping in front of the right shoulder.

C. Twist your body one hundred and eighty degrees to the left and perform an inside block with the right hand by bringing your right fist across the front of the body and stopping front of the left shoulder.

D. Repeat B and C seven more times.

E. Perform a left inside block to the front, followed by a right inside block to the front, eight times with each hand.

F. Repeat B through E once again.

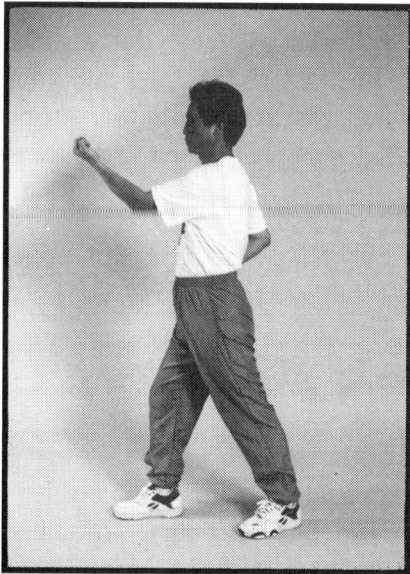

B

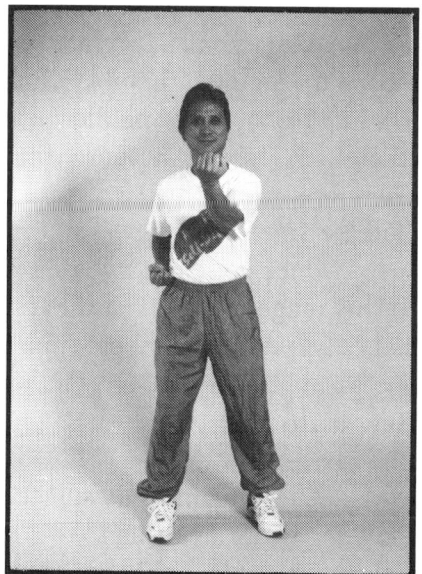

E

343

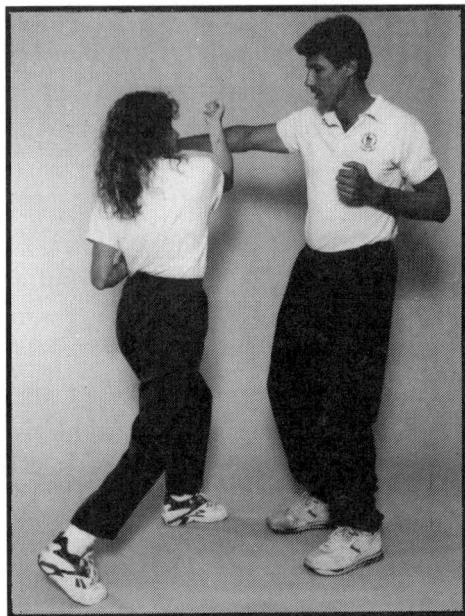

Application

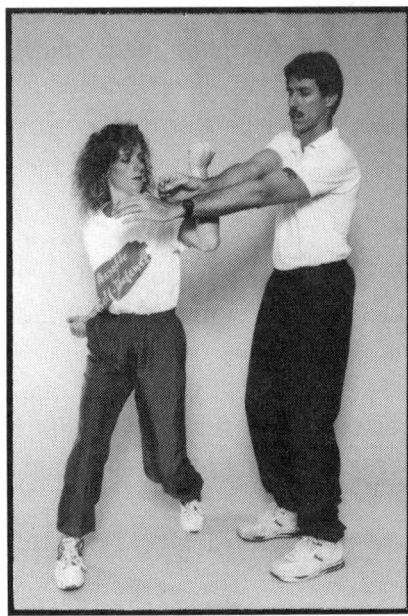

Application

9. Elbow to Chin

When someone grabs you with two hands on one, you can still escape through the thumbs. Since both thumbs face the middle, pull your hand up through the middle. It is possible that your one arm is not strong enough to escape because the attacker has two hands on your one. Therefore, you may have to grab your fist to use your other hand to increase your leverage.

Once you have released your wrist, you will be at very close range. At this range an elbow strike to the chin is very effective, and flows quite naturally out of the escape.

How to do it:

A. Maintain ready stance in guarding position (stand with your legs shoulder width apart and your knees bent. Make a fist with both hands, place your hands in front of your shoulders and your elbows covering your ribs).

B. Lift your left elbow straight up above shoulder level.

C. Lift your right elbow straight up above shoulder level.

D. Repeat B and C fifteen more times.

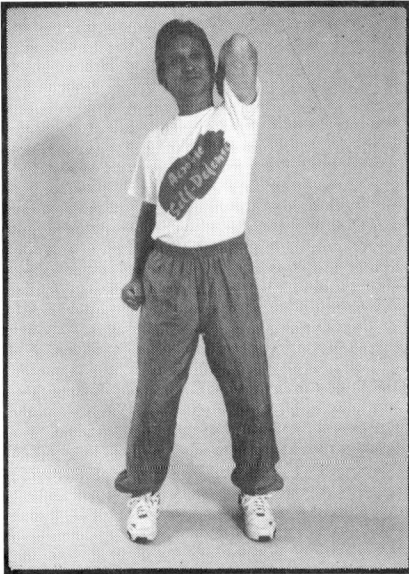

B

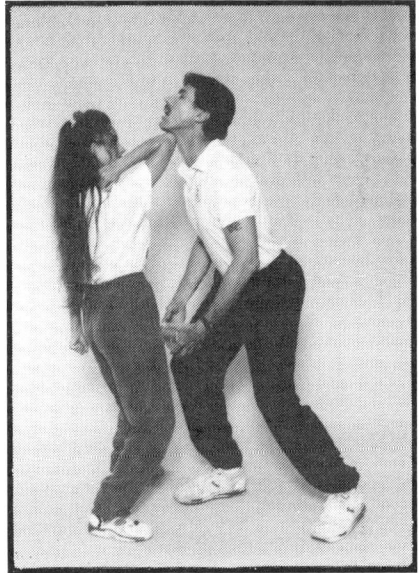

B application

10. Knee Kick

A knee kick allows even a beginner to disable an attacker at close range. When someone attacks from the front and is too close to be kicked or punched easily (for example, he is hugging you), a quick knee kick will render him helpless.

How to do it:

A. Maintain ready stance (stand with your legs shoulder width apart and your knees bent).

B. Extend your left hand straight out in front of your hip, with the palm down. Perform a low knee kick by lifting your left knee to touch your hand.

C. Extend your right hand straight out in front of your hip, with the palm down. Perform a low knee kick by lifting your right knee to touch your hand.

D. Repeat B and C seven more times.

E. Extend both hands in front of your face as if grabbing someone around the back of the head. Pull both hands down to the your left knee kick.

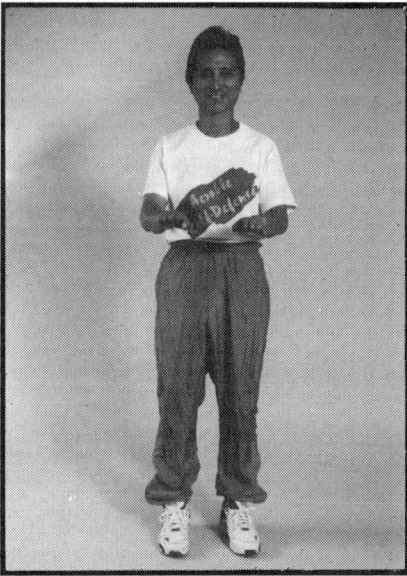

B extend

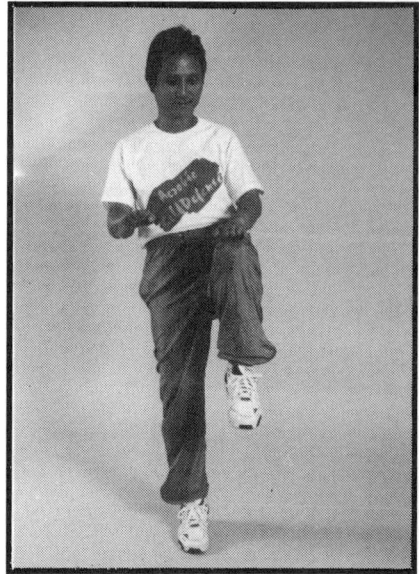

B knee kick

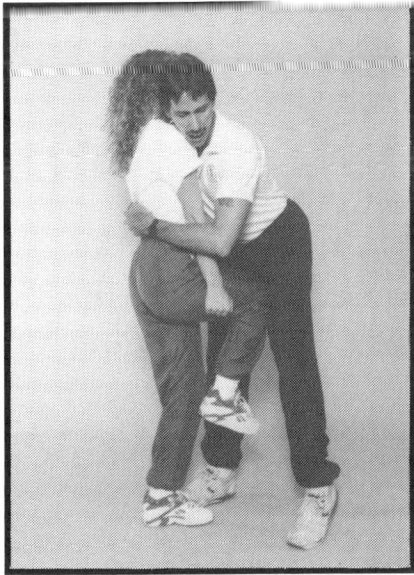

B application

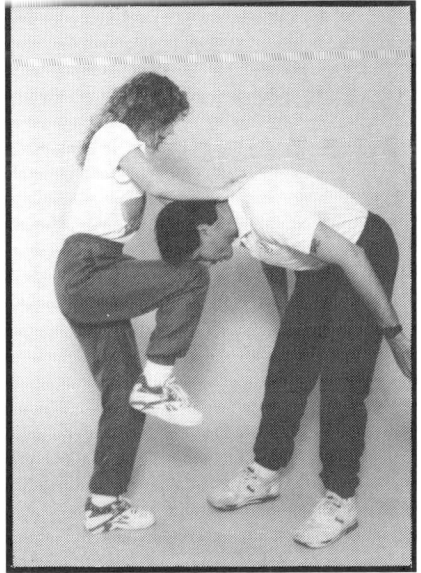

E application

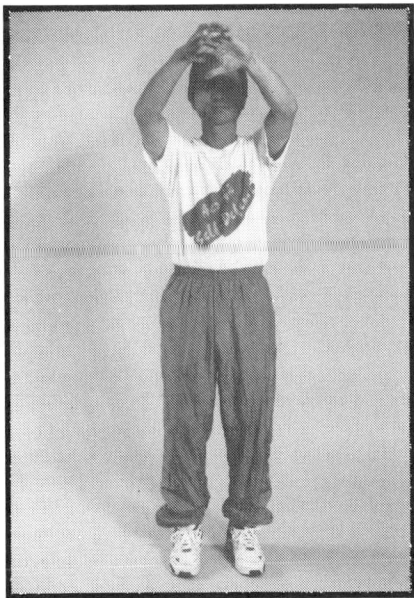

E (extend)

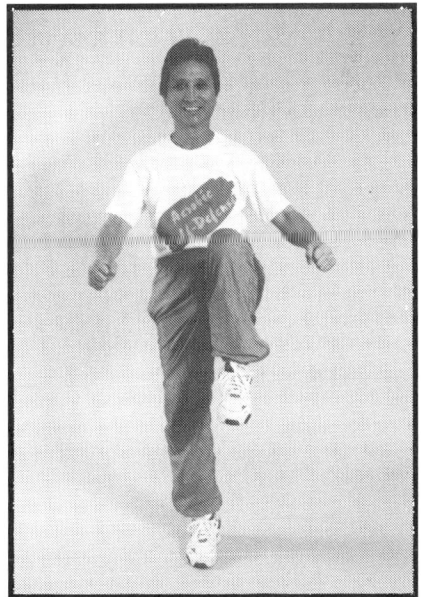

E (pull)

347

F. Repeat E using a right knee kick.

G. Repeat E and F seven more times

H. Repeat B through G once again.

11. Finger Up and Turn

This motion is an exaggeration that moves your shoulders in the correct paths and angles to use leverage to escape from a lapel grab or front choke.

How to do it:

A. Maintain ready stance (feet shoulder width apart but even).

B. Lift your left index finger and point it overhead toward the ceiling.

C. Step your left foot across the front of your right foot so that you turn ninety degrees to the right while dropping your left elbow straight toward the floor.

D. Step your left foot back to position A and lift your right index finger and point it overhead toward the ceiling.

E. Step your right foot across the front of your left foot so that you turn ninety degrees to the left while dropping your right elbow straight toward the floor.

F. Repeat B through E fifteen more times.

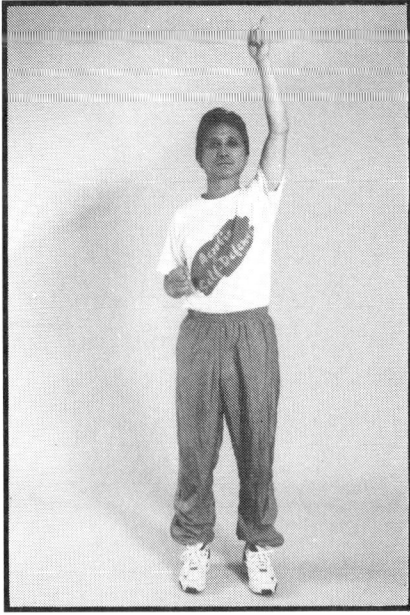

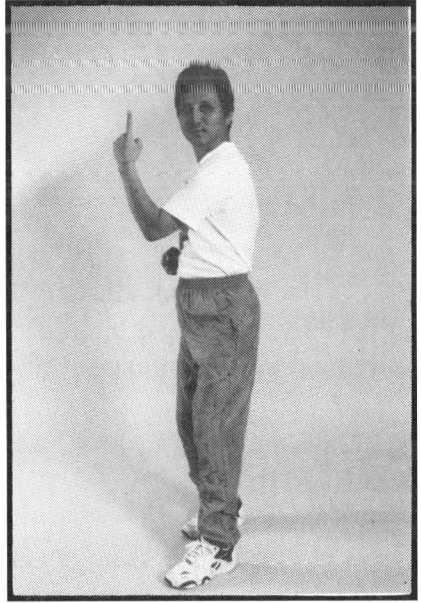

B   C

March

March and check your heart rate. Place your index and middle fingers to the side of the throat and feel for your pulse. Look at a watch with a second counter, and count your heart beats for six seconds. Whatever number you get, put a zero on the end to give you your heart rate in beats per minute (for example, 17 is 170 beats per minute). Look on page 316 to determine if you are within your training range. If your

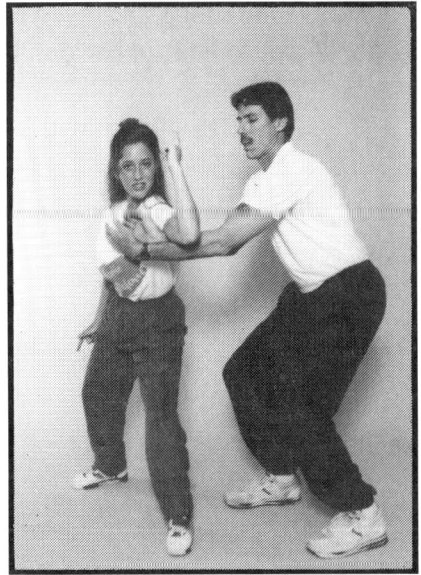

C application

heart rate is too high, slow down your movements or just march in place until you feel better. If your heart rate is too low, try to move stronger and faster to get more out of your workout.

12. Front Kick

The front kick allows even a beginner to utilize the strength of his (or her) legs to defend himself. The legs are a very strong point, and can be used to great advantage against an attacker's weak points.

How to do it:

A. Return to ready stance in guarding position (stand with your legs shoulder width apart and your knees bent. Make a fist with both hands, place your hands in front of your shoulders and your elbows covering your ribs).

B. Low front kick with the left leg by lifting the knee and extending the foot (striking with the ball of the foot) about knee high; inhale and pull the foot back and return it to the floor.

C. Low front kick with the right leg.

D. Repeat B and C seven more times.

E. Middle front kick with the left leg (about groin high).

F. Middle front kick with the right leg.

G. Repeat E and F seven more times.

H. Repeat B through G once again.

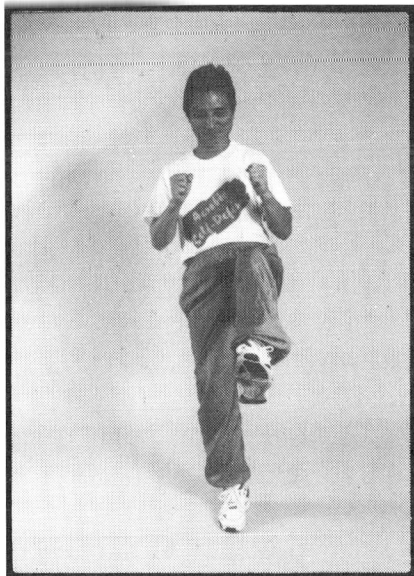

B

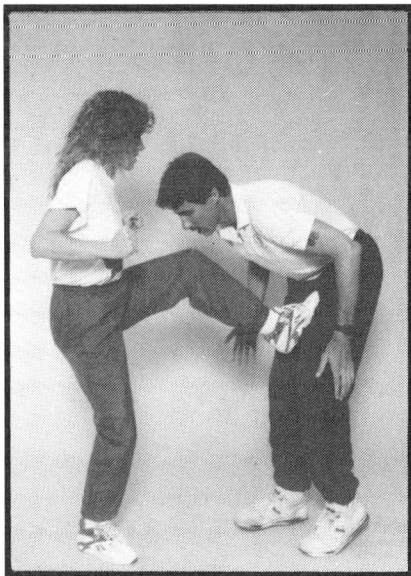

E Application

13. Palm Up Strike

The palm up strike can be used to release a grab to the head or hair. The shock of the strike will cause the grip to be released, while the movement will take the hand away from you.

How to do it:

A. Maintain ready stance in guarding position (stand with your legs shoulder width apart and your knees bent. Make a fist with both hands, place your hands in front of your shoulders and your elbows covering your ribs).

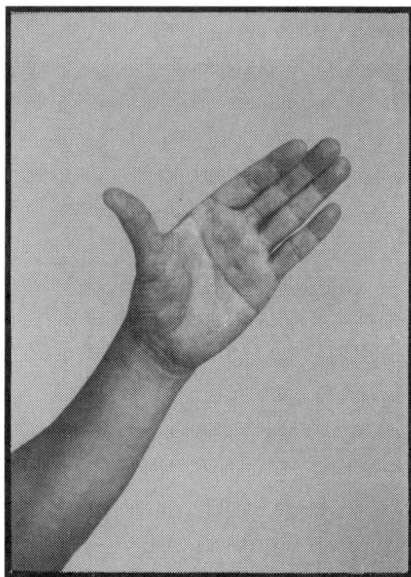

B

B. Open your left hand into an arc hand by separating your thumb from the rest of your fingers.

C. Perform a left palm up strike by extending your left hand diagonally to the right and above your head while straightening your elbow.

D. Perform a right palm up strike.

E. Repeat B through E seven more times.

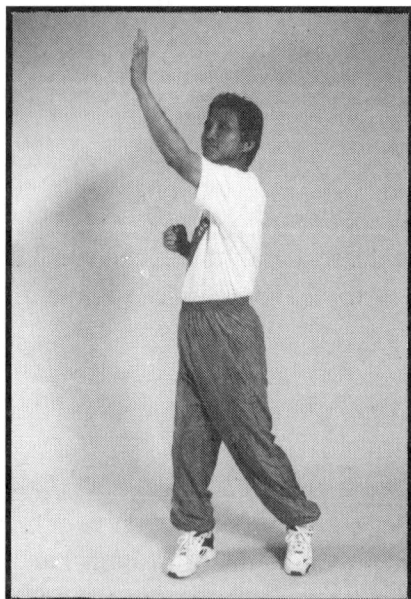

C

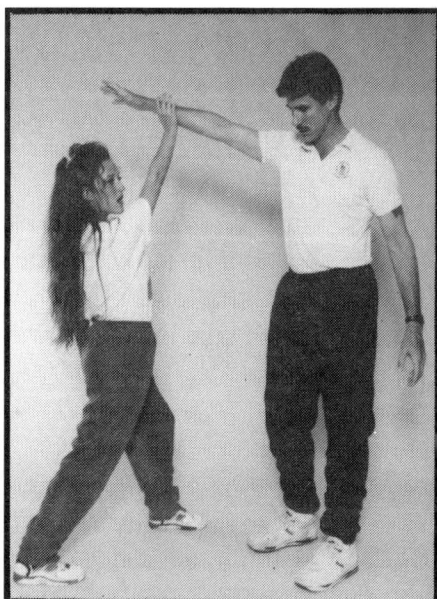

C application

F. Perform a left palm up strike to the front, followed by a right palm up strike to the front, eight times.

G. Repeat B through F once again.

14. Side Kick

The side kick allows even a beginner to utilize the strength of his legs against an attacker who is not in front, but beside him.

How to do it:

A. Maintain ready stance in guarding position (stand with your legs shoulder width apart and your knees bent. Make a fist with both hands, place your hands in front of your shoulders and your elbows covering your ribs).

B. Low side kick with the left leg by lifting the knee, extending the foot directly to the side at shin height, pulling the foot back, and returning it to the floor.

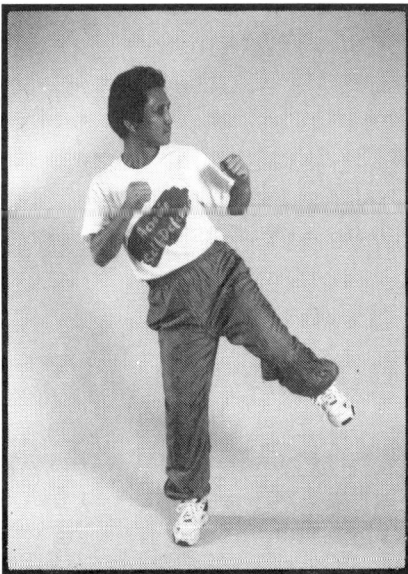

B

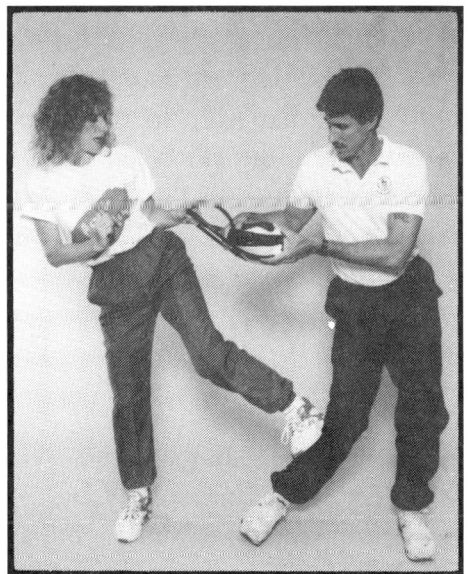

B application

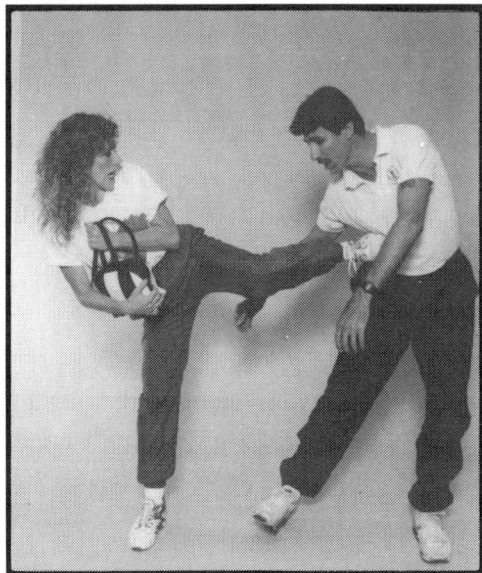

C. Low side kick with the right leg.

D. Repeat B and C seven more times.

E. Middle side kick with the left leg (about groin height), followed by a middle side kick with the right leg, eight times.

F. Repeat B through E once again.

E application

15. Elbow Up and Back Turn

Just like #11, the finger up and turn, which is an easy escape from a front grab, the elbow up and back turn is an easy escape from a rear shoulder grab. In this case, someone walks up behind you and grabs either your shoulders, neck, or clothing with his arms extended.

How to do it:

A. Maintain ready stance in guarding position (stand with your legs shoulder width apart and your knees bent. Make a fist with both hands, place your hands in front of your shoulders and your elbows covering your ribs).

B. Perform a left elbow up and back turn by raising your left elbow directly to the side above your own shoulder height and turning backward to the left, by stepping your left foot backward, and dropping your elbow forcefully toward the ground.

C. Step back to ready stance and clap your hands.

D. Perform and right elbow up and turn, return to ready stance and clap your hands.

E. Repeat B through D fifteen more times.

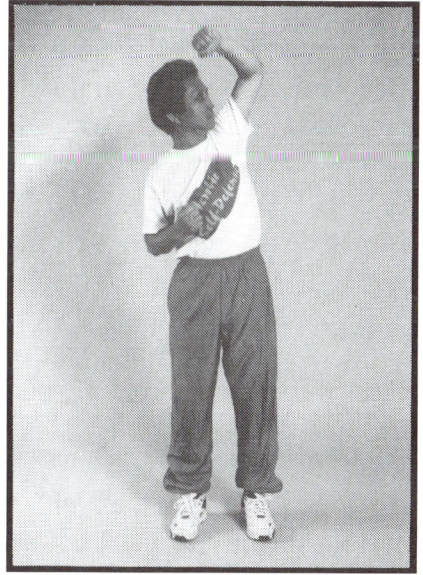

B (raise)

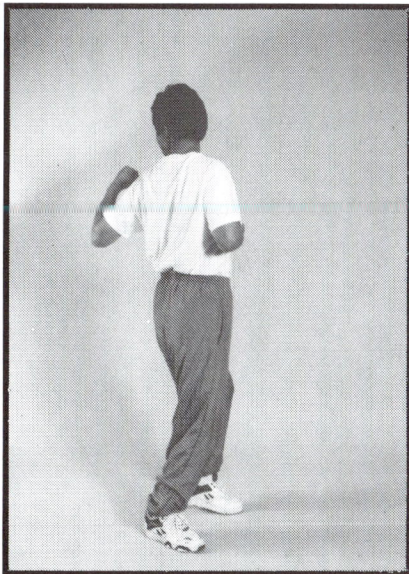

B (turn)

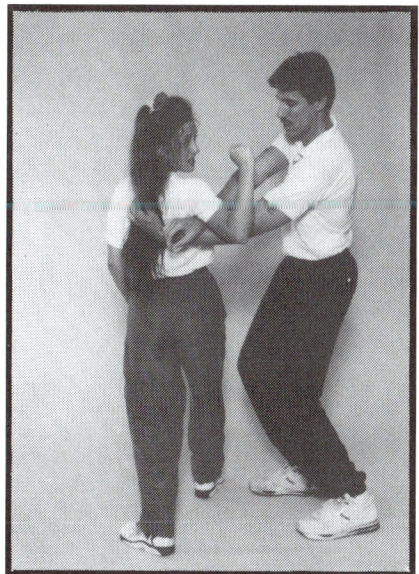

B application

16. Back Kick

The back kick allows even the beginner to use the power of his legs against an attacker who is positioned behind him. It is especially effective because the victim is facing away from the attacker and the kick is usually a surprise.

How to do it:

A. Maintain ready stance in guarding position (stand with your legs shoulder width apart and your knees bent. Make a fist with both hands, place your hands in front of your shoulders and your elbows covering your ribs).

B. Low back kick with the left leg by lifting the knee, extending the foot directly to the back at knee height, pulling the foot back, and returning it to the floor.

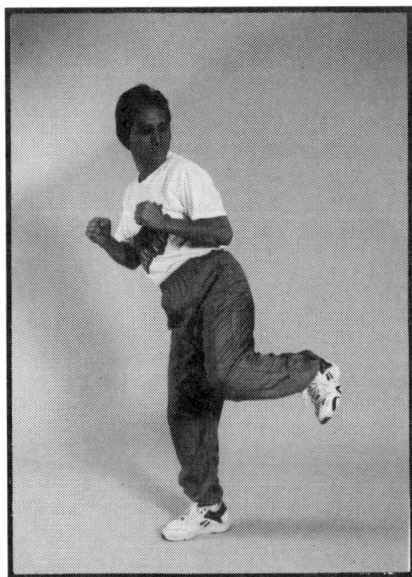

B

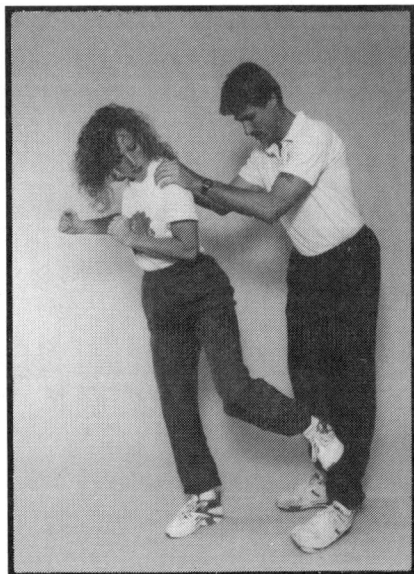

B application

C. Low back kick with the right leg.

D, Repeat B and C seven more times.

E. Middle back kick with the left leg (groin height).

F. Middle back kick with the right leg.

G. Repeat E and F seven more times.

H. Repeat B through G once again.

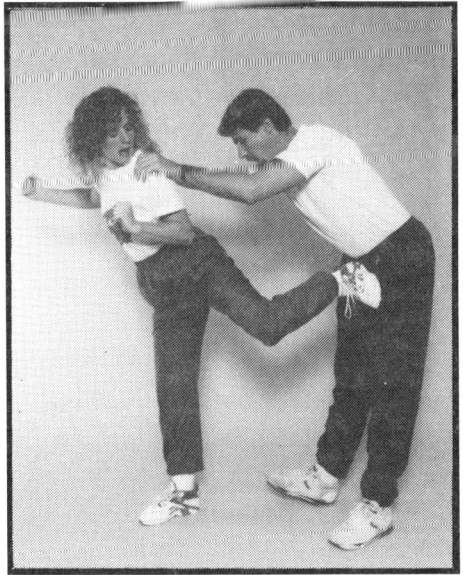

E application

17. Double Arm Wrist Escape

When an attacker grabs both wrists at the same time, you can use the thumb escape effectively on both wrists at the same time.

How to do it:

A. Maintain ready stance in guarding position (stand with your legs shoulder width apart and your knees bent. Make a fist with both hands, place your hands in front of your shoulders and your elbows covering your ribs).

357

B. Perform an outside wrist escape by extending both hands in front of your waist and making a small circle by moving both hands together, upward, and outward.

C. Perform an inside wrist escape by extending both hands in front of your waist and making a big circle by moving both hands outward, upward, together, and then downward.

D. Repeat B through E fifteen more times.

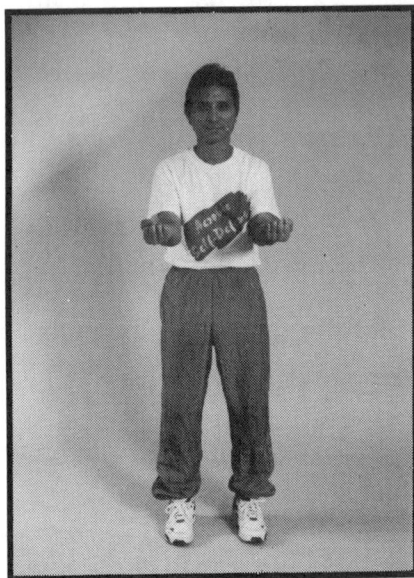

B

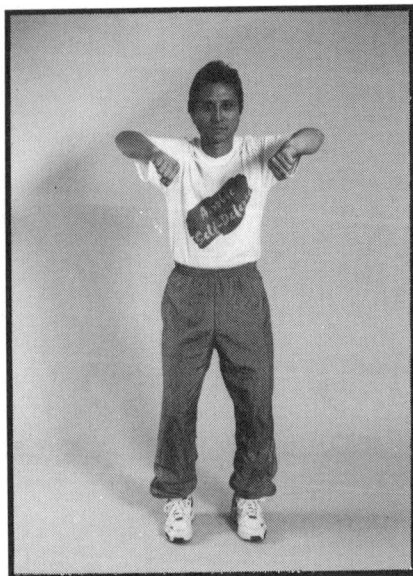

C

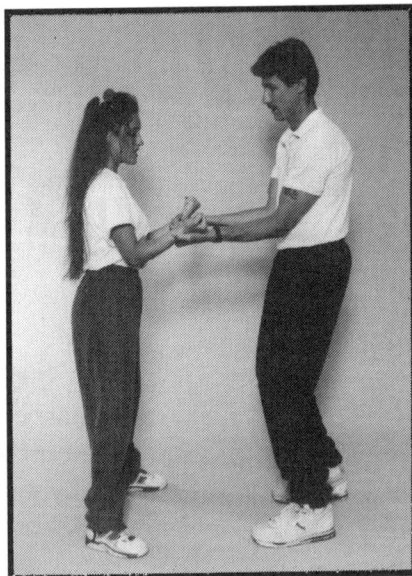

C application

358

18. Pushing Kick

The pushing kick is not intended do disable an attacker. It is intended to push him away. Sometimes you can push the attacker away just long enough to escape, and you don't need to disable him. Other times it is difficult to disable him because he is so close, and you need to push him away in order to disable him. For either situation, the pushing kick allows you to use the strength of your legs to push the attacker away.

How to do it:

A. Maintain ready stance in guarding position (stand with your legs shoulder width apart and your knees bent. Make a fist with both hands, place your hands in front of your shoulders and your elbows covering your ribs).

B. Left middle pushing kick leg by lifting the knee, extending the foot (striking with the whole bottom of the foot) to the groin, stomach, or face, pulling the foot back, and returning it to the floor.

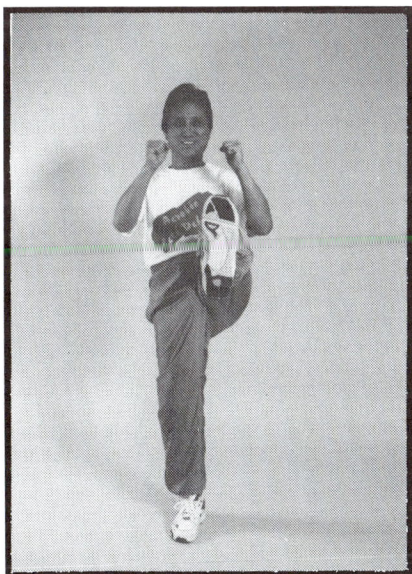

B

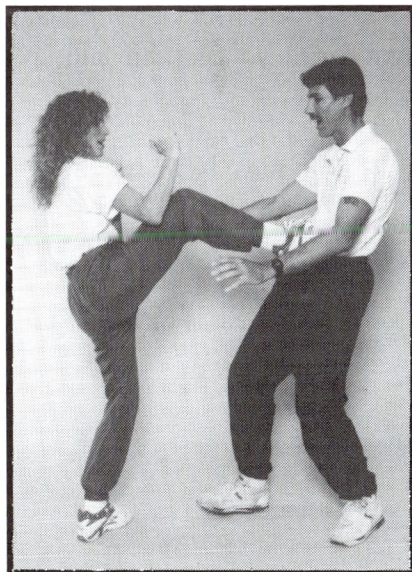

B application

C. Right middle pushing kick.

D. Repeat B and C fifteen more times.

19. Claw Groin, Elbow

This is a combination of two techniques. It is extremely effective when someone grabs you from behind with one arm either around your shoulders or around your throat. Use the opposite side hand to strike the groin, and then elbow either the head or the solar plexus, whichever is an easier target. In the steps below, I will only describe the elbow to the head.

How to do it:

A. Maintain ready stance (your feet shoulder width apart and your knees bent).

B. Position your left hand as if holding a grapefruit. Drop your left hand beside your left hip and use your fingers to strike behind you.

C. Lift your left elbow up to the side, just above shoulder level, and strike with the elbow straight behind you while twisting the hips.

D. Claw to the groin with your right hand then elbow strike.

E. Repeat B through D fifteen more times.

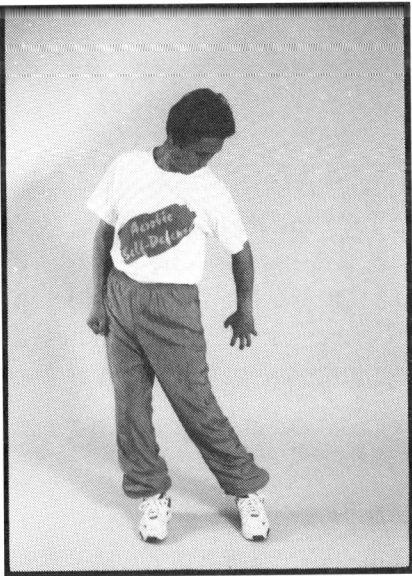

B

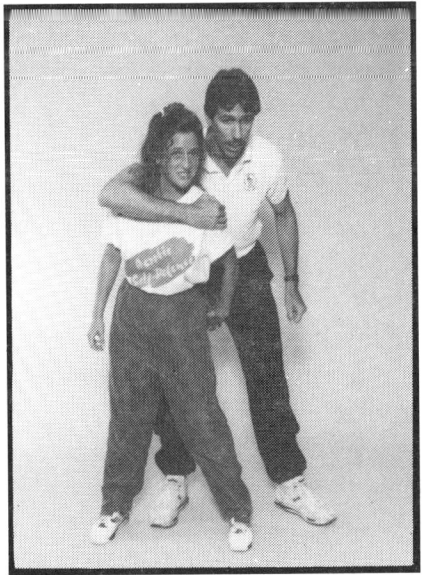

B application

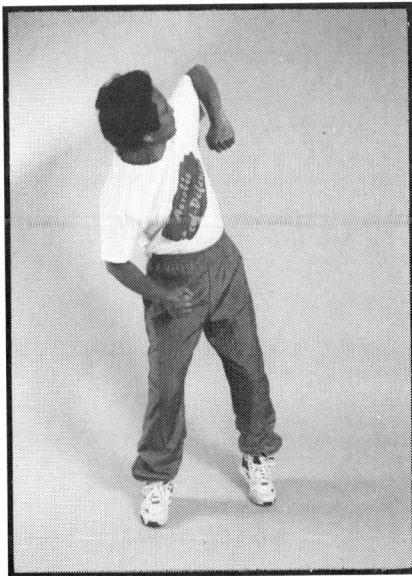

C

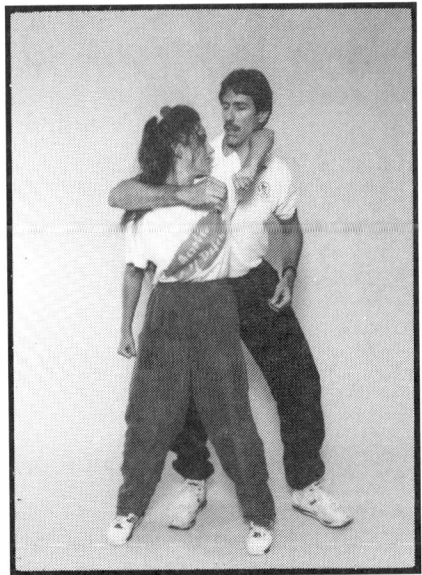

C application

March

March in place for two sets of eight counts.

20. Multiple Kick

The multiple kick is a great exercise for your lower body that will get your heart rate up, improve your balance, and increase the speed and power of your kicks. In this exercise, you kick to the front, to the side, to the back, and to the side again, in rapid succession. It simulates a self-defense situation in which you are defending against more than one attacker.

How to do it:

A. Return to ready stance in guarding position (stand with your legs shoulder width apart and your knees bent. Make a fist with both hands, place your hands in front of your shoulders and your elbows covering your ribs).

B. Low front kick with the left leg (#12, p. 350), followed by a low front kick with the right leg.

C. Low side kick with the left leg (#14, p. 353), followed by a low side kick with the right leg.

D. Low back kick with the left leg (#16, p. 356), followed by a low back kick with the right leg.

E. Low side kick with the left leg again, followed by a low side kick with the right leg.

F. Repeat B through E once again.

G. Repeat B through F using middle kicks in each direction.

H. Repeat B through G once again.

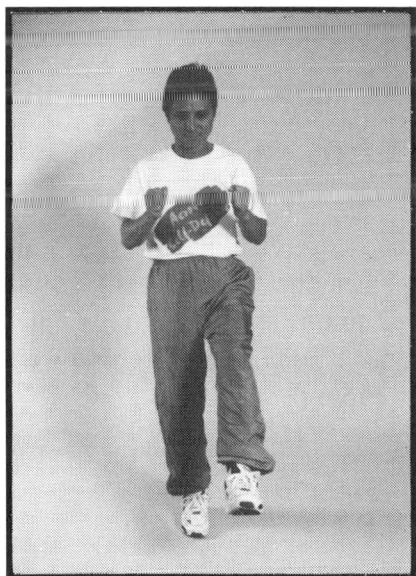

B

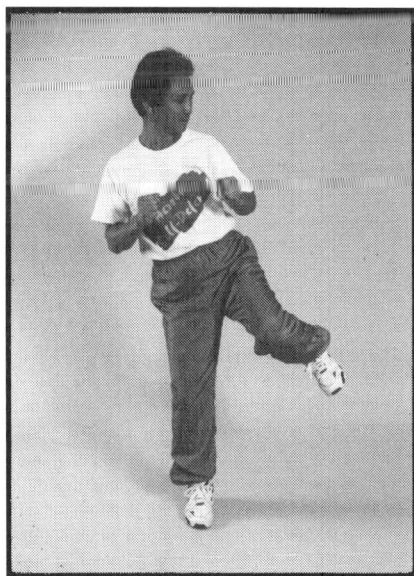

C

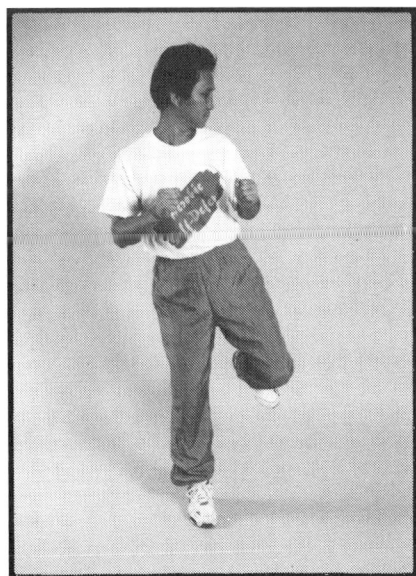

D

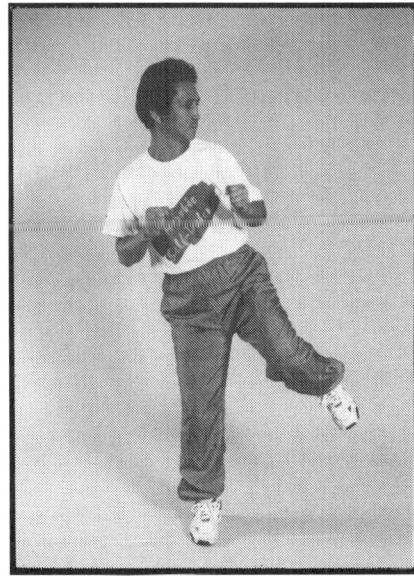

E

363

March

March in place for two sets of eight counts.

21. Multiple punch

A multiple punch is a great upper body exercise that will get your heart rate up and increase the speed and power of your punches. In this exercise, you punch on many different levels to one side, then to the other side, then to the front, in rapid succession. It simulates a self-defense situation in which you are defending against more than one attacker.

How to do it:

A. Maintain ready stance in guarding position (stand with your legs shoulder width apart and your knees bent. Make a fist with both hands, place your hands in front of your shoulders and your elbows covering your ribs).

B. Punch diagonally to the left, first with the left hand and then with the right hand low (groin), left and right middle (solar plexus), left and right middle-high (throat), and left and right high (face).

C. Punch diagonally to the right, first with the right and then with the left, low, middle, middle-high, and high.

D. Punch directly to the front, first with the left and then with the right, low, middle, middle-high, and high.

E. Repeat B through D once again.

F. Punch to the front double time (twice as fast), low, middle, middle-high, and high; then high, middle-high, middle, and low.

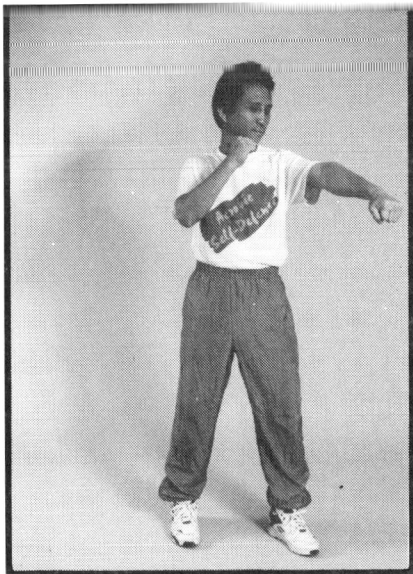

B

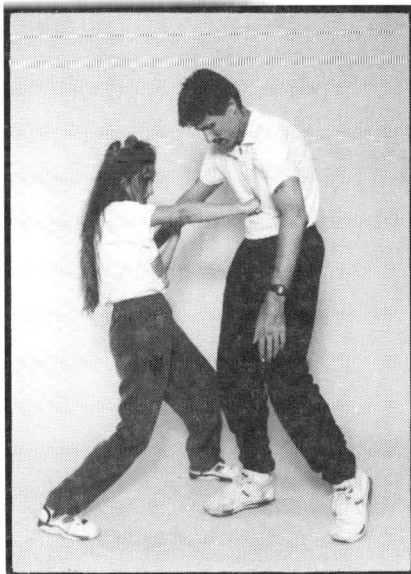

Application

22. Two Knife-Hand Strike

When an attacker grabs you by the lapels with both hands, you can release yourself and counter attack in two quick moves.

How to do it:

A. Maintain ready stance in guarding position (stand with your legs shoulder width apart and your knees bent. Make a fist with both hands, place your hands in front of your shoulders and your elbows covering your ribs).

B. Bring both hands together in front of the chest, as if praying. As you straighten your knees and rise up on your toes, forcefully extend your hands up over your head and allow them to separate about shoulder width.

C. As you drop your body weight by bending your knees and letting your whole foot touch the floor (do NOT let your heels hit hard and jar your body), bring your hands forcefully down as if to strike with the knife edge of both hands on the collar bones of an imaginary attacker in front of you.

D. Repeat B and C fifteen more times.

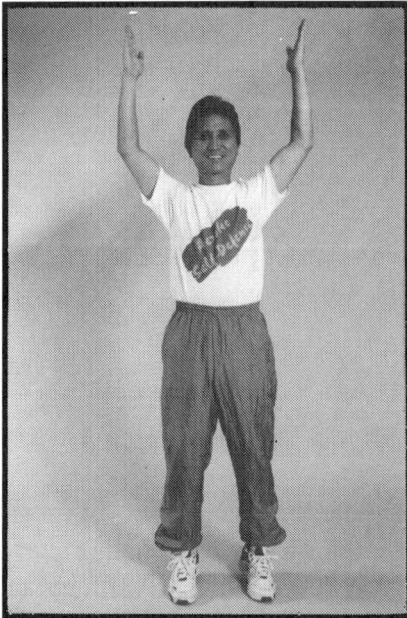

B

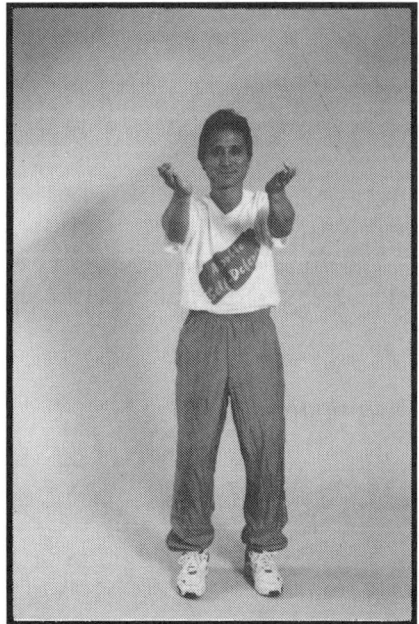

C

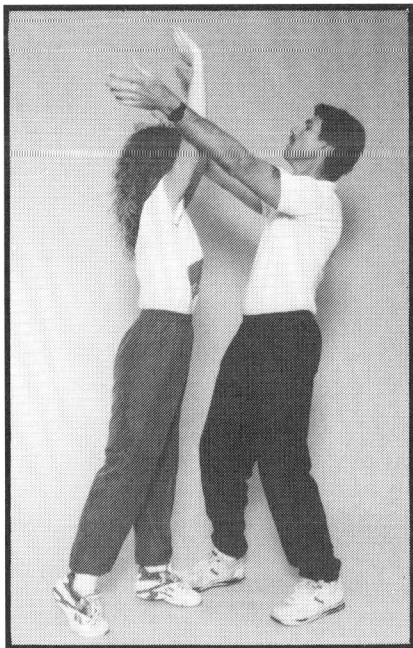

B application

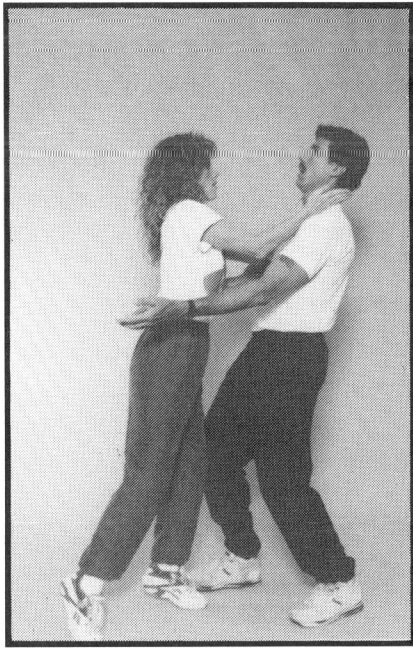

C application

23. Claw Groin and Double Arm Up

The groin is a weak point for any male attacker. It can be struck by either the foot or the hand, depending on the kind and angle of attack. The claw is an effective defense for an attacker who grabs from behind with a bear hug, pinning the arms so they are not free. Once you have struck to the groin, you can free yourself by lowering your body and raising your arms.

How to do it:

A. From ready stance (legs shoulder width apart and legs bent), sidestep left by stepping your right foot to your left, then stepping your left foot two shoulder widths to the left into a horse riding stance.

B. Sidestep right by stepping your left foot to your right, then stepping your right foot to the right into a horse riding stance.

C. Repeat A and B seven more times.

D. Continue to sidestep, but when your feet are together, claw the groin (as in #19) by dropping your left hand beside your left hip and using your fingers to strike behind you. As you step to the left, bend both knees even more, and lift both elbows straight out to the side to shoulder height.

E. Continue to sidestep right, clawing with the right hand and raising both elbows.

F. Repeat D and E fifteen more times.

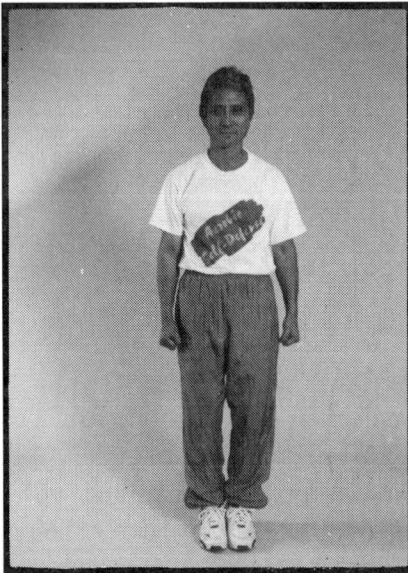

A together

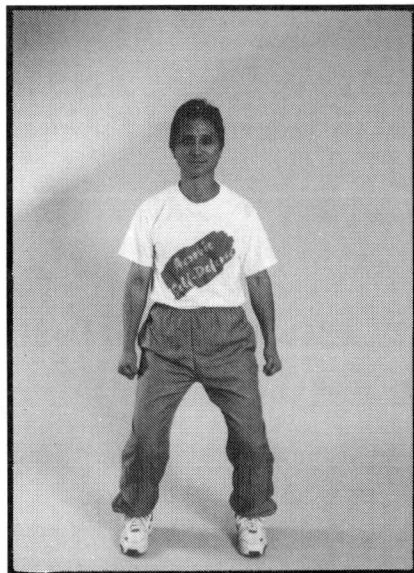

A horse riding stance

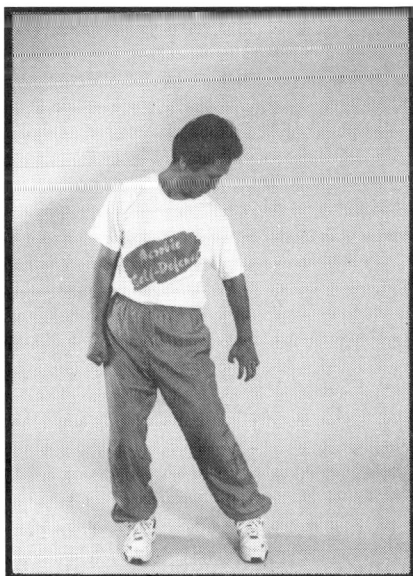

D claw

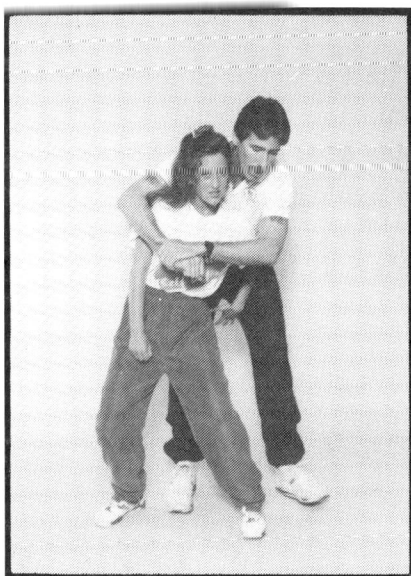

Claw application

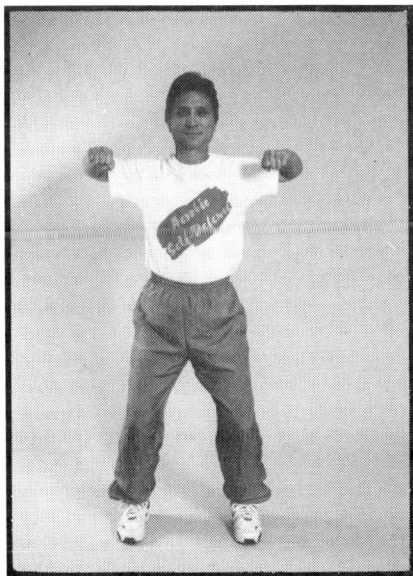

D raise elbows

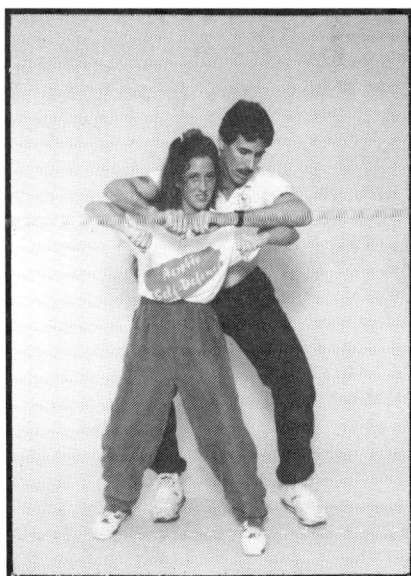

Raise elbows application

24. Elbow Strike

The elbow is an extremely effective weapon to use when the attacker is too close to kick or punch. When the attacker is behind you, probably grabbing you with a bear hug with your arms free so that you do not have an open strike to the groin, the elbows can be used to great advantage.

How to do it:

A. Return to ready stance in guarding position (stand with your legs shoulder width apart and your knees bent. Make a fist with both hands, place your hands in front of your shoulders and your elbows covering your ribs).

B. Left elbow strike low by lifting your left elbow up to the side just below shoulder level and twist the elbow back, using the hip and shoulder for power.

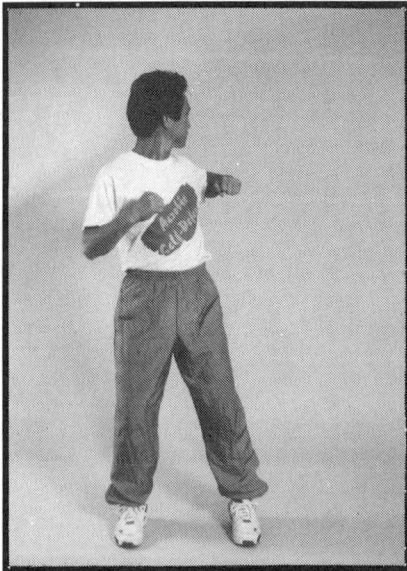

B

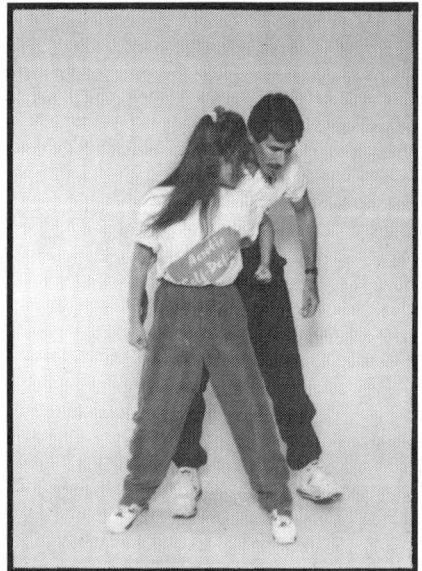

B application

370

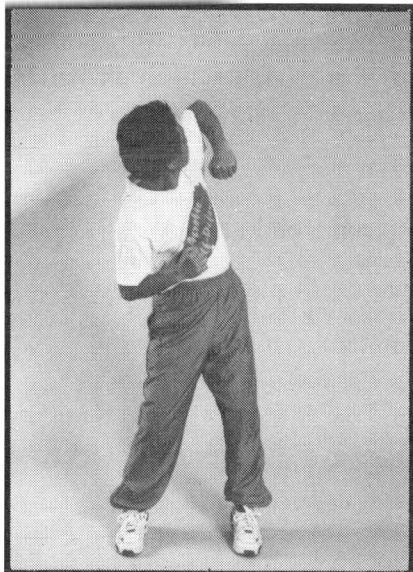

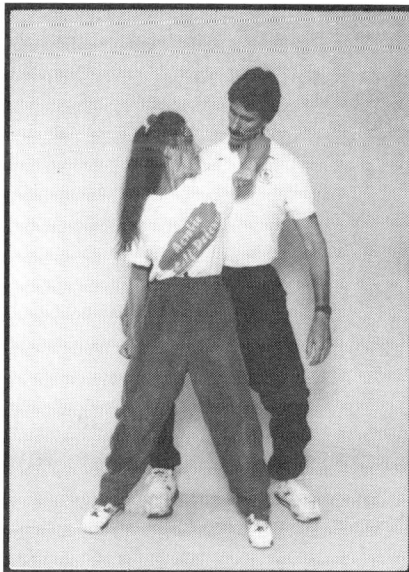

C   C application

C. Left elbow high strike by lifting the elbow above shoulder level and twist the elbow back, using the hip and shoulder for power.

D. Right elbow strike low, followed by right elbow strike high.

E. Repeat B though D fifteen times.

25. Low Block

The low block is designed to protect you from a low attack, usually a kick. It allows you to defend your groin and abdomen (weak points) with the speed and dexterity of your hands.

How to do it:

A. Maintain ready stance in guarding position (stand with your legs shoulder width apart and your knees bent. Make a fist with both hands, place your hands in front of your shoulders and your elbows covering your ribs).

B. Sidestep left, followed by sidestep right, eight times.

C. Sidestep left and perform a left low block by circling your left hand downward and sideways in a clockwise semi-circle.

D. Sidestep right and at the same time perform a right low block by circling your right hand downward and sideways in a counter-clockwise semi-circle.

E. Repeat C and D seven more times.

F. Return to ready stance in guarding position. Perform a left low block to the front, followed by a right low block to the front, eight times.

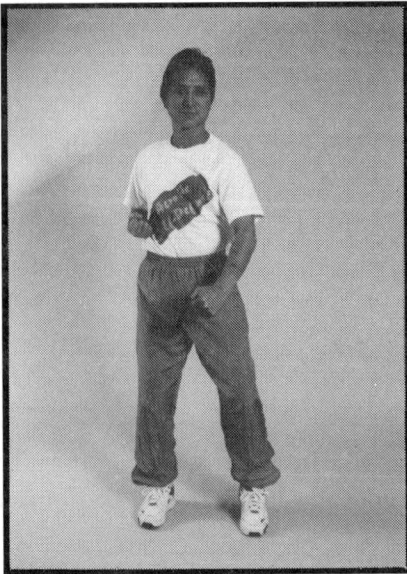

C

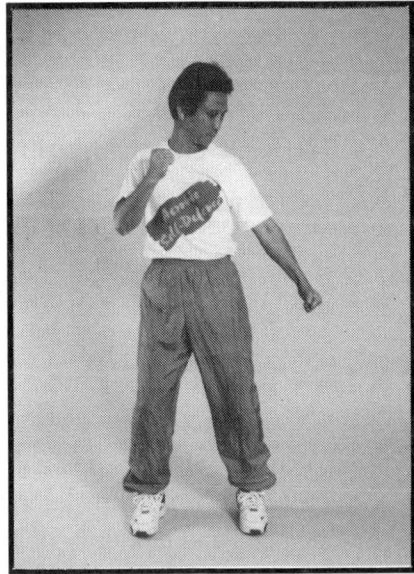

F

26. Stomp

The stomp is nothing more than a very low back kick. It is not directed at the knee or groin, it is directed at the arch of the foot or possibly the low shins. It is not a disabling move as much as it is a distracting move. It hurts badly enough to divert the attacker's attention while you escape. Once you escape you can either run or disable the attacker, depending on the situation.

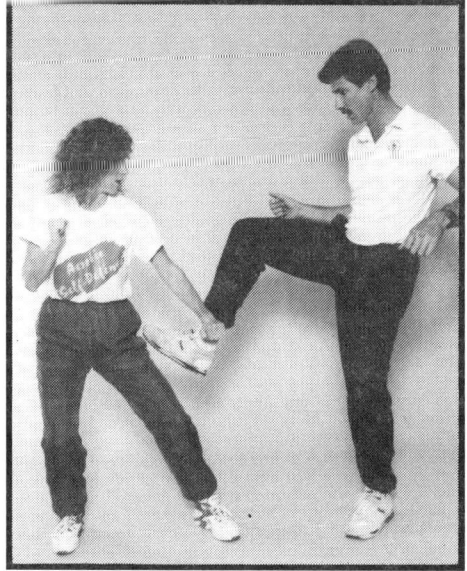

low block application

How to do it:

A. Maintain ready stance in guarding position (stand with your legs shoulder width apart and your knees bent. Make a fist with both hands, place your hands in front of your shoulders and your elbows covering your ribs).

B. Left stomp by lifting the knee, extending the heel at a slight angle to the back and to the floor, pulling the foot back, and returning it to the floor.

C. Right stomp.

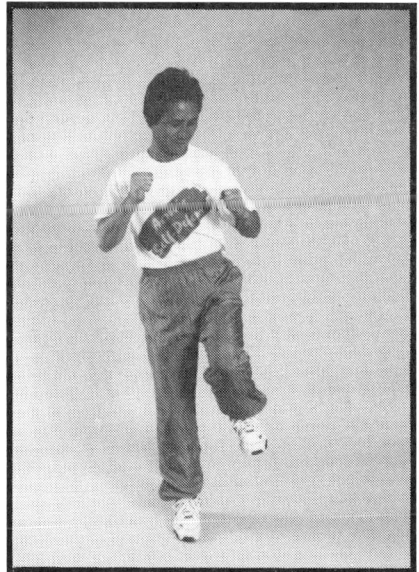

B

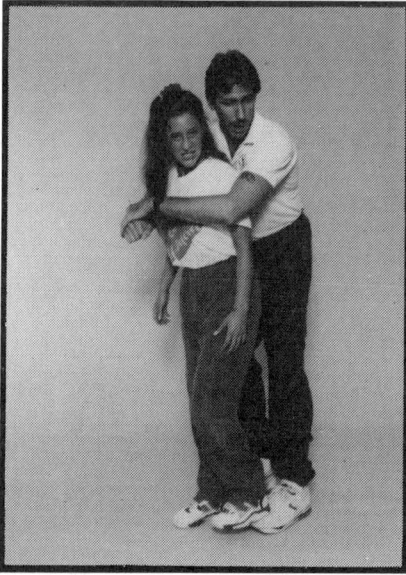

B application

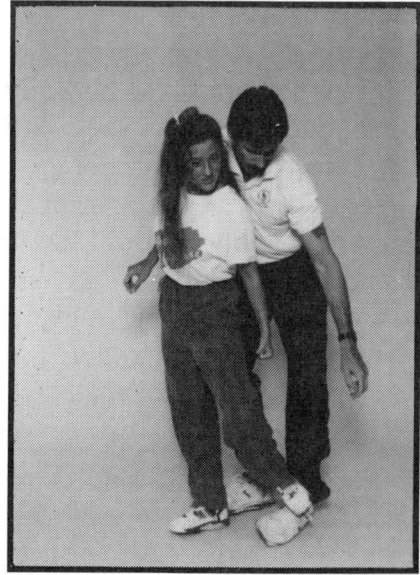

E application

D. Repeat B and C three more times.

E. Left stomp using the knife edge of the foot, followed by a right stomp using the knife edge of the foot, four times.

F. Repeat B through E once again.

March

March for two counts of eight.

27. Side Step and Shake

The side step and shake will help you cool down and loosen up your muscles after an exciting workout.

How to do it:

A. Maintain ready stance (legs shoulder width apart and your knees bent) with your arms hanging loosely.

B. Sidestep left and shake your shoulders and arms gently, to loosen up.

C. Sidestep right and shake your shoulders and arms gently.

D. Repeat B and C three more times.

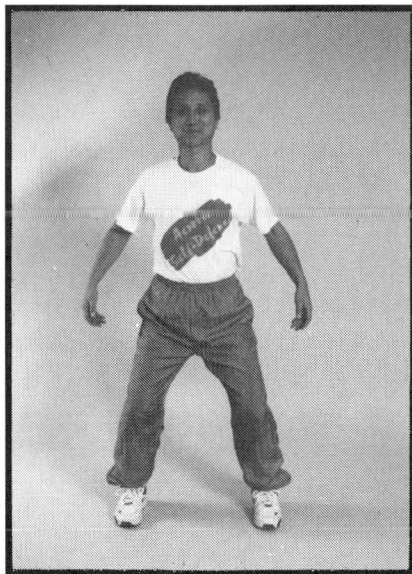

B

28. Deep Breathing

Deep breathing will restore oxygen to your body and help you bring your heart rate back down.

How to do it:

A.   Bend your knees slightly, with your feet approximately shoulder width apart.

B. Open your hands, cross your arms in front of you and slowly circle your arms up and over your head as you inhale through your nose into your lower abdomen.

C. Continue the circles outward and backward as you continue to inhale and expand the chest.

D. Slowly exhale through your slightly opened mouth as your hands move downward and inward. Gradually straighten your knees and bend forward while pulling in or tightening your stomach and stretching your back to push out all the remaining carbon dioxide and stale gas.

E. When your hands come together at the bottom, slightly bend your knees and slowly inhale through your nose again, but this time keep your hands at waist height and open them outward and backward in a half circle.

F. When you have circled outward as far as is comfortable, slowly exhale through the mouth and bring your hands inward. Gradually straighten your knees and bend slightly forward while pulling in or tightening your stomach and stretching your back to push out all the carbon dioxide.

WARM DOWN (3 min.)

1. Rhythm Power Breathing   (see pages 271-273 for description and illustrations)

2. Finger Chain Breathing   (see pages 273-275 for description and illustrations).

3. Open Leg Stretching (see pages 263-267 for description and illustrations).

4. Sit-ups   (see pages 284-285 for description and illustrations).

5. Single Leg Pull (see pages 286-288 for description and illustrations).

6. Inverted Butterfly Pull   (see pages 288-289 for description and illustrations).

7. Adjust the Spine (see pages 290-292 for description and illustrations).

8. Full Body Stretch (see pages 292-295 for description and illustrations).

9. Power Meditation (see pages 178-188 for description and illustrations).

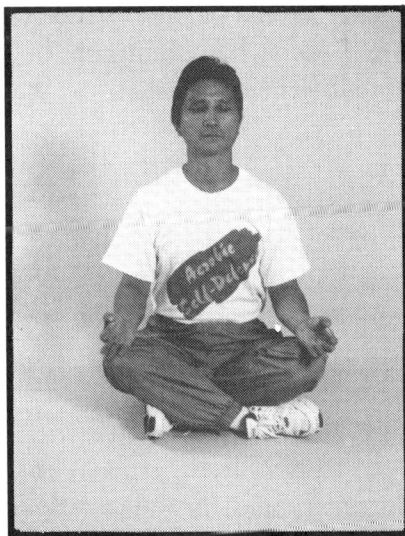

Light Energy Exercises

What are Light Energy Exercises? Are they the same as regular energy exercises except that they contain fewer calories? Well, sort of. They burn fewer calories, because they were not designed as a full exercise session that might make you sweaty.

Light Energy Exercises are a quick few exercises to give you energy at a time or in a place where you can't do a full exercise session. They will wake you up, give you more energy, relax tight or tense muscles, and clear your mind.

Your body is designed to move. At least once a day you need a full exercise session to release tension and clean some of the toxins out of your muscles. In addition, during the day you may need some light exercises to counteract bad posture, stress, or lack of movement. Whenever you feel a minor headache coming on, or your muscles tightening up, or a negative attitude developing, do some light energy exercises.

Especially if you must work in an awkward position, you need to let the muscles relax and go to back to their rightful place. Choose a few of the appropriate Power Exercises that will relax and refresh the right muscles. Do not worry about the other people around you or what they may say or think.

Light Energy Exercises are much better for you than aspirin, cigarettes, and the other solutions that they probably use for the same discomforts.

Office Energy Exercises

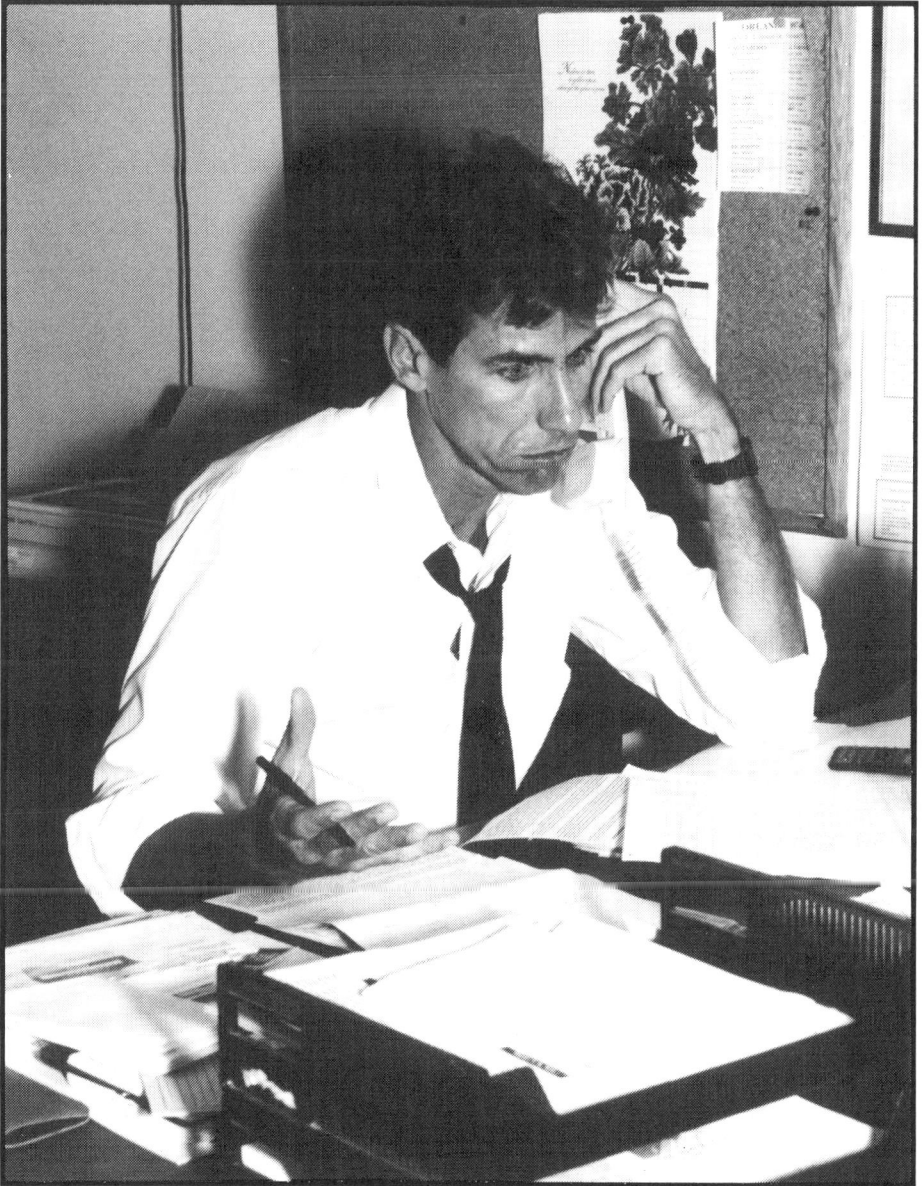

*Office exercises will save your health
and strengthen your company.*

379

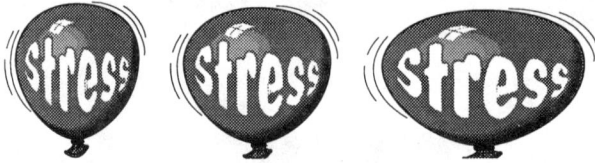

Most modern sicknesses are caused by stress. Most of the stress in our lives comes from our office environment.

Why? It is obvious:

* we do very little physical work (maybe our fingers work) and a lot of brain work. This is definitely not a good balance.

* we sit with bad posture all day long typing, writing, drawing, and talking on the phone.

* we have a bad relationship with our boss or co-workers.

* as bosses, we have problems with employees, financial pressures, deadlines, production, marketing, etc.,

Whether you are the employer or the employee, you end up eating stress and storing tension. You can develop a very nasty attitude, depression, confusion, and overall weakness, which will allow you to get sick. You hurt your company because you are less productive; you make your family worry; and most important of all, you destroy yourself. You become part of the $800 billion health care problem in the U.S. You may be the one out of every five Americans who gets cancer.

Just remember: without your health, nothing in the world matters. Your health is your top priority. Without it you cannot take care of your family. So what do you do? Do you quit your job or close down your business? No. Really, you don't have to worry at all. Just continue to do your job well and find a healthy way to release that stress. I will show you an easy and convenient way, and it will be up to you whether or not you do it. If you want to make yourself sick, lose your job or company, hurt your family, and destroy yourself, do not follow my advice. If you want to be healthy and strong, able to support your beloved family, and happy at work without worrying about lay-offs, just follow my advice.

First, during work you can do internal exercises. No one will notice anything different, even in a crowded office. Do Basic Breathing #3 (see page 64) or Intermediate Breathing #3 (see page 79), or toe exercises (see page 391). Take at least five to ten minutes four times a day, or whenever you feel uncomfortable. If you do them properly, you will feel the difference right away. After ten days, you will notice a difference in your whole day, not just the time after you practice your breathing, and after one hundred days they will become a healthy habit that comes as naturally as . . . well . . . breathing. You will be more energetic. You will have a fresh mind. You will enjoy your work more, and build up a better relationship with your boss and co-workers.

Second, while you are working and need more energy, take three to five minutes to do Relaxation Meditation (see page 390). After that, shake your body by practicing Rhythm Power Breathing (see pages 100 and 390) to recharge yourself.

Third, if you need more energy for yourself while doing work, you can do some light exercises at your desk without really taking a break. Your health is more important than anything else, and these quick exercises will allow you to keep working without a break when necessary. If you have the self-confidence to do them without worrying what others think, I admire you. When people notice you have a better attitude and more energy, they will naturally begin to ask how, or just figure it out for themselves and copy your movements. Don't be ashamed to share something good with others. Don't be afraid to become a leader.

Try these very simple exercises that will take three to five minutes:

381

1. Finger Chain Breathing

How to do it:

A. Sit comfortably in your chair but keep your body erect so that you can breathe into your lower abdomen. The best posture is to move your back away from the back support of your chair, but, if that is not comfortable, at least sit up straight.

B. Place your palms in front of your chest as if praying.

C. Interlock your fingers into a finger chain and extend your hands up over your head with your palms up as you inhale.

D. Release your fingers and bring your extended arms down each side as you begin to exhale.

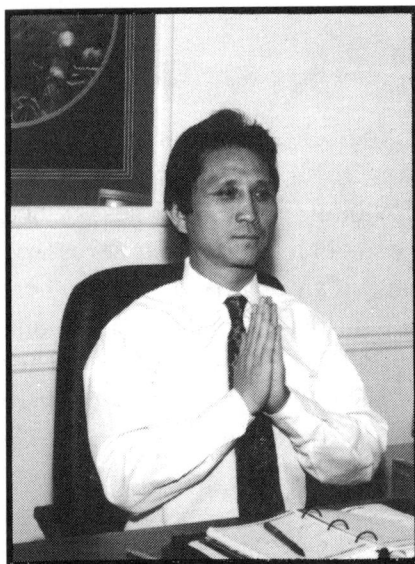

A, B

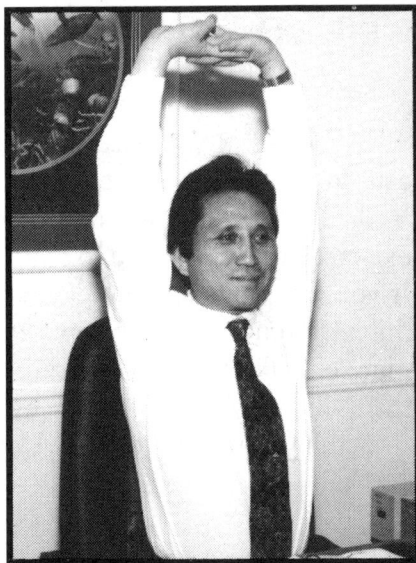

C

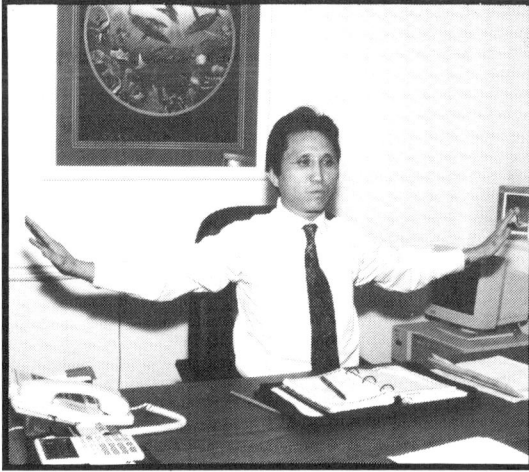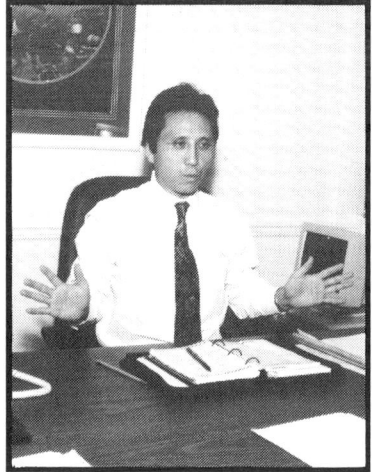

D	E

E. When your hands reach waist level, begin to inhale and bring your hands forward into position B.

F. Repeat B through E three more times.

2. Seated Shoulder Exercise:

How to do it:

A. Sit comfortably in your chair but keep your body erect so that you can breathe into your lower abdomen. The best posture is to move your back away from the back support of your chair, but if that is not comfortable at least sit up straight.

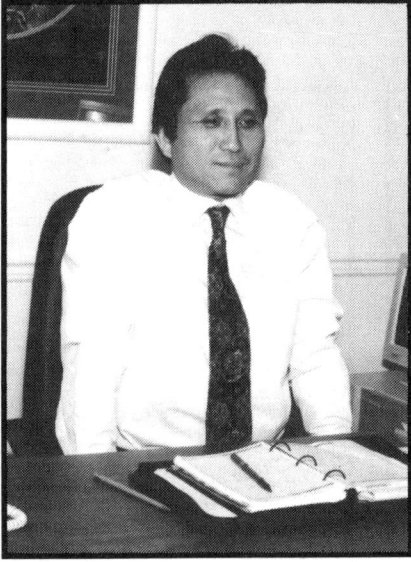

2 B (up)

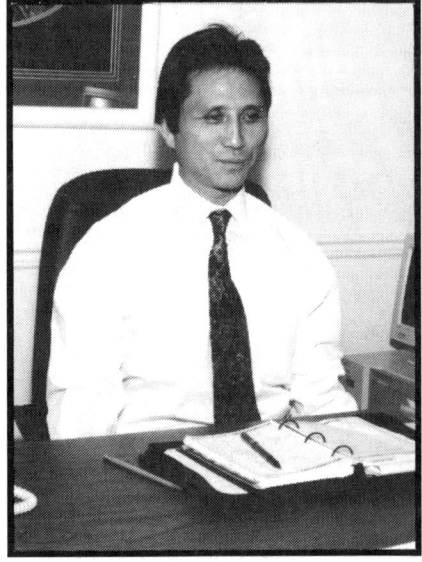

2 B (down)

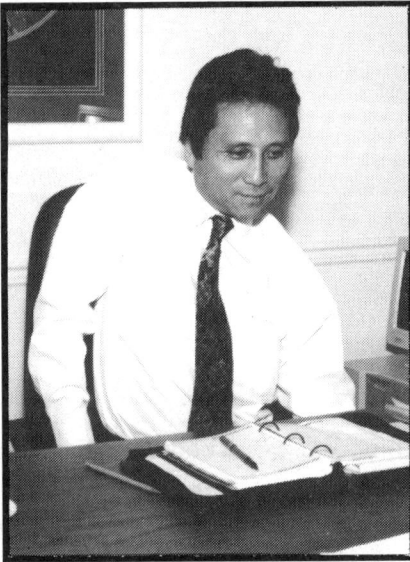

2 C & D

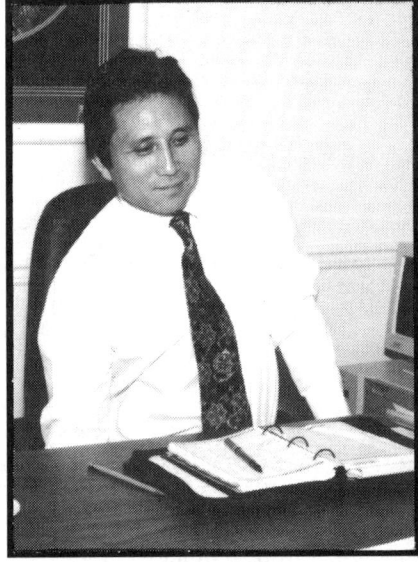

2 C & D

B. Shrug your shoulders all the way up to your ears, then let them relax (8 repetitions).

C. Alternately roll your shoulders back and up, then front and down; first roll the left shoulder forward, then the right (4 ea.)

D. Alternately roll your shoulders front and up, then back and down; first roll the left shoulder backward, then the right (4 ea.)

Caution:

Do not tighten the muscles during B; it will stop the circulation and increase the blood pressure.

3. Seated Neck Exercise

How to do it:

A. Sit comfortably in your chair but keep your body erect so that you can breathe into your lower abdomen. The best posture is to move your back away from the back support of your chair, but if that is not comfortable, at least sit up straight.

B. Inhale without moving. Exhale and slowly bend the head forward. Inhale as you bring head back up.

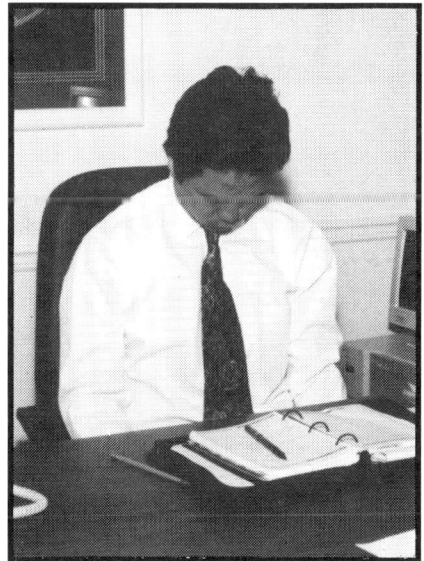

B

385

C. Exhale and slowly turn the neck to look left. Inhale and turn the head to face front.

D. Exhale and slowly turn the neck to look right. Inhale and turn the head to face front.

E. Exhale and slowly lean the head to the left shoulder. Inhale and bring head back up.

F. Exhale and slowly lean the head to right shoulder. Inhale and bring head back up.

Caution:

Neck exercises should be done very slowly.

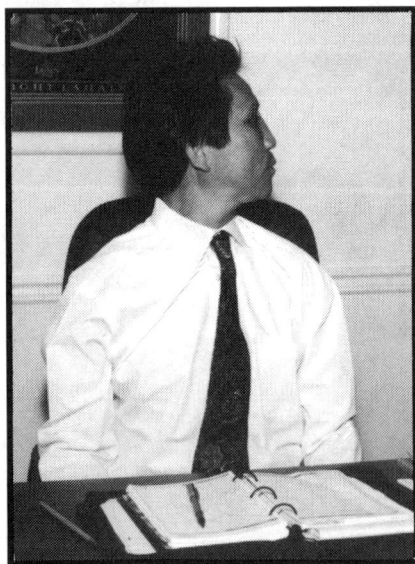

C

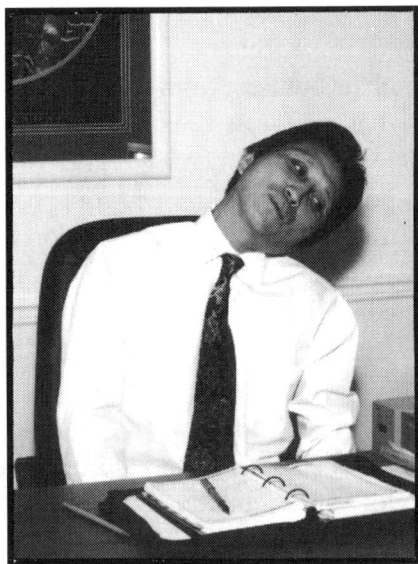

E

4. Seated Face Exercises

How to do it:

A. Sit comfortably in your chair but keep your body erect so that you can breathe into your lower abdomen. The best posture is to move your back away from the back support of your chair, but if that is not comfortable at least sit up straight.

B. Tighten all your different face muscles by:

> 1) chewing and moving your tongue over each gum, inside and outside the teeth, top and bottom,
> 2) blinking,
> 3) moving your nose and ears, separately and together in random sequence.

C. While making faces, rub your palms together to build up some heat in your hands.

D. Stop making faces and rub the *trapezius* muscles and the back of your neck with your hands.

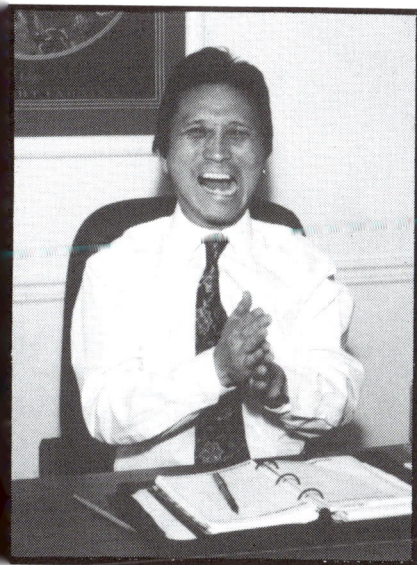

B & C

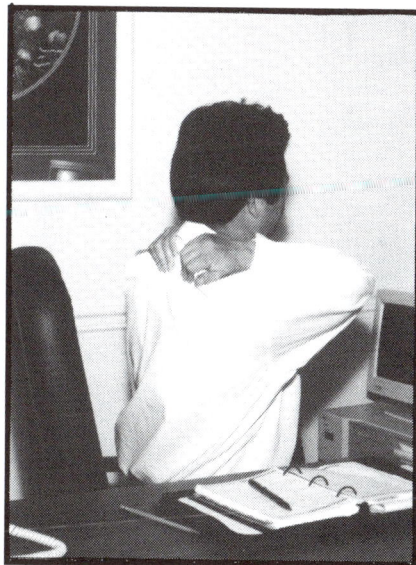

D

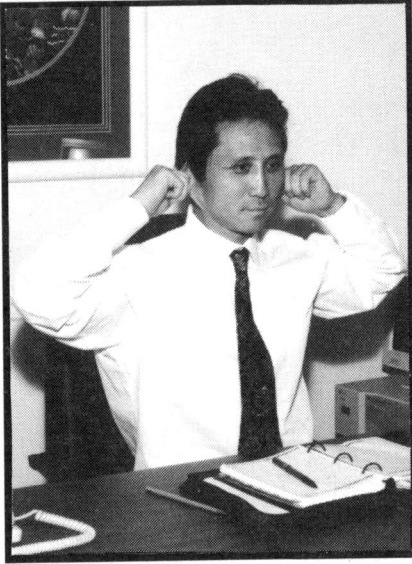

E

E. Continue to move your hands to grasp your ears between your thumb and index finger, pull lightly and massage them.

F. Rub your palms together again to build up heat, press the heel of your palms to your eyes, nose and cheeks.

G. Wash your face with air, while breathing in and out through the mouth very quickly.

H. Continue to rub and wash your scalp while breathing in and out through the mouth very quickly.

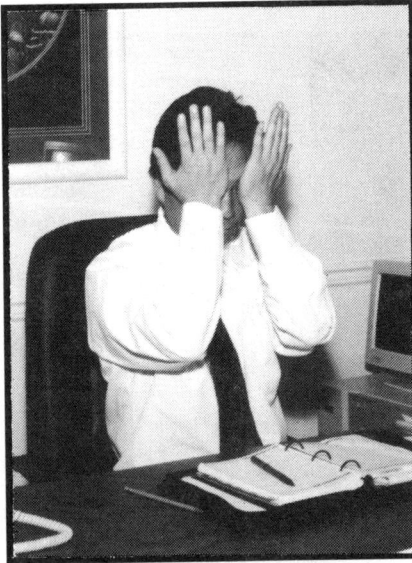

F

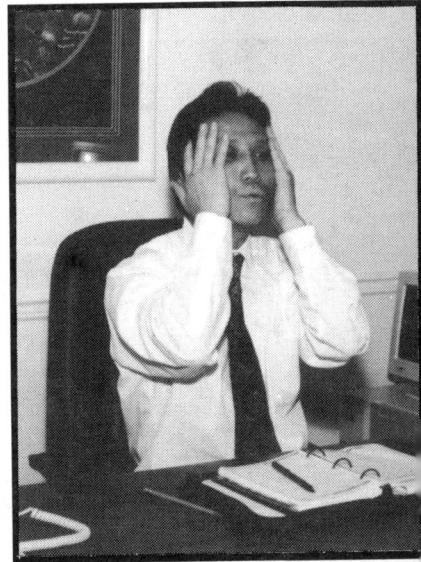

G & H

5. Seated Pull Down Exercise and Loosen Up

How to do it:

A. Sit comfortably in your chair but keep your body erect so that you can breathe into your lower abdomen. The best posture is to move your back away from the back support of your chair, but if that is not comfortable at least sit up straight.

B. Reach above your head as if grabbing a wide trapeze. Pull both hands straight down while keeping your shoulders as far back as possible. You should feel the muscles get tight across your upper back and shoulder (8 repetitions).

C. Loosen up the muscles you just tightened by placing your right hand on your left upper arm and pulling the arm across the chest. Use your left hand to pull your right upper arm across the chest. Relax and shake your shoulders a little.

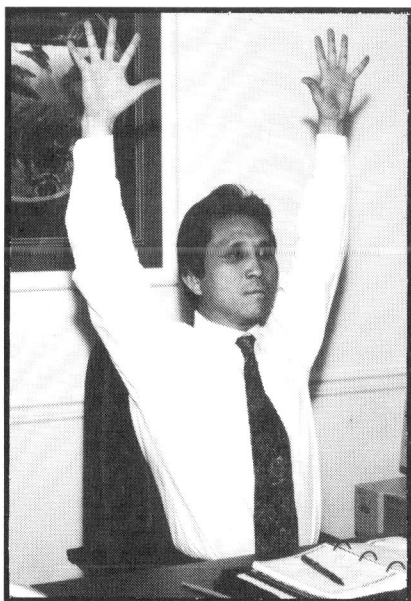

B (reach)

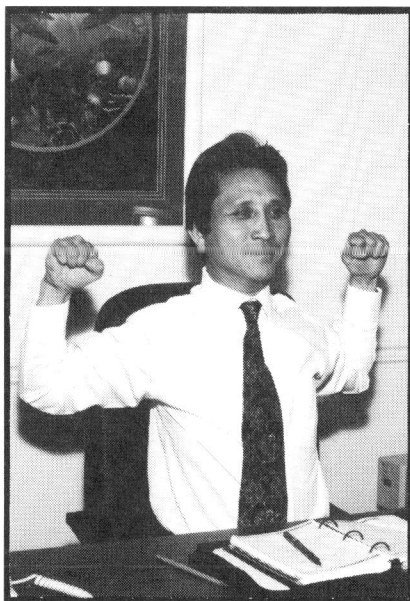

B (pull)

389

Caution:

People with bad or weak shoulders should not pull back too far; it is possible to pull a weak shoulder out of socket in this exercise.

6. Rhythm Power Breathing

How to do it:

A. Sit comfortably in your chair but keep your body erect so that you can breathe into your lower abdomen. The best posture is to move your back away from the back support of your chair, but if that is not comfortable at least sit up straight.

B. Place both hands on your lower abdomen (or on your knees, or on the chair). Inhale through the nose as deeply as possible, pulling the energy all the way to the bottom of your body.

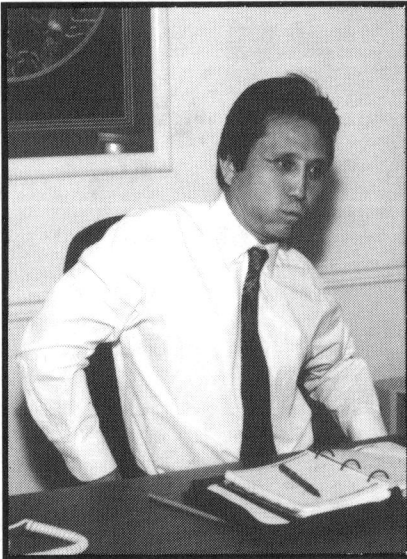

6 C (left)

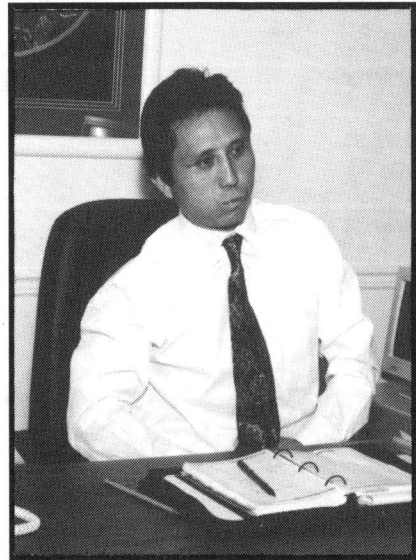

6 C (right)

C. Exhale through the mouth as long as possible (practicing either Basic or Intermediate Breathing). Keep your head still and rock your lower abdomen left to right. Continue rocking until you have exhaled all the way.

D. Repeat A and B once again, and whenever you feel indigestion, sleepy, stress, or tension.

7. Seated Toe Exercises

How to do it:

A. Sit comfortably in your chair but keep your body erect so that you can breathe into your lower abdomen. The best posture is to move your back away from the back support of your chair, but if that is not comfortable at least sit up straight.

B. You may take your shoes off or leave them on, but in either case rub your big toe against your second toe up and down eight times.

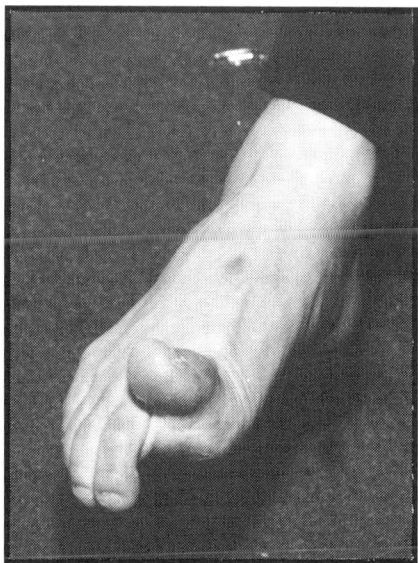 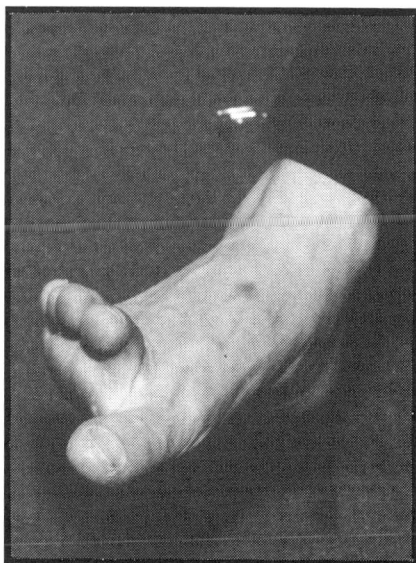

7 B (up)   7 B (down)

C. Tightly curl all your toes against the sole, then extend them as far as possible toward the instep eight times.

D. Point your toes and straighten your ankle, then flex your ankle as far as possible eight times.

E. Inhale and tighten your whole leg, from your toes to your hip, and then exhale and relax two times.

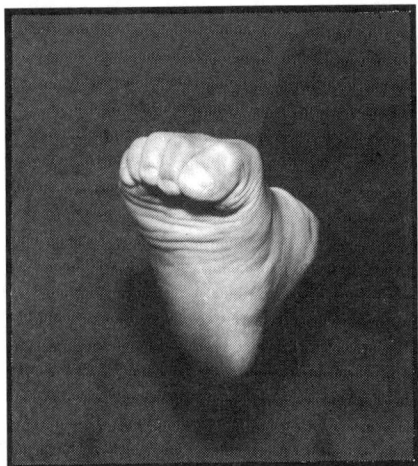

7 C (curl)

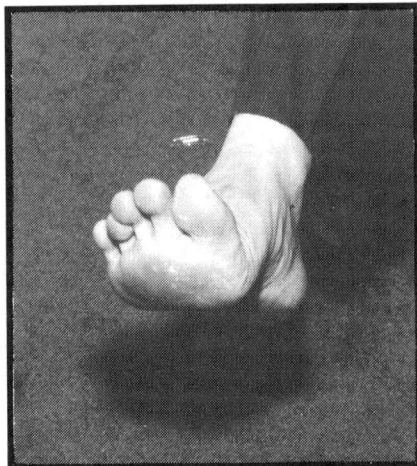

7 C (extend)

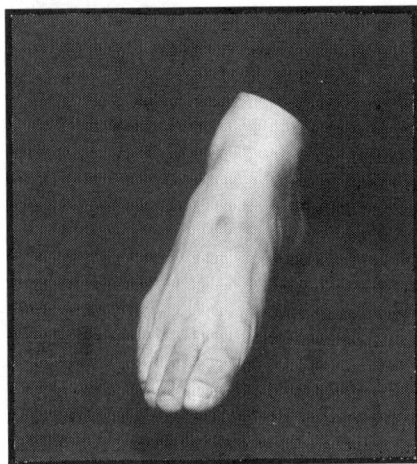

7 D (point)

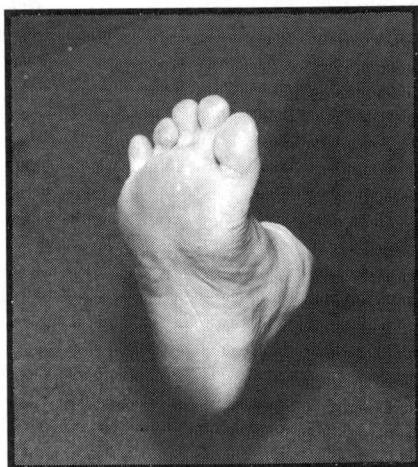

7 D (flex)

8. Seated Adjust the Spine

How to do it:

A. Sit comfortably in your chair but keep your body erect so that you can breathe into your lower abdomen. The best posture is to move your back away from the back support of your chair, but if that is not comfortable at least sit up straight.

B. Inhale and cross your right leg over your left. Look over your right shoulder, exhale, and turn as far as possible to the right, grasping the arm and back of the chair for support.

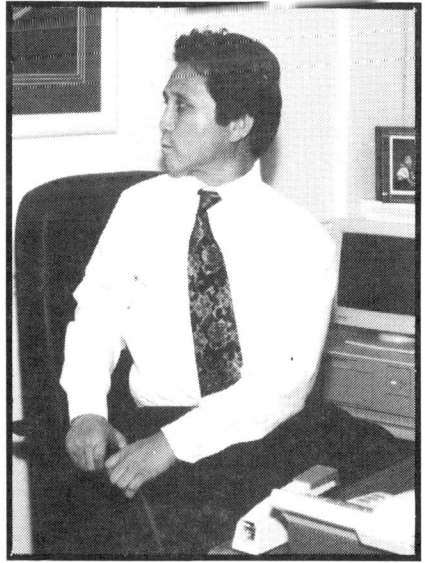

B

C. Inhale and face the front. Cross your left leg over your right.

D. Look over your left shoulder, exhale, and turn as far as possible to the left, grasping the arm and back of the chair for support.

E. Inhale and return to the front.

9. Standing Breathing Exercise

How to do it:

A. Stand up at your desk with your feet approximately shoulder width apart and your knees slightly bent.

393

B. Open your hands, cross your arms in front of you and slowly circle your arms up and over your head as you inhale through your nose into your lower abdomen.

C. Continue the circles outward and backward as you continue to inhale and expand the chest.

D. Tighten your lower abdomen and slowly exhale through your slightly opened mouth as your hands move downward and inward, while pulling in your stomach to push out all the remaining carbon dioxide and stale gas.

E. When your hands come together at the bottom, slowly inhale through your nose again, but this time keep your hands at waist height and open them outward and backward in a half circle.

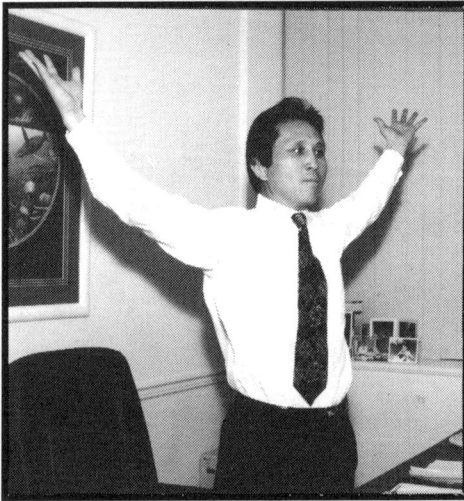

8 B

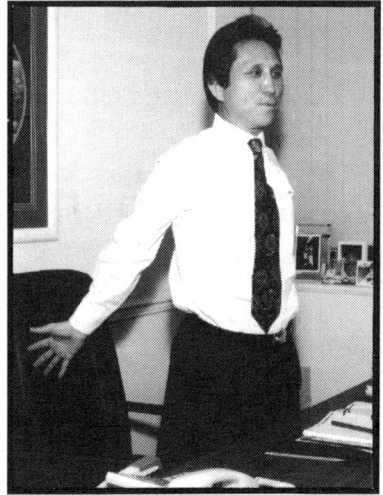

8 C

F. When you have circled outward as far as is comfortable, slowly exhale through the mouth and bring your hands inward, while pulling in your stomach to push out all the remaining carbon dioxide and stale gas.

G. Repeat B through F.

For more details on the benefits of any of these exercises, see the similar Standing Power Exercises on pages 206-237, and the Seated Power Exercises on pages 269-273.

Finish up with Basic Breathing #3, and relax. You can do these exercises in a few minutes that you might spend daydreaming. They will release a lot of tension from sitting, plus they will relax your spine, back, and legs, and massage your internal organs. They will clear your mind and give you a new burst of energy. You can add or substitute any of the Power Breathing or Power Exercises that you find work particularly well for you. You will feel great.

Fourth, if you work continually on the phone or otherwise talking with people, you will not be able to change your breathing pattern or perform Power Exercises without taking a break. When you get really tight and need to take a break before you bite off the corner of your desk, do it. Take a five to ten minute exercise break instead of a coffee or cigarette break. It will be much healthier for your body and mind, and much better for your company as your work time will be more productive. Find some spot in the hallway, in the parking lot, or anywhere and do a short version of Standing Power Exercises (see pages 206-256). Another solution for people who use the phone all the time is to get a headset -- it will save your neck and help your posture.

Finish with a Concentration Meditation (p. 166-170). You will return energized and relaxed. You will have released all your stress and tension. It will be good for you personally, good for your family, and good for your company. Invest a few minutes in your health before a problem starts. When it comes to sickness, prevention is much better than cure.

The first day you may feel a little awkward or self-conscious, depending on whether or not you can find a quiet place to begin your exercises or not. Once you begin, though, I know you will feel the difference, and continue to do it. Soon you will be telling others how to relax and get energy. You will become the office expert. With a little sharing, you will make your whole office environment healthier and happier.

Finally, I would like to recommend to you the best single exercise program I know: the martial arts. If you can find a class to attend during lunch or after work, you will not regret it. Not only will you release all the day's stress and tension before you go home, you will get physically stronger, more flexible, and aerobically fit. Mentally you will improve your self-control and concentration, and, from the mental discipline, gain better judgement. Martial arts training builds a sound body and a sound mind. It will re-charge you physically as well as mentally. It will give you self-confidence, and help you achieve your goals.

Search your area to find the best expert to teach you a complete curriculum, including traditional martial arts physical, mental, and philosophical training, as well as self-defense. Find an instructor who will really care about you, and help you balance the four corners of the foundation of your health. You will have a lot of fun and be able to enjoy your life more.

Airplane Energy Exercises

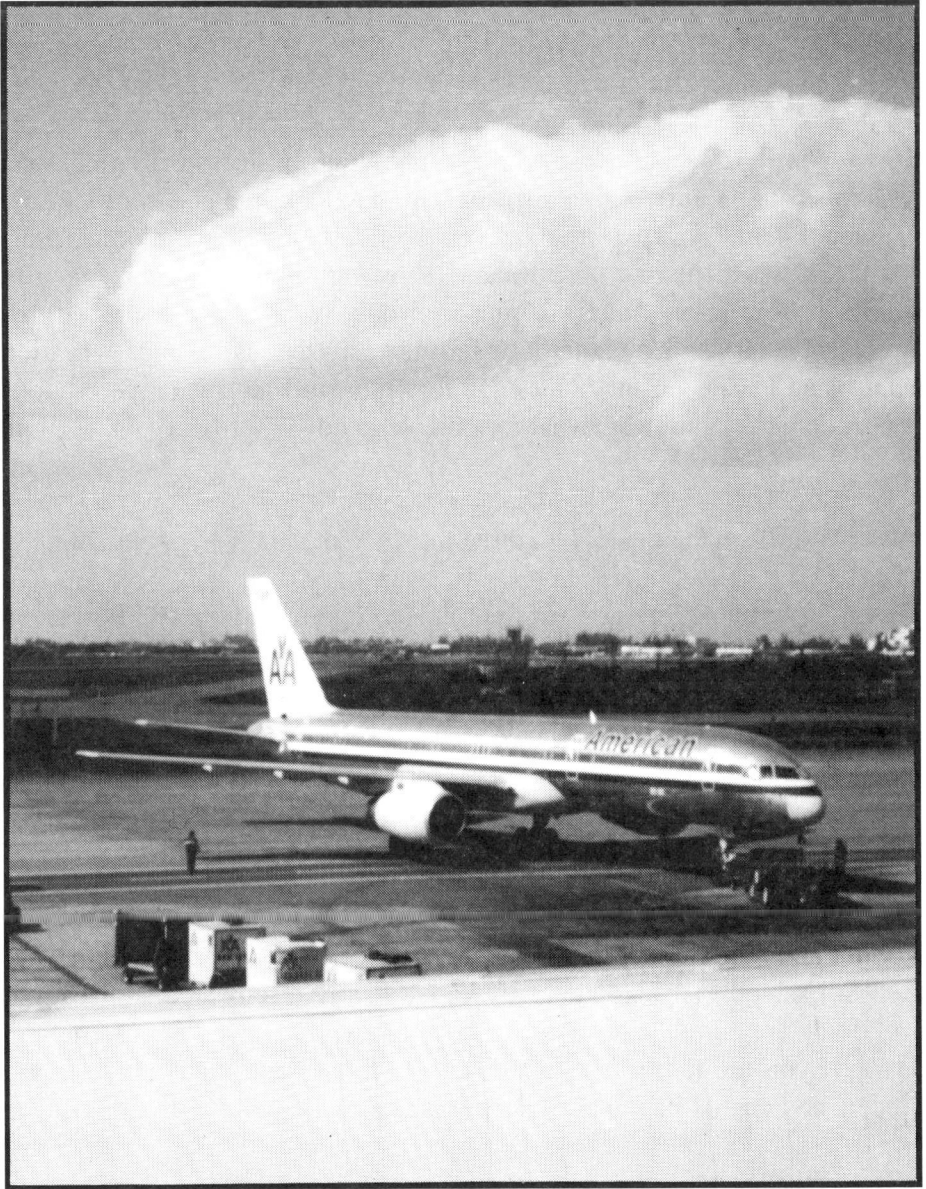

Enjoy your airplane trip and get in shape.

I've heard many times from traveling businessmen (and even vacationers) that after a long airplane trip they feel tired and bored, or that they feel like they are getting old, even though they are only middle aged.

I've seen people on airplanes showing signs of discomfort after sitting for four or six hours -- some after only two or three hours. I love long airplane trips. No matter how far the trip, I feel like I am on vacation, even when I work on the plane. Before the trip I always prepare books, pens, notebooks, and whatever work I have to do.

While on the plane, I do three things to make my trips pleasant:

1. Airplane Energy Exercises (including meditation, and Power Breathing),

2. Work or study (read and write), and

3. Sleep.

If you sit for a long time without doing anything, of course you will be tired and bored. If you are tired, do some Power Breathing to relax, and then fall asleep. At least this way you will arrive refreshed and ready to go. If you are bored, read, write, or do some work. Try to learn something new. If you are tense, do your Power Exercises and meditate. Time is golden, and cannot be replaced once it is lost.

Whenever I am in an airplane I usually see people work, read, talk, or sleep, but I never see anyone exercise. Airplanes are not a good place to jog or do high impact aerobics, but there are some simple exercises you can do to help you enjoy your trip and get in shape.

Exercises for short trips (one to three hours)

1. Seated Finger Chain Breathing (p. 382)
2. Seated Shoulder Exercise (p. 383)
3. Seated Neck exercise (p. 385)
4. Seated Face Exercises (p. 387)
5. Seated Pull Down Exercise (p. 389)
6. Rhythm Power Breathing (p. 390)
7. Seated Toe Exercises (p. 391)
8. Concentration Meditation (p. 166)

You will feel energetic and you can clear your mind for fresh ideas and thoughts to improve yourself. You will have a great mini-vacation on the airplane.

Exercises for long trips (over three hours)

1. Seated Finger Chain Breathing (p. 382)
2. Finger and Wrist Exercises (p. 210) in your seat
3. Shoulder Exercises (p. 214) in your seat
4. Neck Exercises (p. 216) in your seat
5. Face Exercises (p. 218) in your seat
6. Chest Exercises (p. 220) in your seat
7. Pull Down Exercise (p. 234) in your seat
8. Rhythm Power Breathing (p. 100)
9. Bending Power Breathing (p. 103)
10. Deep Breathing (p. 207)
11. Concentration Meditation (p. 166)

Stand up and walk around the airplane.

This Power Exercises routine will relieve all your stress and tension. You will feel much more energetic -- like you are flying. You will be able to work, sleep, or do whatever you want. If you are on a very long trip and get stiff or tense again, you can choose a few exercises and refresh yourself, or

1. Practice Power Breathing (Basic, Intermediate, or Advanced -- whichever you know), or

2. Meditate (Relaxation Meditation #3, p. 173, or Power Meditation #4, p. 178).

Wherever you go, you can always take your Power Exercises, Power Breathing, and Meditation with you. Many people say they have no time to exercise, and then they tell you that airplane trips are boring. Utilize your time. You can buy and sell the world, but you cannot buy your health. Once you lose it, it cannot be replaced. Invest your time in your health, so that you can have a future.

Do not even think about other people who might look at you or what they might think or say. As long as you do not directly bother them, your health is more important than their narrow mindedness. Airplane Energy Exercises are better than aspirin, and much better than being tired, bored, or depressed. You will have more energy, and a more positive, worthwhile airplane trip.

I hope when you read this section you do not just say, "That makes sense," and do nothing about it. I believe you will do it whenever you take a trip. Some day I hope all of the airline companies will take Y. K. Kim's advice and supply directions for Airplane Energy Exercises whenever there is a long trip. It will make the flight healthier and happier, with more smiles per mile.

You can also use these exercises on a train, a bus, a ship, or in a car whenever you have to travel long distances.

Driving Energy Exercises

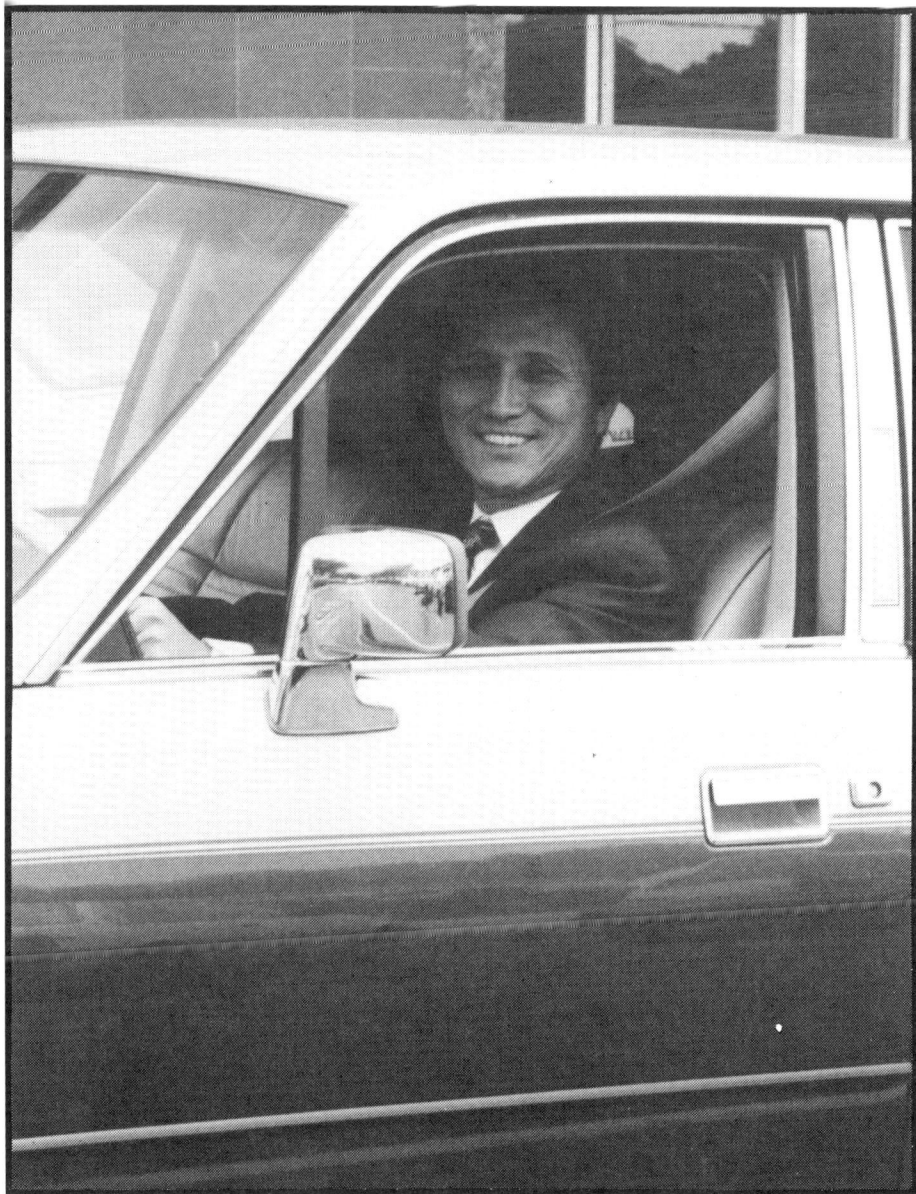

Exercise creates energy for healthy living.

Long drives make you sleepy. Watching the white lines pass by in such a consistent rhythm can even hypnotize you. Your body is still, so you do not get good circulation. This is not a healthy situation. How can you make the best of it, especially if you travel a lot in your job?

First of all, remember that the automobile is the most deadly weapon in America. Cars kill more people than guns, knives, and explosives all put together. If you catch yourself falling asleep, PULL OFF THE ROAD and take a short nap. It is better to be 10 or 20 minutes late than to not show up at all. This is a life or death decision. If you really feel you can't spare the 10 minutes, stop the car, get out, and do some quick Power Exercises to get the blood circulating again.

Second, plan to keep your mind occupied during long drives. You obviously can't read while driving, but it is no great trick to listen to educational, motivational, or inspirational tapes and still pay attention to the road. Your local library probably has a large section of cassette tapes including books on tape, motivation and self improvement, foreign language, comedy, and even good music. With a little planning, a long drive can be a restful and enjoyable experience.

Even short drives are a good opportunity to practice Power Breathing. It will refresh and relax you, and improve your internal health. If you can remember to practice Power Breathing (obviously with your eyes open) whenever you drive, it will soon become second nature. Your health will improve without taking even one second out of your busy schedule. Remember that your worst enemy is you, but your best friend is also you. You can destroy yourself or improve yourself by the simple choices you make. Make the good choice.

Here are some exercises you can do while driving. Do not attempt to do anything but drive in high traffic situations. Only do exercises on open, uncrowded roads that do not demand your full attention, or at stop lights, or on the side of the road when you pull over.

For short drives (10 to 30 minutes):

1. Do Basic Breathing #2 (p. 60) or #3 (p. 64), or Intermediate Breathing #2 (p. 76) or #3 (p. 79), with your eyes wide open and on the road.

2. Do Rhythm Power Breathing (p. 100, 390) with your eyes wide open and on the road.

3. Do the Seated Shoulder Exercise (p. 383) while keeping both hands on the steering wheel.

You will release tension and stress and get in shape while you are driving. You will feel very energetic.

For longer drives (more that 30 minutes):

1. Do Rhythm Power Breathing (p. 100, 390).

2. Do Seated Shoulder Exercise (p. 383) with both hands on the steering wheel.

3. Do Seated Neck Exercise (p. 385) in your seat as long as you keep your eyes on the road (do not turn sideways).

4. Do Seated Face Exercise (p. 387), except do not rub your hands together or massage yourself; keep your hands on the wheel.

5. Do Power Breathing while keeping your eyes wide open and on the road.

6. Stop the car at a rest stop, convenience store, or on the side of the road and do five to ten minutes of your favorite standing Power Exercises, especially those that loosen the shoulders and neck.

In our busy culture, you need to utilize your time wisely. Do not waste time during short drives: do Power Breathing and drive yourself to better health. Get the most out of long drives by making them enjoyable and educational, rather than boring. The automobile has taken away our natural exercise of walking, but it need not take away our health. Plan to get the most out of this time we spend on a regular basis.

Whenever I drive alone, I release all my stress and tension and generate lots of energy and ideas by:

1. Power Breathing.
2. Driving Energy Exercise.
3. Yelling loudly (it makes me feel fresh).
4. Laughing loudly (it makes me feel happy).
5. Rehearsing speeches.
6. Reflecting on myself and concentrating on new ideas.
7. Listening to motivational, educational, and inspirational tapes.

Whenever I am driving alone I feel like I am on a mini-vacation. When I take a long drive of more than three hours I stop the car and get out to do some light Power Exercises. I really don't care when other people look at me, as long as I know I am not bothering them. I hope you can adopt the same attitude.

Once you realize how to use your time this way, you can no longer say "I do not have time to exercise." You have plenty of time to exercise while you are doing other things, and that will give you more time to enjoy your life.

Walking Energy Exercise

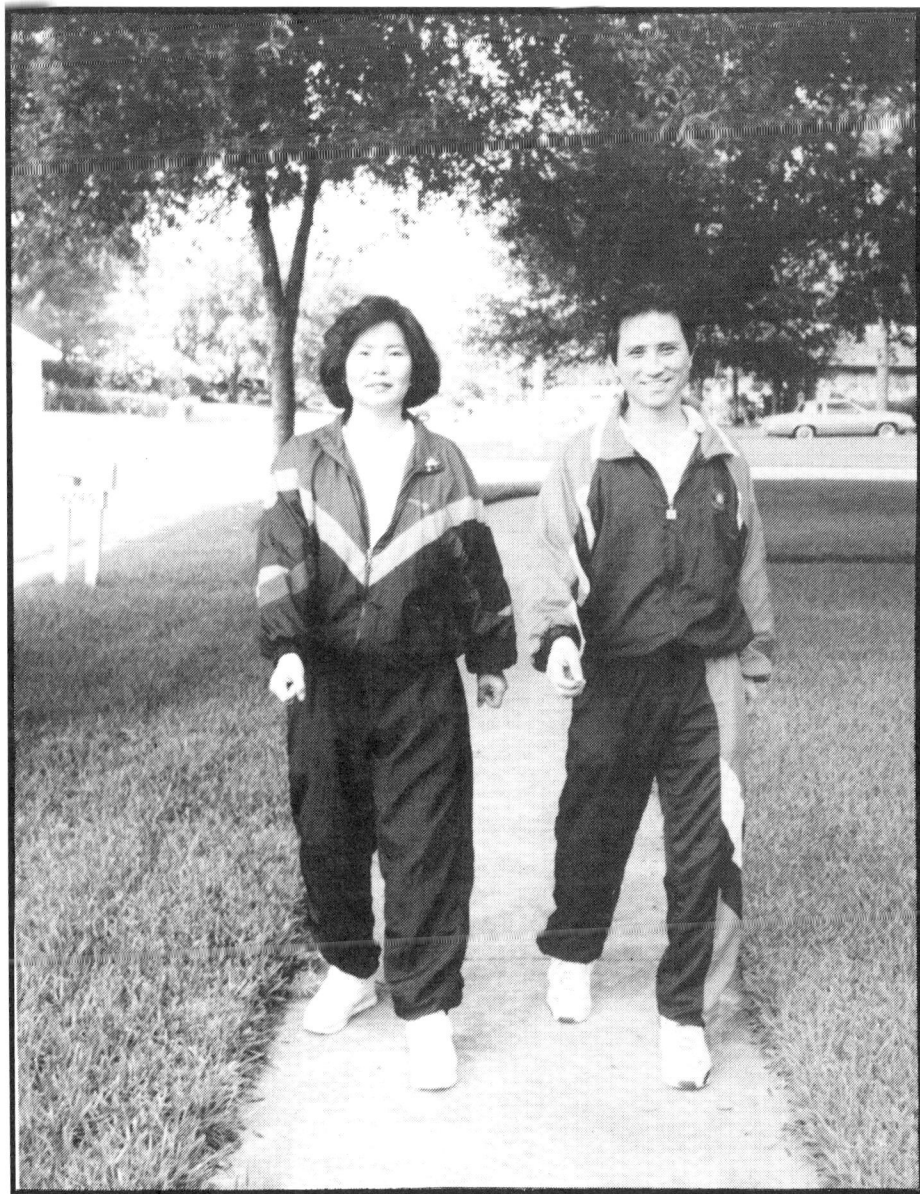

Exercise enlivens your daily life.

Walking and jogging are very popular exercises and they are good for your health because they increase the circulation and allow you to breathe fresh air while relaxing your mind. Where you walk or jog is very important, though. If at all possible, choose a time and location that will allow you to see trees and flowers, and breathe the fresh oxygen that these plants produce. If these choices are not possible, walking or jogging in the city is better than not walking or jogging at all. Just wear good shoes (modern technology has gone a long way to help us walk and run on asphalt.)

I personally walk every day. It is my vacation time. It clears my mind, and allows me to come up with some of my best ideas. It helps relieve tension and stress, builds stamina, and gives me energy. I have solved many of my business and personal problems with ideas that I had during a walk. I also practice Tae Kwon Do during my walks. It gives me a positive attitude and builds my confidence. I really don't care if somebody watches me or not. It is good for me, and it would be good for them if they would try it, too. I hope you, too, can make some time to walk every day. You will be healthier, happier, and more confident in yourself.

If you cannot schedule a separate time for walking, you can practice Power Breathing when shopping, walking to or from work, or going anywhere else. Walking is a great exercise, but we do not walk enough because of our modern technology. We drive cars, ride buses, take escalators and elevators. Not many people use their legs and feet.

If you drive somewhere, don't drive around in circles trying to find the absolute closest parking space. Intentionally park a little farther away, and get a little more exercise. It will be good for you, good for your family, and good for your company. The legs and feet were designed to walk, and when they don't, the health of the rest of the body begins to suffer. If your legs lose their strength, your whole body gets weak and subject to disease.

Walking and jogging are great natural exercises. Power Breathing and doing Power Exercises while walking or jogging will dramatically increase the benefits of both.

How to do it:

A. Inhale and open your chest, as you take two or three steps (maybe more, depending on your lung capacity.) If you are walking comfortably, breathe through the nose; if you are walking very fast you will need to breathe through your mouth. You may do Basic Breathing or Intermediate Breathing, depending on your development.

B. Exhale for the same number of steps as your inhale. Bend forward only slightly to get more air out of your lungs.

C. Repeat and continue throughout the length of your walk. You may also add many arm exercises from Standing Power Breathing (pp. 206-256) or Aerobic Self-Defense (pp. 314-377) while you are walking, or you can stop and do a short session of Aerobic Self-Defense, and then continue your walk.

Benefits:

Walking will:

* increase your circulation.
* freshen your mind.
* increase your energy level.
* reduce your weight.

I sincerely hope that when you read this section you do not just shake your head and agree with me, but put your belief into action. You can get the health benefits for yourself, and you can share the knowledge with people close to you so they can become more healthy, too.

Once again, I have to emphasize that you cannot worry what other people are thinking, or even if they say dumb things to you. As long as you do not bother anyone else, get as much benefit as you can out of your walk. If you really believe health is the most important thing in your life, do not let a little shyness get in your way.

Y. K. Kim's Walking Method

Park far away.

Use the stairs instead of the elevator.

Power Breathe while walking.

Do upper body exercises while walking.

Morning Energy Exercises

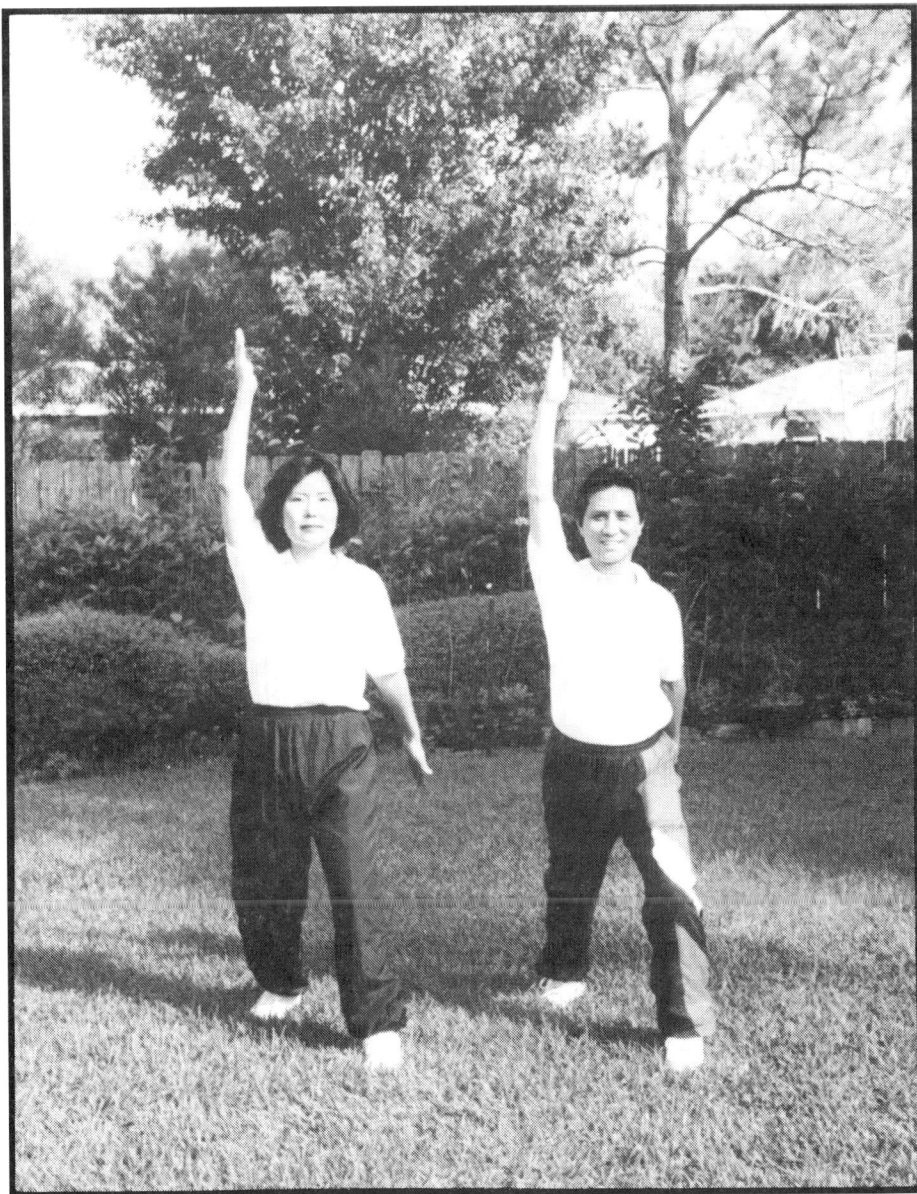

*Most successful leaders in the world
do some form of morning exercises.*

Most successful, respected, and energetic leaders in the world have one thing in common: they wake up before sunrise and do some morning exercises. Before the sun comes up you can have the most clean air (and *ki* energy) because all the dust is down on the ground.

First thing in the morning when you wake up, make yourself positive, energetic, and smile. How?

1. Go to bed before midnight, wake up before sunrise (there are many exceptions, depending on your work schedule).

2. Before you go to bed, do Night Relaxation Exercises (later in this section).

3. When you wake up, the first thing you should do is say to yourself with a big smile,

"I feel good this morning. I will have a wonderful day."

Repeat it three to five times, until you believe it. If anybody else is in your room, say,

"Good morning, _____. I feel good this morning,"

also with a big smile. Then you will have a positive attitude for the rest of the day. (It's easy to imagine what kind of day you will have if you tell yourself, *"What a lousy day. I feel terrible. I don't want to get up."*) You create your own world. Create a good one.

When you wake up, drink one third of a cup of pure water and begin your morning exercises before you do anything else. After your exercises you can drink more to begin flushing out your system.

If you ever watch a wild animal wake up, it will usually stretch it's muscles. Most of us have the same tendency, because it is a natural transition for the muscle from the resting state to the ready state.

410

Whenever you wake up, while you are still lying on your back, stretch your body like so (see pp. 293-294 for pictures):

A. Put your fingers into a finger chain,

B. Extend your hands horizontally over your head,

C. Inhale, point your toes, and stretch your whole body,

D. Exhale, release your fingers, and relax.

E. Repeat steps A through D a few times.

The most important thing is your mind, because your mind controls your body, and your body and mind have to work together. While you are stretching, you must say to yourself positive things like,

"I feel good.

"I feel wonderful this morning.

"I feel strong.

"I will have a great day today."

The first time you do it, it may feel strange. Continue to practice, and after ten days it will seem like normal, and after one hundred days it will be your healthy morning habit.

Occasionally, you will find it difficult to get out of bed. Sometimes your body wants more sleep, but you have to wake up to go to work, to school, or to honor a commitment you made. Maybe you stayed up too late working, playing (even drinking), or maybe you just feel lazy.

Have you ever noticed that if you get out of bed quickly and start the day energetically, you set the pace and have energy all day? Or have you noticed that when you sleep an extra five minutes, stumble and grumble out of bed, you set the pace and are tired all day?

The following Power Exercises will help you get your motor running so you can accomplish whatever goals you have set for the day. The most important thing to decide is how much time you will make to exercise. If you do a heavy workout later in the day, just do a short exercise session in the morning. If you do not have a vigorous workout planned later in the day, do a full exercise session first thing in the morning.

If you are only doing a short session:

Light Morning Power Exercises (approximately five minutes)

1. Deep Breathing (p. 207)
2. Finger and Wrist Exercises (p. 210)
3. Shoulder Exercises (p. 214)
4. Neck Exercises (p. 216)
5. Face Exercises (p. 218)
6. Chest and Back Exercises (p. 220)
7. Knee and Thigh Exercise (p. 225)
8. Ankle and Shoulder Exercise (p. 227)
9. Pull Down Exercise and Loosen Up (p. 234)
10. Abdomen and Back Exercises (p. 237)
11. Push-Up Stretch (p. 277)
12. Meditation (p. 163)

If you have 10 to 20 minutes:

Do a full session of Standing Power Exercises, 1-19 (pp. 206-256).

If you have 15 to 30 minutes:

Walk one to two miles with Power Breathing and upper body Power Exercises. Finish with meditation.

If you have 20 to 40 minutes:

Run one to three miles, then do a full session of Power Exercises and Meditation.

If you have 30 to 60 minutes:

Do Aerobic Self-Defense or Tae Kwon Do training and Meditation.

Following your exercises, get rid of all the junk in your system by using the toilet. Then brush your teeth, shave (if appropriate), and shower. You can get an extra internal cleaning during your shower by massaging your muscles as you wash. Don't just spread soap over the skin, but squeeze each muscle to wash the stale blood out and move fresh blood in. After cleaning your whole body with warm water, rinse with cold water. You can rinse again with warm water, and again with cold water, one, two, or three times -- whatever you feel is right.

Have a great breakfast of natural, nutritional food. You will have a great day with a positive attitude and energetic feeling every day.

Whenever you travel, please take your walking shoes and a warm-up suit with you so you can exercise during your trip.

By making a conscious effort you can change your outlook every morning to a positive and healthy one. If you share your experience with others, we can begin to make our collective dream come true: a healthier and happier world. I hope some day soon all neighbors in all towns, all cities, all states, all nations, all over the world, will get up before sunrise and come out doors and exercise together for better health every day. We can build health and smiles around us, and build a healthier America and A Healthy World.

Night Relaxation Exercises

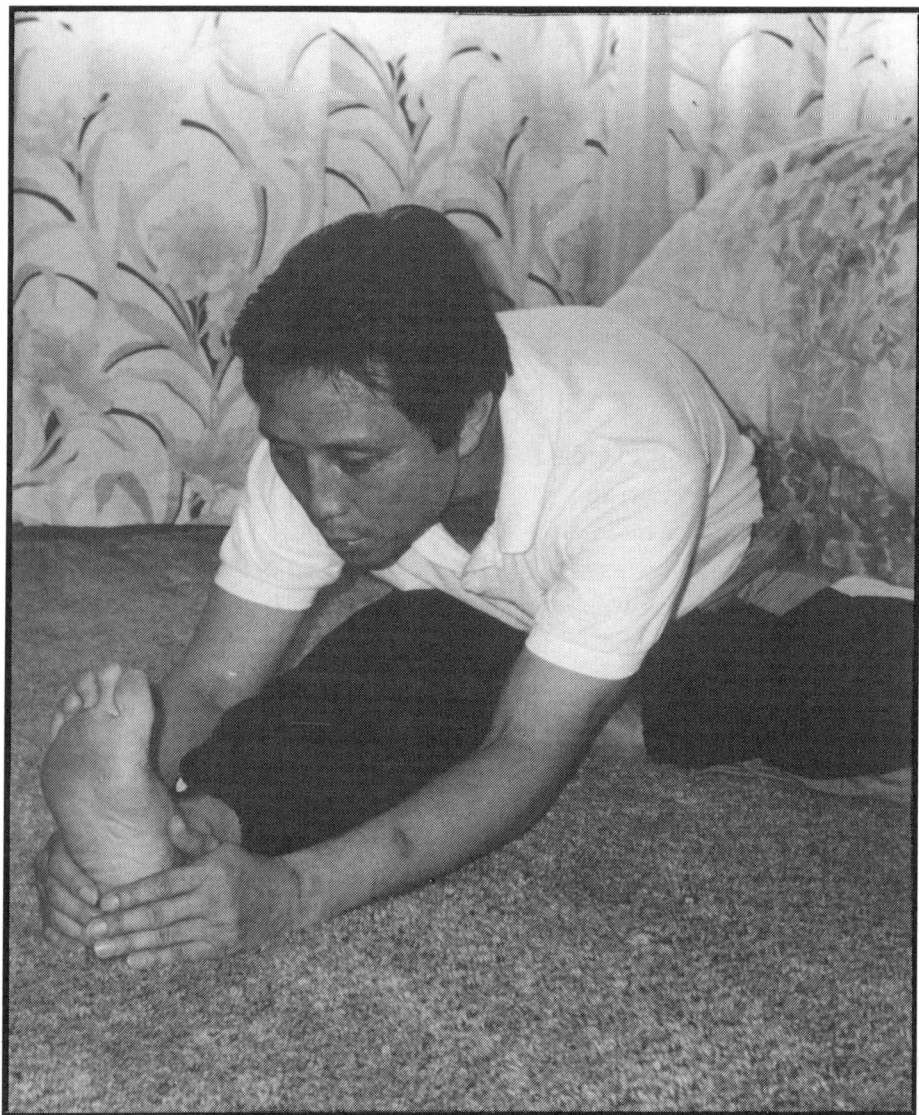

Deep, peaceful sleep is one of the best tools for relaxation and the release of stress; it will help you generate energy.

Deep and peaceful sleep will release your tension and stress and recharge your body and mind. You will be more positive and energetic.

Before you go to bed, clean your body and brush your teeth.

In order to have deep and peaceful sleep, you need:

1. A sturdy, supportive bed,

2. A good pillow, depending on your sleeping position,

3. Cool (but not cold) temperature,

4. Quiet,

5. Before you go to bed, do some exercise and meditation.

Here are some specific exercises you can do from the Seated Power Exercises:

A. Foot Massage (p. 258)
B. Single Leg Stretch (p. 260)
C. Butterfly (p. 262)
D. Open Leg Stretch (p. 263)
E. Double Leg Stretch (p. 267)
F. Seated Adjust the Spine (p. 269)
G. Rhythm Power Breathing (p. 271)
H. Finger Chain Breathing (p. 273)
F. Bending Power Breathing (p. 103)

Finish with Reflective Meditation (#2, p. 170) and Concentration Meditation (#1, p. 166), to review today and plan tomorrow.

You will have deep and peaceful dreams and the next morning when you wake up you will feel like you can fly. You will be fresh and positive, confident and energetic in what you will do today.

Once you go to bed, you can do Relaxation Meditation (#3, p. 172), Reflective Meditation (#2, p. 170), Concentration Meditation (#1, p. 166), and Power Breathing. Your mind will be relaxed, and you will be able to sleep like baby. You can become your own alarm clock, and wake up with lots of energy.

The whole idea of insomnia strikes me as nonsense. I wish I could have insomnia every night so that I could do more work. If you cannot sleep tonight, do some work. Read a book and learn something. If you are tired all day tomorrow, you will be able to sleep tomorrow night. No more insomnia.

Actually, I know I'm exaggerating, and it's not that simple. Insomnia usually means you are worried about something (although it can mean you took too much caffeine late in the day). If your mind is overworked but your body is not really tired, you will not sleep comfortably. You need to make your body as tired as your mind so that you are balanced and able to sleep.

The best exercises to do in the middle of the night are Power Exercises with Power Breathing. You can do them right in your bedroom and they will calm your mind (and take it off of whatever you are worried about). The improved circulation will restore your system to balance, and let you sleep.

When you finish your power exercises, lie down on the bed and do Relaxation Meditation and Concentration Meditation. You should be relaxed and fall asleep quiet easily.

Another thing to do is read a book while doing deep breathing exercises. The breathing will relax your body and mind, and the reading will take your mind off of your worries and tire your eyes. You will drift off soon enough.

416

The best prevention for insomnia is to work out hard during the day. People who do physical labor or who practice an extremely active sport or martial art like Tae Kwon Do rarely have trouble sleeping. Intense exercise is the best medicine for insomnia

Whatever you do, do not take sleeping pills or potions. I see television advertisements for insomnia medicine almost all the time. We could save a lot of money that we spend on these medicines and get in better shape at the same time by practicing Power Exercises, Power Breathing, or Tae Kwon Do.

I hope you have deep sleep and peaceful dreams starting today. You will be able to relax and recharge your energy.

HEALING POWER

Generally speaking, we create our world with our minds. If we see ourselves as healthy, we take the steps necessary to become healthy. If we see ourselves as sickly, we notice every little ache and pain and turn it into a plague. We've all heard stories of people who heal themselves of terminal diseases like cancer through positive thinking. They believe they will get better, and they do. The doctors can only call it a "miracle." I call it the power of positive thinking.

Fortunately, I never had cancer, but my living nightmare was as close as I ever want to come. I was as stiff as a board, stuck in my bed, and suffering excruciating pain. I didn't know if I would ever recover enough to walk, much less regain my full health. If I did not believe in myself, and if I did not think positively, I might never have recovered.

In order to heal ourselves, we first need to have a positive or healthy mental attitude. We have to want to be healthy. If we want to heal ourselves, another important factor is our past, and the foundation we have built our health upon. If your health has been built by balancing the four corners of the foundation of health, and you have developed the positive habits of the nine steps to health, you will have a strong body that will heal quickly from any disease. If your body is weak from misuse and abuse, it will not heal quickly, if at all.

We know that prevention is better than cure, but if sickness has already struck, what can you do to heal it as soon as possible?

To utilize your body's natural healing power:

1. Find the cause of your problem.
2. Stop or otherwise remedy the cause.
3. Balance the four corners of the foundation of your health.
4. Develop the positive habits of the nine steps to health.
5. Achieve and then maintain harmony with your nature.

1. Find the cause of your problem.

How can we diagnose internal sickness?

If you already know what is the cause of your sickness, you can move on to step two and try to remedy the cause. If you feel sick but cannot identify what is wrong, the following information may be useful to you:

In Eastern medicine each organ has positive or negative energy, and the balance between the organs and their positive and negative *ki* will affect your total health. Any imbalances will show up in specific symptoms, especially in the face. Please understand that I am not trying to make sweeping generalizations about people with yellow, white, or black skin because of their race. The tints I mention are in addition to whatever skin color a person may have when he is healthy. Caucasians with weak lungs are not just naturally white, but unnaturally pale. Even an Oriental's skin, which is yellow to begin with, turns a dull, sickly yellow when he has spleen problems.

Here is a very brief summary of this kind of diagnosis:

A. A person whose face has a blue tint, has a bad temper, has weak eyes, and neck pain may have a weakness in the liver or gall bladder.

B. A person whose face has red blotches, who feels weak during hot weather, and whose tongue is weak or clumsy may have a weakness in the heart or small intestines.

C. A person whose face has a yellow tint and no shine, who dislikes moisture so that rainy days are uncomfortable, and who thinks too much may have spleen and stomach problems.

D. A person whose face is pale and has no color from healthy blood circulation, who is depressed, and who suffers during times when the air is dry (especially in the autumn) may have lung problems.

E. A person whose face has a black tint and no shine, and who is uncomfortable in cold weather may have a kidney problem.

If you recognize any of these symptoms in yourself, see your doctor right away and follow his advice. In the mean time, follow the nine steps to health and establish a balance in the four corners of the foundation of your health to begin healing your sickness.

Later in this chapter I address some specific common health problems like headaches, back pain, and stomach aches. I examine each one for its individual causes. If you are suffering from one of these problems, perhaps I can help you identify the cause.

As I mentioned earlier, the leading cause of most modern sicknesses is stress. If you are suffering and cannot find the cause, ask yourself if you could be suffering from some form of stress.

2. Stop or otherwise remedy the cause.

If you can identify the cause as something that you are doing (for example, eating too much), then simply stop doing that.

If you can identify the cause as something you are not doing, (for example, not exercising at all), then simply start doing what you need to do.

If you can identify the cause as something that is a result of your environment (for example, stress), then change the environment to a more healthy one.

If you can identify the problem as something internal (for example, a vertebrae out of place), then get someone who can put it back in the right place.

Whatever you have identified as the cause, just fix it. However, be careful that you identify the real cause. The cause of your headache may be tight muscles in your neck. Loosening up those muscles may relieve your headache, but unless you go one step farther and find the cause of the tight muscles (like stress) and remedy it, the muscles will just get tight again.

420

3. Balance the four corners of the foundation of your health.

A. Release all your mental fat, which is your negative thinking, and build up a positive, healthy mental attitude through self-discipline. Meditate and send more *ki* to the specific area of your sickness to begin the cure (see pp. 178-188). It will help heal you much more than you expect.

B. Increase the supply of fresh oxygen and blood circulation throughout your body to strengthen your internal organs and quiet your nervous system through Power Breathing.

C. Nourish your body so that it can fight off the sickness and rebuild healthy tissue by eating natural, nutritional food.

D. Release stress and tension, and get rid of all waste products from your body, while you strengthen your joints and muscles by doing Power Exercises. Begin the day with morning exercises, do a full Power Exercises with gentle movements sometime during the day, and do the Night Relaxation Exercises before you go to sleep.

4. Develop the positive habits of the nine steps to health.

Identify the good and bad habits that affect your health. Take your bad habits and change them into good habits, one at a time. Step by step improve yourself and your health until you have reached harmony with your nature.

5. Achieve and then maintain harmony with your nature.

Once you have balanced the foundation of your health, and changed your bad habits into good habits, you will have the best prevention and healing power on earth on your side: nature. Unfortunately, you can throw your body out of balance, create bad habits, and unbalance your foundation very easily, if you are not careful. Health is a lifelong process. You do not achieve it once and enjoy it forever. You must constantly be aware of what you are doing and what is happening to you in order to maintain it. If you do, you will remain healthier, stronger, and more confident, and live a long, happy life.

How to Quit Smoking

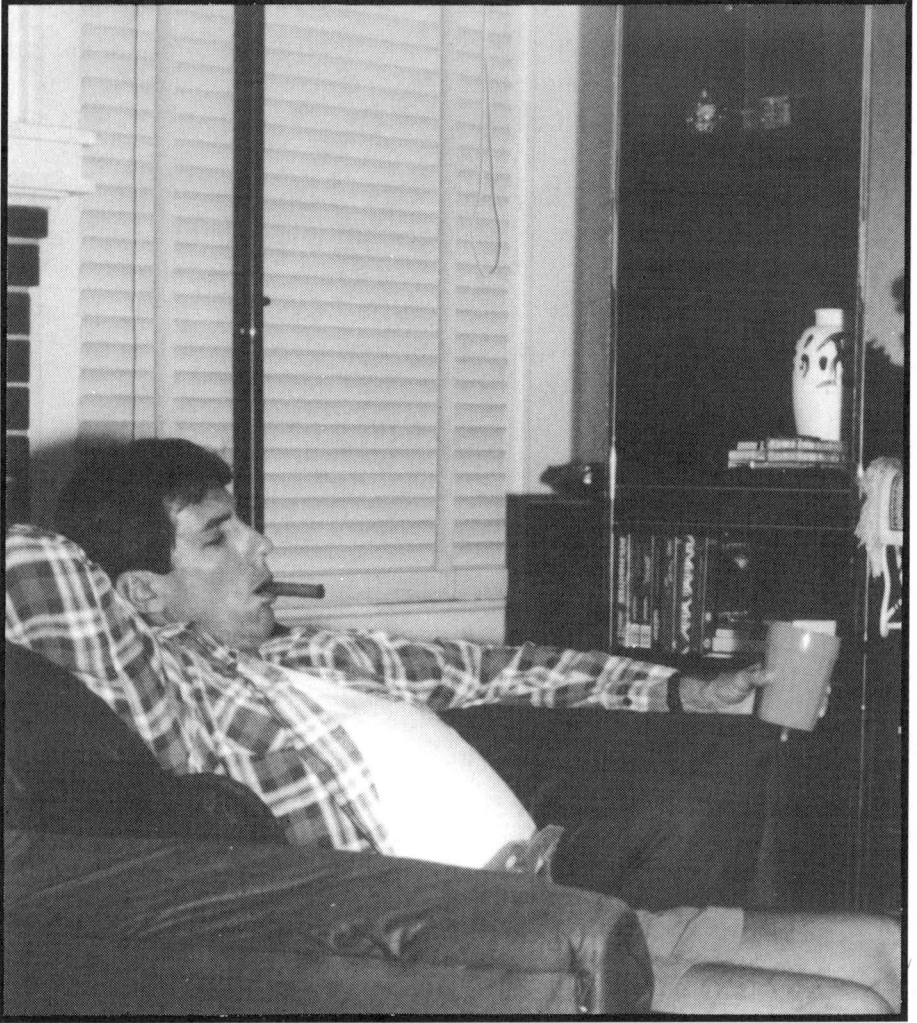

"Throw away your cigarettes, lighters, and ash trays NOW. Do not beg, borrow, or buy any more.

"Kick out your bad habits, and get in shape. Become a winner in your life."

-- Y. K. Kim

Quitting smoking is fun and exciting.

If you want to quit, you are already a non-smoker. If you do not want to quit, you will never quit. If you are afraid to quit, you will smoke more than before.

To quit smoking you have to quit now. I mean RIGHT NOW. Throw away all the cigarettes that you have, all the lighters, and all your ash trays.

Instead of smoking, do Power Breathing:

1. Exhale through the mouth, and count from one to seven.
2. Inhale as deeply as possible through the nose and count from one to seven.
3. Repeat for about five minutes.
(See "Power Breathing", p. 178-188, for more details.)

Whenever your body wants a cigarette, do Power Breathing. It will clean out your lungs and strengthen your internal body.

I was once dumb enough to smoke three packs of cigarettes a day. I was slowly destroying myself with cigarettes. I am glad that I am a non-smoker, now.

Let's look at why you need to quit smoking:

1. Smoking is a dirty, unhealthy, and rude habit. It does not make you look sexy. It does not make you more attractive to others. It makes you smell bad, and gets that smell all over other people's food, clothes, and hair. Is that something worth dying for?

Instead: Quit now and do Power Breathing whenever you feel the urge for a cigarette.

2. Smoking has been established beyond reasonable doubt to be connected with bad health. The nicotine is a foreign substance to the body that acts as a stimulant. The tar builds up on the lungs to prevent them from absorbing oxygen. Most commercial tobaccos contain large amounts of sugar, which some believe contributes more to lung cancer than either

the tar or nicotine. No matter how you look at it, smoking reduces the amount of oxygen available to the body, and, therefore, reduces the effectiveness of the blood circulation. Plus, the white blood vessels of the immune system are greatly reduced, lowering your ability to fight off diseases. One recent study has even established a link between smoking and lower back pain. If this sounds like a good health program to you, I recommend you start smoking double the number of cigarettes you are smoking now. You can spend the rest of your life in bed or in the hospital.

Instead: throw away all cigarettes, don't buy any more, and don't borrow any more. Begin practicing Tae Kwon Do to improve your self-image and physical health.

3. Smoking costs you a lot of extra money and extra bother. You always need to have a pack of cigarettes and a lighter in your pockets. You always need to look for ashtrays. There are many places that are designated non-smoking areas, and you feel like a third class citizen, sneaking into bathrooms or going outside to smoke. This gives you a lower self-image and unnecessary emotional trouble. In addition, you are contributing to the pollution of the environment of our beautiful earth. If these are the things you want, then do not even bother to read this book any more.

Instead: Spend your money on self-improvement: for example, join a Tae Kwon Do school or a fitness center. Increase your freedom and build your self-esteem.

In order to quit smoking, the main thing is to WANT to quit smoking. If you don't want to quit, nothing will make you quit. Once you have a good reason, then you can do it. What exactly is a good reason? That varies for different people. Some people cannot quit for themselves, but they can quit for someone else. For example, a lot of young ladies quit smoking when they become pregnant, because of the research that has shown what smoking can do to the unborn child. Oddly enough, once the baby is born, they start smoking again. Other people quit when someone they know dies of lung cancer. Others just make the decision and do it. Whatever is a good reason for you, you have to find a good reason to break the habit.

If you can picture yourself without cigarettes, and you believe you can successfully quit, you can. If you tell yourself you'll never be able to quit, you'll believe yourself and make your belief come true.

One complicating factor is that nicotine is addicting. You actually go through withdrawal. You become tense, irritable, and your body "gets hungry" for a cigarette. On the other hand, sugar is also addicting; so is alcohol. If you have a good reason to quit, you can do it. Just throw away all your cigarettes. Don't buy any more, don't borrow any more. Practice Power Breathing to calm yourself down and clean out your lungs. Your body will return to its natural state of health and balance.

I am very glad to have helped many people quit smoking. Quitting smoking is an opportunity to become a winner or a loser in healthy living. Quitting smoking is very simple, yet it is a fun and worthwhile endeavor. It is fun because it is a chance to compete within yourself, and worthwhile because it is a chance to embark on a constructive lifestyle.

How to quit:

Do not try to reduce smoking and do not wait. Quit right now and throw away all your smoking paraphernalia: lighters, ash trays, etc. Start doing Power Breathing whenever you feel the need to smoke. The first five to ten days the nicotine will still be in your body and you will have to fight with yourself. How can you win?

1. Create a clear mental picture of yourself as a non-smoker, free from cigarettes and their addiction.

2. Meditate. Intentionally visualize that you are throwing away all nicotine from your body. Create a clear mental picture that you are drawing all of the nicotine to your lungs and then breathing it out. Do this visualization meditation for ten minutes at least three times a day (see p. 178).

3. When your body wants a cigarette, drink a glass of pure water.

4. Avoid drinking alcohol, eating fatty foods, and any other substances that will weaken your resolve and stimulate your desire to smoke.

425

5. Develop new habits: keep your mind busy by doing physical activities: exercising, walking, cutting the grass, cleaning the house, climbing mountains, swimming, etc. Another option, if you are at home, is to shower with cold water. The best form of exercise for your body, mind, and spirit is Tae Kwon Do.

6. Tell yourself and tell as many other people as possible, especially those who care about you, that you have quit. Get your pride involved, so that you will be ashamed to tell these people that you have started smoking again.

Say things like,

"I am glad I am a non-smoker.

"How could I have smoked like that before? It is a dirty, unhealthy habit that puts smoke and ashes everywhere. Plus, many people die of lung cancer."

Think of all the negative things you can about smoking, and say them out loud. Then say some positive things about the future like,

"I am so happy and proud I am now a non-smoker.

"I am a winner and can do whatever I believe in. I am strong."

7. Avoid spending time with friends who smoke and avoid going to smoking areas like lounges, smoking movie theaters, smoking sections of restaurants, etc., until the nicotine is gone from your system.

8. Whenever you get the urge to smoke, think about all of the things that you dislike about yourself. Think of all the reasons you should be ashamed of yourself. Think of all the things you most hate in life. Go beyond that and think of the worst, most vile, and disgusting things you can possibly think of, and associate all of these things with smoking. Say things in your own mind like,

"When I smoke, it is like having sex with my mother -- totally against nature."

426

When you do this, you will associate smoking with all these negative thoughts and disgusting feelings, and your desire to smoke will go away.

After forty to one hundred days the nicotine will be completely gone from your system, and you will not have to deal with the physical addiction any longer. The desire to smoke will go away forever.

If you do not stick to your promise to yourself and to the people you love, you will be ashamed. You will suffer stress because you did not live up to your own expectations. You will be embarrassed to see the people you told, and ashamed when you are alone, because you know you gave up. You will have the quitting habit. You will spend the rest of your life in fear of other people and of your own weakness. You will think negatively about your future because you know you are weak and cannot finish what you set out to do. You will be unhappy with yourself and your life.

On the other hand, when you succeed in quitting smoking, you will have the knowledge that you changed your whole life. You will have a well-deserved confidence in yourself and your strength of will. You will not only be proud of yourself, you will believe in yourself. It will give you the winning habit and a positive mental attitude throughout your life. You will not be afraid to meet any challenge for the rest of your life because you will know you have the strength to succeed in anything you set your mind to. You will be happier with yourself and happier with your life.

Kick your bad habits and get in shape!

How to Quit Drugs, Alcohol,
or other addictions

I have never personally suffered from drug addiction or alcoholism, but the principles of overcoming any bad habit, even a physically addicting one, are the same as smoking. You can kick all your bad habits, one at a time, following the procedure I outlined to quit smoking.

Relieving Lower Back Pain

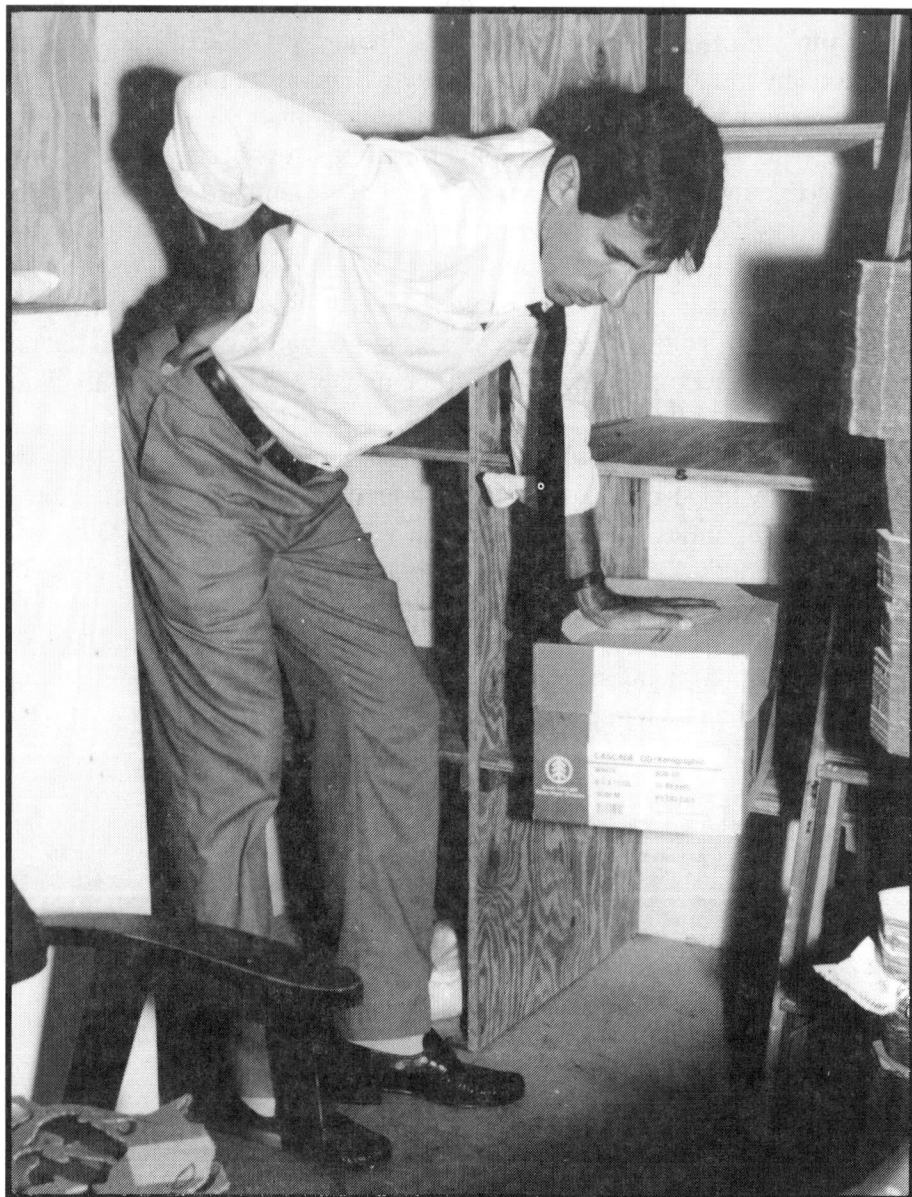

You must do your back exercises every day or the pain will come back.

Lower back pain is the most common health problem in the U.S.A. today. One health magazine has reported that seventy-five per cent of American citizens suffer from lower back pain.

I believe it because I was one of them. I still have my lower back pain, and I know it will never go away for the rest of my life. I have to live with it, but it does not bother me because I know how to keep myself strong.

The lower back is the center of the body. It is vitally important because every major movement of the body involves the lower back. If you lose the mobility of the lower back, you will be bedridden. Your mind will still move, but your body will not follow it.

If you currently suffer from lower back pain, do not worry. You will be O.K., just like me. I was worse than anybody I know. I could not work because I had to stay home in bed; I could not move . . . I could not even go to the bathroom. I still have the problem, but it does not hinder me at all. I have recovered and I lead a normal life. I work harder than ever. I can even do jump spinning kicks again. This is one of the biggest reasons I worked day and night to write this book: I want to share my experience with each one of you. I believed I had the power to heal myself. If you believe you have the power to heal yourself, you will be more than O.K. for the rest of your life, as long as you take the necessary steps to heal and stay healthy. Just like eating: if you don't eat every day, you will lose your health; if you eat the wrong food, you will get sick. If you do not do your back exercises every day, you will lose your mobility; if you do the wrong exercises, you will hurt yourself. Follow my simple program every day and you will be very happy, like I am.

If you are suffering from lower back pain, here's what to do:

1. You have to find the cause of the lower back pain. If the pain is muscle related, you may be able to discover it in the following pages. If there is a structural problem in the bones, you will need to consult a medical doctor, chiropractor, or other specialist.

2. Remove the cause to allow your back to heal.

3. Strengthen your back to prevent future pain.

If you do not find the cause, you can hide the pain with pain killers, but the pain will come back soon enough. I was dumb enough to suffer lower back pain for years without realizing that stress was the cause. I took pills and kept adding more stress, and did not do the right exercises to relieve it. It was a one way street that went the wrong way.

Lets look at some common places where lower back pain can start or be aggravated, so that we can find the cause and fix it:

1. Your bed: the mattress is too soft or not supportive.

Solution: change your bed. Get a new bed, new mattress, or put a support under your mattress. If you cannot afford any of those options, just sleep on the floor until you can.

2. Your shoes: heels can create an unnatural arch in your back; any unpadded shoe on concrete can jar your spine.

Solution: change your shoes. Wear flat shoes as much as possible. Wear padded, supportive shoes for walking, running, or playing sports.

3. Your posture: leaning forward or slumping backward instead of sitting straight can strain back muscles.

Solution: Sit straight. Gravity pulls consistently downward. If you keep your back straight, with your head directly on top, you can cooperate with gravity to balance your body. If you lean in any direction, you must fight gravity to keep upright.

4. The way you work at home:
        A. Bending too long to clean the house.
        B. Leaning forward to wash the dishes.
        C. Lifting heavy objects.
        D. Carrying children.

Solutions:

A. Do not bend at the waist; stand straight when vacuuming, etc. Use the proper equipment: brooms, mops, and other tools with long enough handles.

B. Wear cushioned shoes and balance on one foot (shift from one foot to the other every once in a while) while washing dishes.

C. Bend your legs, not your back, in order to use the large muscles in your legs to lift, rather than the smaller muscles of the back.

D. When carrying the baby, shift the baby and your own weight on to one foot (shift from one foot to the other every once in a while).

5. The way you work at your job:
    A. Using only one side, like a golfer or a carpenter.
    B. Lifting heavy objects with the back.
    C. Sitting too long with bad posture.
    D. Working with bad posture.

Solutions:

A. Whenever possible, learn to work with both sides. When impractical (like golf), do a proper warm-up and stretch before you use your back, and do other exercises to balance your muscular development.

B. Get a support belt to support your lower back if you do a lot of lifting, and always bend your knees and not your back to use the large muscles in your legs instead of the small muscles in your back.

C. Sit straight and do Office Energy Exercises (see p. 379)

431

D. Use good posture whenever possible. When not possible, warm-up before you begin, and every five or ten minutes, stand up and do a light loosening up exercise.

6. Your weight: excess weight strains your back.

Solution: Lose weight through diet and exercise (see Natural Nutritional Food, p. 121 and Aerobic Self-Defense, p. 314).

7. Your exercise program:
   A. Moving cold, stiff muscles too hard, too fast.
   B. Improper stretching or warm-up exercises.
   C. Letting the heel strike the ground when walking, running, or jumping.

Solutions:

   A. Always warm-up before doing intense exercise.

   B. Do Power Exercises as a warm-up and follow the cautions for each exercise.

   C. Run and jump on the balls of your feet. Whenever the heel strikes the ground with any force, it jars the bones of the back.

8. Your body development: just recently doctors have been noticing that a substantial number of people have one leg longer than the other, causing uneven pressure on spine.

Solution: Consult your health care professional to get the appropriate size lift to make your legs even.

9. Your sleeping conditions: if you sleep in cold temperature, your muscles become hard and tight with the cold.

Solution: Either sleep in warmer conditions (turn up the heat or use more blankets) or do Morning Energy Exercises (see p. 409) to loosen up.

10. Your pregnancy: carrying a baby can strain your lower back.

Solution: Strengthen your lower back in the early stages of your pregnancy, in preparation. If you did not prepare, stretch and strengthen the lower back by gradually increasing to a full Power Exercises program every day.

11. Your temper: losing your temper makes your body tense.

Solution: control your temper. If you still get too tense, Meditate, or do Power Exercises or Aerobic Self-Defense to work off some of the anger.

12. Your travel patterns: you spend too long in a car, bus, train, or airplane.

Solution: Sit with good posture and do Airplane Energy Exercises or Driving Energy Exercises.

13. Your gear: you carry a bag, whether it's a briefcase, suitcase, lunch box, book bag, or gym bag.

Solution: switch hands, so that you carry it half of the time in each hand.

14. Smoking: a recent research project has linked smoking with lower back pain.

Solution: quit smoking (see pp. 422-427).

15. Stress: is the greatest cause of back pain in modern cultures.

Solution: relieve stress by Power Breathing, meditation, Power Exercises, and proper nutrition.

16. <u>Unbalanced exercise program</u>: you only develop one side in your exercise program -- for example, a martial artist who kicks mostly with one leg, or a weight lifter who only develops his upper body.

Solution: always follow a balanced training regimen, doing equal exercises with the left and right sides, and the upper and lower halves.

You must realize that there is probably one main cause for your back pain, but, like most people in modern American society, you probably have several contributing factors that further aggravate your problem.

Solution: Remove as many of the above mentioned causes from your daily routine as possible. Do Power Exercises and Power Breathing daily. You will release stress and tension, and strengthen your lower back.

Warning:

1. When you have bone-related lower back pain, you need to consult your doctor, chiropractor, or other qualified professional.

2. Do not take muscles relaxers -- they are bad for you. They may give you temporary relief, but they do not solve the problem; they only hide the symptom.

3. When you have sharp pains, don't try to do any physical exercise.
> A. Just relax.

> B. Do Power Breathing to restore lots of oxygen to the muscles, and relax the mind.

> C. Massage your back from your neck to your tail bone.

> D. Alternate hot and cold. Use hot towels for ten minutes, followed by cold towels for two minutes.

> E. When the pain goes away, try some gentle Power Exercises to get the muscles back in shape.

How I recovered from debilitating back pain:

As I described earlier in this book, I once was flat on my back for several weeks from back pain. I had the worst case of anyone I know, yet I now feel my back is stronger than it ever was in my life. If I can recover this far, you can, too. Here's what I did:

First, I decided that I wanted to recover. I believed in myself and I believed that I could recover. In other words, I developed a healthy mental attitude due to positive thinking.

Second, I discovered what caused my pain: stress, further aggravated by bad diet, improper exercise, and shallow breathing.

Third, I learned how to release my stress and stop the cause of my pain through balancing the four corners of the foundation of my health with positive thinking, deep breathing, a healthy diet, and proper exercise. I developed the new positive habits of the nine steps to health, and have maintained these positive habits on a daily basis.

Since then I have been improving consistently. I still have stress in my life, but whenever I feel my back begin to stiffen I immediately do some Light Energy Exercises (p. 378) and I release the stress before it builds up on me.

Power Exercises release stress and tension.

You have to do your Power Exercises every day. Power Exercises were specifically designed as whole body exercises, including the internal organs, from fingers to toes, from face to feet. They will especially loosen up your neck, your upper back, the muscles connecting the spine, and the lower back.

Power Exercises are a lower back pain killer.

Just because you ate a big meal yesterday, do you not need to eat today? You eat every day of your life. The same is true of back exercises. You must do them every day, or your back will begin to hurt again.

435

If you only do lower back exercises, though, your body will not be balanced. Remember, the plan of nature is harmony. Your entire body must be in harmony for every part, including your lower back, to be strong. A balanced health program utilizes the four corner foundations:

1. A Healthy Mental Attitude

2. Power Breathing

3. Natural Nutritional Food

4. Power Exercise, including

> Morning Energy Exercises,
> Night Relaxation Exercises, and
> Light Energy Exercise whenever you feel tension.

and adopts the positive habits of the nine steps to health.

If you are a victim of lower back pain like I was, follow my simple plan for recovery. I could not write this book without the benefits I received from a healthy attitude, Power Breathing, natural foods, and Power Exercises. My lower back is now stronger than ever. I want you to try this four-fold plan for total health.

Power Exercises will save your lower back.

Once you begin it, though, you must have the strength to continue, and never give up. Do not pay attention to other people who look at you or even say things about your exercises. As long as you don't bother them, do not let them bother you. Wherever you feel stiff or tense -- at the office, in the mall, walking down the street -- don't be afraid to do some of the simple Light Energy Exercises to loosen up and release the stress and tension. I do Power Exercises every day and Light Energy Exercises whenever I need to release stress, regardless of place or time, as long as I do not bother anyone else.

When I walk, I also practice

A. Power Breathing (p. 39),
B. Neck Exercises (p. 216),
C. Face Exercises (p. 218),
D. Chest and Back Exercises (p. 220),
E. Finger Chain Stretch to the side (p. 232), and
F. Pull Down Exercise and Loosen Up (p. 234).

Sometimes I will stop walking and practice

G. Hip and Abdominal Exercises (p. 223),
H. Elbow and Hip Exercise (p. 229),
I. Finger Chain Stretch to the front (p. 233),
J. Abdomen and Back Exercises (p. 237),
K. Hamstring and Back Stretch (p. 244),
L. Balance Stretch (p. 246),

and then continue walking with Power Breathing.

At work, I do Light Energy Exercises at my desk. For example, I will practice:

A. Seated Neck Exercises (p. 385),
B. Seated Face Exercises (p. 387),
C. Seated Finger Chain Breathing (p. 273),
D. Seated Pull Down Exercise (p. 389),
E. Rhythm Power Breathing (p. 100, 390),
F. Bending Power Breathing (p. 103), and
G. Power Breathing (p. 39).

When my back begins to bother me, I will practice:

        A. Power Breathing (p. 39),
        B. Finger Chain Stretch (p. 231),
        C. Pull Down Exercise and Loosen Up (p. 234),
        D. Abdomen and Back Exercises (p. 237),
        E. Shoulder and Lower Back Exercises (p. 240),
        F. Hamstring and Back Stretch (p. 244), and
        G. Power Breathing (p. 95).

If you ever go back to your old habits, you will go back to your old pain. If you are dedicated, you will be strong and healthy for the rest of your life. It worked for me. It will work for you.

Power Exercises will strengthen your lower back.

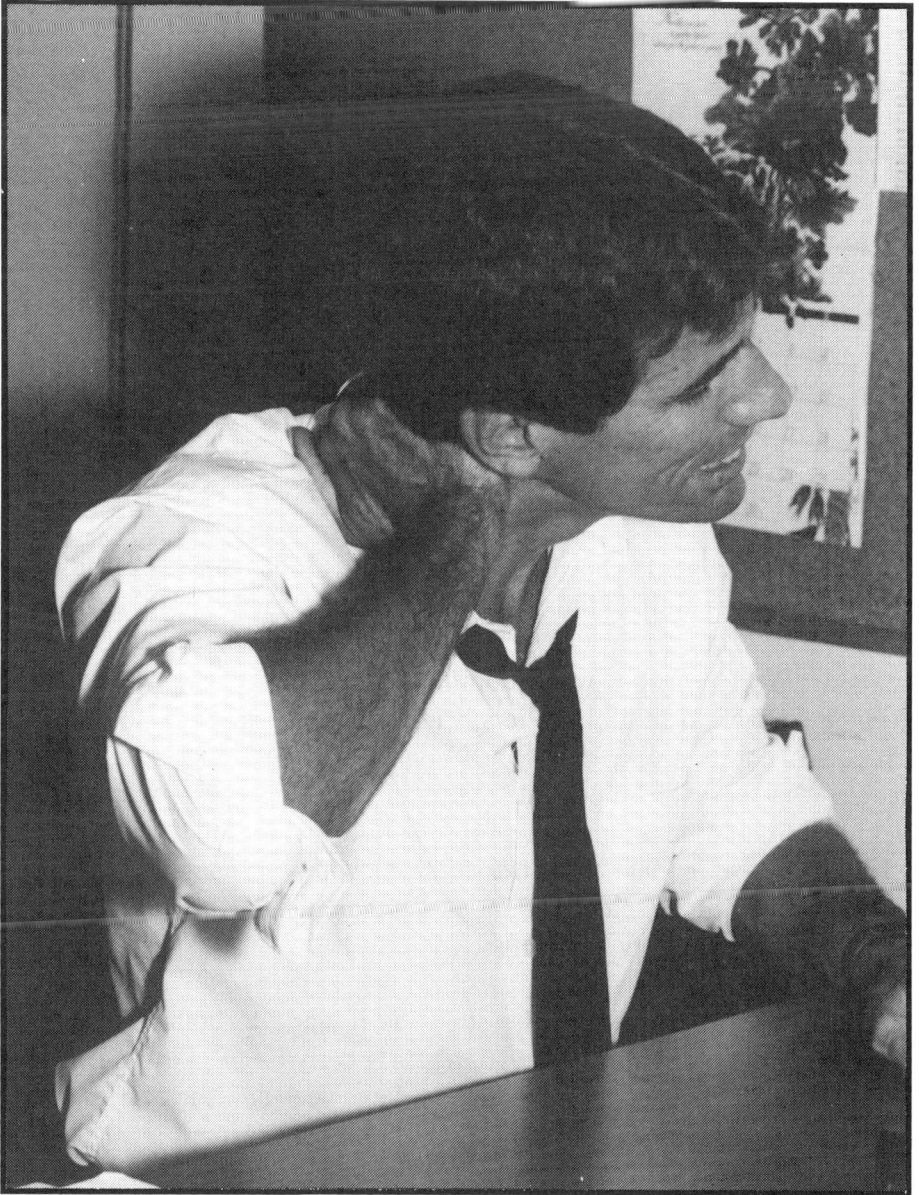

Release your back pain and free yourself to enjoy life.

Neck and upper back pain are very common complaints in our culture. These aches cause a lot of suffering and they generate a lot of headaches. If you suffer from neck and upper back aches, you do not need to worry from now on. Just find the cause of the pain, take the cause away, and strengthen the muscles to prevent it's return.

Common causes of neck and back ache:

1. Stress and tension. The first sign of stress in many people is a stiff neck.

2. Bad posture.

3. Long hours working in an awkward position (bad posture).

4. Sleeping in a bad position (with or without a pillow).

Most people do not have a single cause for their neck and upper back pain, but a combination of the above causes. Here's what to do:

1. You probably won't eliminate stress and tension in your life, even if you win a million dollars. The answer is to learn to deal with stress, and not let it pile up on you. You need to put things into focus and decide what is really important. Most of the things we worry ourselves sick about could be eliminated from our lives without hurting us. If you don't want to eliminate that stressor from your life completely, at least eliminate the attitude that it is a life or death matter. Put it in proper focus and don't literally worry yourself sick.

You can also relieve the stress as it starts to build up by doing Power Exercises and Power Breathing on a daily basis. Power Exercises were specially designed to prevent and relieve neck and back aches. Many of the exercises concentrate on loosening the muscles and increasing the blood flow in this area. Whenever you feel stressed, take a few minutes to do some Light Energy Exercises to relax your body and your mind.

Some Light Energy Exercises that specifically help the neck and upper back are:

1. Deep Breathing (p. 207)
2. Neck Exercises (p.216)
3. Face Exercises (p. 218)
4. Chest and Back Exercises (p. 220)
5. Finger Chain Stretch (p. 231)
6. Pull Down Exercise and Loosen Up (p. 234)
7. Rhythm Power Breathing (p. 100, 390)
8. Power Breathing (p. 39)

You can do these special Power Exercises in your home, in your office, indoors, outdoors, even in an airplane. With minor adjustments for safety, they can even be done while driving a car. The old excuse, "I don't have time" just does not apply here. These exercises will help you loosen tense muscles and strengthen weak ones, so that your upper back and neck will be strong.

2. To adjust your posture you must become aware of how you are standing, sitting, and reclining. Your back is a group of bones stacked much like poker chips. When you keep your head straight over your back bones, the bones support the head. When you lean your head or shoulders forward, backward, or to the side, the muscles must work against gravity to keep the head up. Do not work against gravity, work with it. Stand and sit as straight as possible, to cause the least strain.

Unfortunately, most of us have had bad posture for such a long time that our bodies have adapted to it. We feel "normal" (not really comfortable) in our bad posture. It will take time to re-adjust the muscles back to where they should be. One of the best ways to re-adjust these muscles is through Power Exercises. It will take time to break your old bad habits, but if you do the Power Exercises every day, you will soon become more comfortable and healthier.

3. If you are not forced to work in an awkward position, don't choose to work that way. Move yourself to a more comfortable and better supported position. If you must work in an awkward position, take a break every hour and do two to five minutes of Light Energy Exercises and Power Breathing to loosen up and re-balance your body.

4. If your problem stems from your sleeping position, change your sleeping position. A high pillow is not good for you when you sleep on your back; use a flat pillow or none at all. If you sleep on your side, you need enough pillow to make up the difference between your shoulder and your head. Changing your sleeping position or pillow may be uncomfortable for one or two nights, but then you will adapt to the new and more natural position.

Warning:

1. Do not take pain killers to deal with these symptoms. The side effects are too unhealthy. Deal with the problem itself, and free yourself from pills, powders, and potions.

2. Do Power Exercises and Power Breathing every day to keep stress and tension under control. Power Exercises were specifically designed to relieve neck and back aches.

3. You must continue to do Power Exercises and Power Breathing on a regular basis not only to keep your neck and back supple, but for the health of your internal organs. Our bodies were designed to breathe, eat, exercise, and sleep every day. You wouldn't think of not breathing, eating, or sleeping every day. Why do people think they can stay healthy without exercising every day? When you don't do Power Exercises, the neck and back aches will come back.

Neck and back aches used to be my best friends. They would come to visit me almost every day. Medical doctors X-rayed me and found nothing wrong. Chiropractors adjusted me, but my friends came back. At times, the only way I could turn my head was to turn my whole body. Pain pills and muscle relaxers would chase them away for a short while, but they would always come back. In the mean time I was destroying my internal organs by taking these drugs.

Since I have developed the Power Exercises and practiced them every day, my friends have gone away.   I'm not sorry to say I don't miss them. I'm saving a lot of money that I used to pay to doctors and drug stores. I still deal with a lot of stress every day. Every once in a while I can feel the warning signs in my neck, and I just do my Power Exercises and Power Breathing, and the tension goes away. If you are suffering from stress related neck and back pains, do what I did: release the tension and get rid of that pain in the neck. You will be healthier and much happier.

If you have friends who are suffering from the same problem, share the good news with them. A great deal of people suffer from stress and tension in our modern, scientific culture. We don't give ourselves a chance to work off or walk off our stress. Don't blame anybody else. Just take responsibility for your own health.   Do Power Exercises and Power Breathing daily to release your stress and prevent a problem before it has a chance to develop. Balance the four corners of the foundation of your health and develop positive habits by following the nine steps to health.

Relieving Headaches

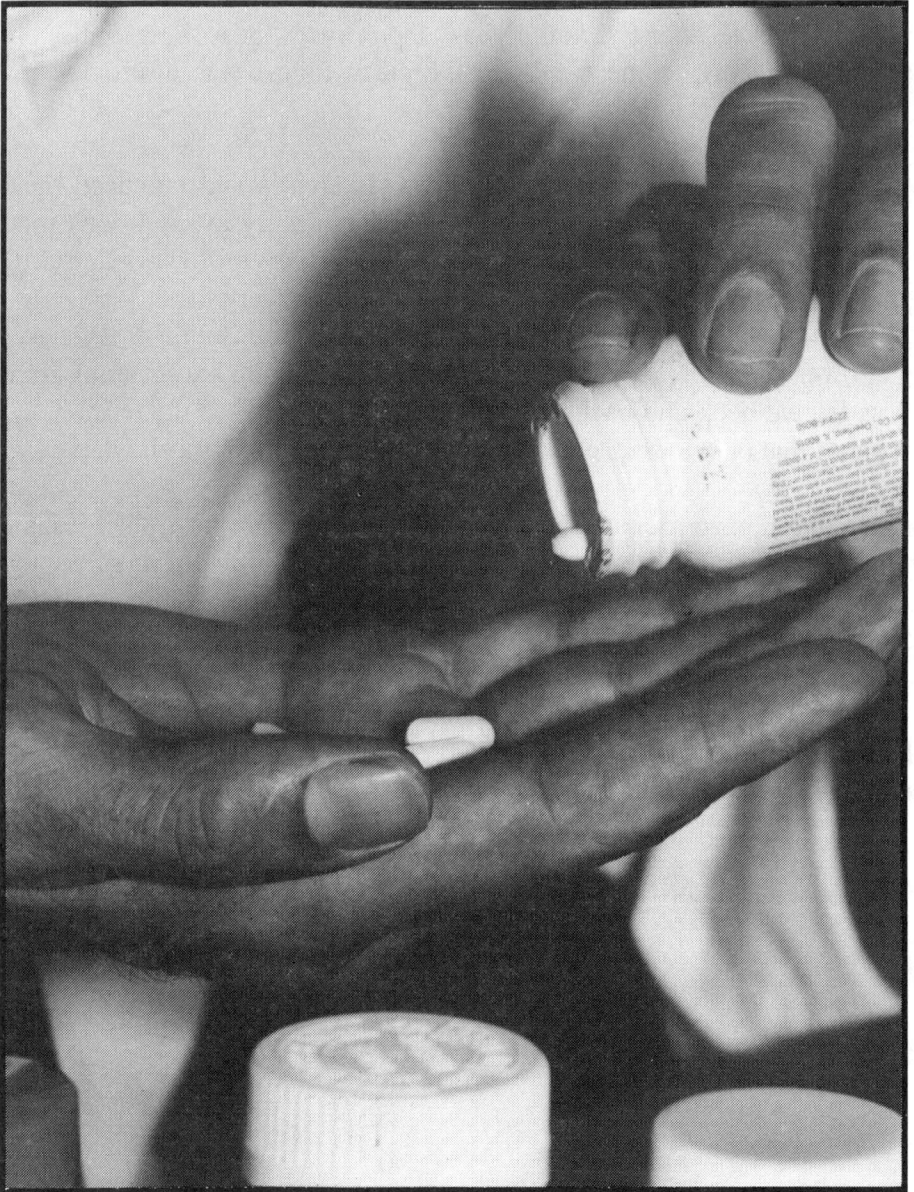

Throw away those pills and build up your health naturally.

Most minor headaches are caused by insufficient oxygen flowing into the head. When the flow of blood is restricted, fresh blood cannot get in and stale blood cannot get out. The body sends you a signal in the form of pain that something is wrong.

Restricted blood flow is usually caused by a muscle (or group of muscles) that is too tight, often in the neck. These muscles usually tense up as a reaction to stress. This is where the term "tension headache" originated.

To Relieve Minor Headaches:

1. Massage shoulder and neck muscles and practice Power Breathing.
    If that's not enough,

2. Do some shoulder and neck Power Exercises while Power Breathing.
    If that's still not enough,

3. Do these Light Energy Exercises and Power Breathing.
    A. Deep Breathing (p. 207)
    B. Neck Exercises (p. 216)
    C. Face Exercises (p. 218)
    D. Chest and Back Exercises (p. 220)
    E. Pull Down Exercise and Loosen Up (p. 234)
    F. Rhythm Power Breathing (p. 100, 390)
    G. Bending Power Breathing (p. 103)

    If that's still not enough,

4. Do a full set of standing Power Exercises with Power Breathing,

5. Do a full Power Exercise routine, including standing, sitting, and lying down, or

    If you have time and space, walk while Power Breathing and perform Walking Energy Exercises (p. 405).

This prescription will relieve ninety-nine percent of minor headaches. It will open your blood vessels and generate oxygen in the blood stream. It will make your headache go away.

You may also be suffering from a lack of sleep. If possible, take a short "cat nap" to refresh yourself.

Another possibility is that you may have eaten too much food. A full stomach will make you sleepy and may even give you a headache because all the blood that could be going to the brain is going to the stomach to digest the food. Next time do not eat so much and try to eat healthy food.

Warning:

1. If your headaches continue, they may be caused by something other than stress and tension. For example, a headache is one of the main symptoms of a food allergy. The next time you get a headache, make a list of the foods you have eaten in the last six hours. After a few headaches, compare lists to see if there is a common food, and try eliminating that food from your diet for a week and see if your headaches go away. Consult an allergist if there is a reasonable suspicion of food allergy.

You also may be getting headaches from back bones that are out of alignment. A chiropractor would be the one to solve this problem. There are hundreds of other possibilities. Try to determine, as best you can, the cause of the headaches, and consult the appropriate health professional.

2.   Do not take headache tablets or powders. They usually work because they contain vasodilators, which means they chemically open your veins and let the blood flow. These chemicals also have other effects on the body. Doesn't it make more sense to open the veins naturally with massage and exercise, and attack the cause of the problem (stress) rather than the symptom? When the body sends a pain message, it is not saying, "There's not enough aspirin in the body. . . send more aspirin." It is saying, "There's not enough oxygen in the head . . . send more fresh blood." Give your body what it needs, not what is easy.

Whenever you feel a headache starting, do not continue to work if at all possible. Take a five to ten minute break to refresh yourself with Power Breathing and a few Power Exercises, or even some quiet meditation. Which is better: a five to ten minute break to stop the headache before it gets intense, or trying to work with a pounding headache for the rest of the day?

If you allow the stress to get a hold, it will be harder to release it. It will try to spread down your neck and into your back, and do to you what it did to me.

I used to have intimate relationships with aspirin and other pain pills. When I realized that they were hurting my other internal organs, I kicked them out of my body. I have never gone back, and if I have the choice, I never want to see them for the rest of my life. Now, when a headache starts, I solve the cause of the problem naturally. This success encouraged me to write this book. I hope you can gain the same freedom I have.

When this natural remedy works for you, I hope you can share it with a lot of other people around you. Your family and friends will not only thank you, they will be healthier, happier, and more positive. This can only make your life more enjoyable.

Relieving Stomach Aches

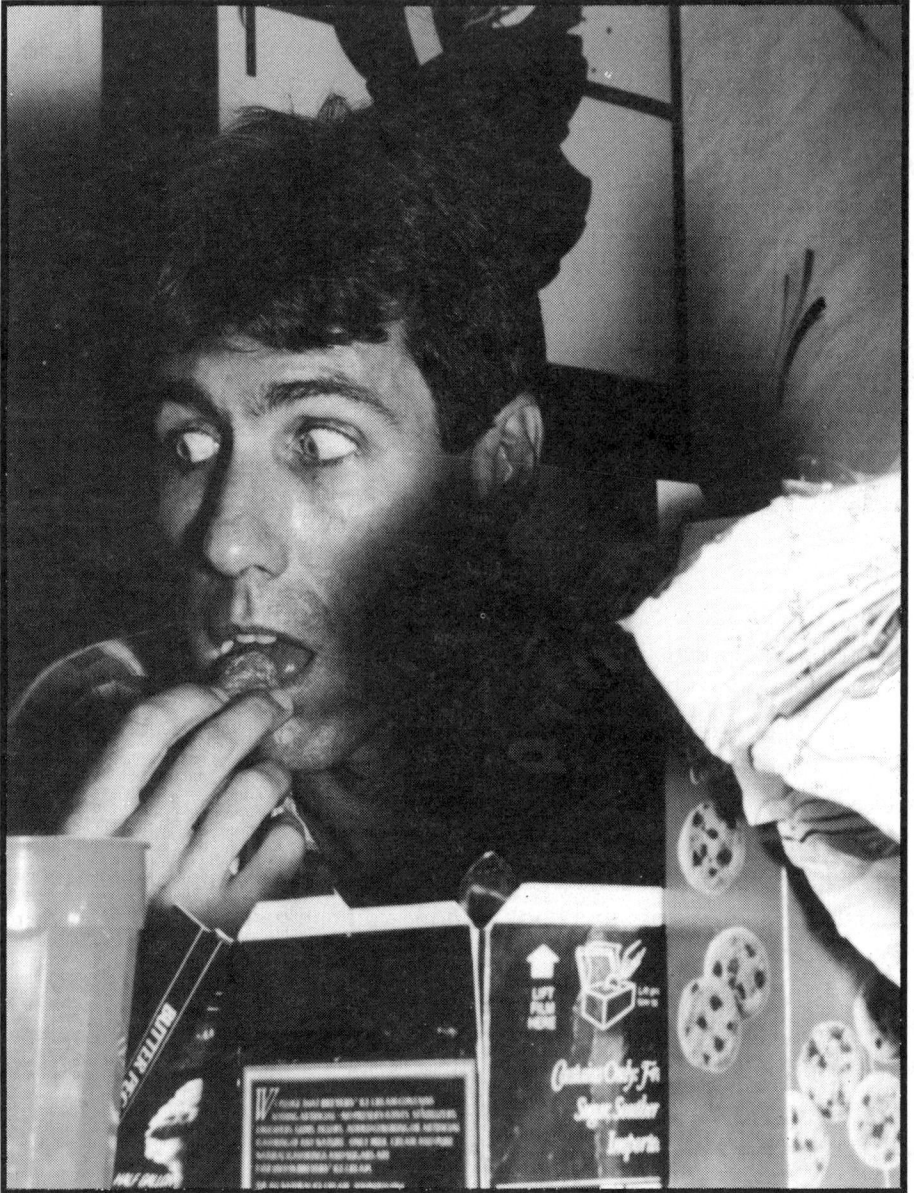

Garbage In -- Garbage Out

You should not suffer greatly from a stomach ache. Under normal circumstances, a stomach ache is a warning from the stomach that you have done something wrong. Once you have been made aware of the situation, you should correct it and the ache should go away. If the ache doesn't go away, you need to re-think what is causing the problem and solve it. If you keep making the same mistake over and over again, you deserve to be in pain. It can expand to become diarrhea, constipation, ulcers, gastritis, and hemorrhoids.

Some of the common causes of stomach aches are:

1. Eating junk food.

2. Eating too much at one time.

3. Eating food for which you have an allergy.

4. Stress.

Solving these problems is reasonably easy:

1. Don't eat junk food. Junk food means foods that either have little or no nutritional value or so-called foods that are actually poisons. Alcohol is an example of a poison that is regularly consumed as if it were a food. Other junk foods include any processed foods in which the natural ingredients have been removed, like "pure" sugar, polished white rice, most pastas, breads, and cereals. Caffeine and other chemical additives like sugar replacements or dairy replacements, as well as chemical preservatives should be avoided. Finally, fatty foods, especially red meats should be avoided. See the "Nutrition" section (p. 121) for more details.

2. Do not eat too much food, even good food, at one time. When food tastes good, especially at a feast or celebration, it is easy to over eat. When there is too much food in the stomach, the digestive juices cannot do their job, and there is sure to be trouble. The food stays in the stomach too long and starts to ferment.

The sensors that connect the brain and the stomach have a lag time, and the brain doesn't give you the "full" feeling until twenty minutes after the stomach has enough. So you cannot wait until you feel "full" to stop. You must use your un-common sense. Your stomach will thank you if you do.

3. Many people have allergies to certain foods. You may be allergic to chocolate, milk, bread, oranges, or any number of other foods, even natural nutritional foods. One of the allergic responses to foods occurs at the place of contact: the stomach, in the form of a stomach ache. This is your body's way of telling you something is not right. See the nutrition section for more about food allergies, or consult an allergist.

4. Do Power Breathing and Power Exercises to reduce stress. Stress causes digestive acids to be released into the stomach. If there is no food in the stomach, or acid-foods already there, the stomach becomes too acid and the juices begin to digest the stomach lining. This is what causes ulcers.

Power Breathing and Power Exercises will help you channel the stress out of the stick points in your body. It will relax your mind, so you do not feel so stressed. It will also help regulate your autonomic nervous system, which controls the flow of digestive juices.

Two of the best Power Breathing exercises to relieve stomach pain are Rhythm Power Breathing and Massage Power Breathing. They will adjust your stomach, release trapped gasses, and balance the flow of digestive juices.

Another thing you can do from a psychological standpoint is to change your attitude. If you smile when you eat, and appreciate the food you have been given, you will be able to digest it much better. If you are tight, angry, and unappreciative when you eat, it should be no mystery that you will get indigestion.

450

I marvel at how stupid I was just a few years ago. I would always eat too much at one time (usually late at night, because it fit my work schedule). I was teaching Tae Kwon Do, so I would be ravenously hungry and eat anything and everything. I slowly destroyed my stomach and began eating digestive "medicines" on top of the bad foods.

Nowadays I do not like junk food even near me or my family. I tell all my friends and students to stop digging their own graves with their teeth. I no longer take medicines for digestion and pain, and I hope you, too, can experience the same freedom. I want you to learn more about nutrition, so you can be healthier and happier. I want you to share what you learn with your family and friends, so that America will be the world's health leader.

Warning:

1. Do not take pills and potions that may have side effects. Instead of taking medicine, take precautions to prevent the need for medicines. If you get stomach pains, do Power Breathing to move and massage your abdominal organs, and restore balance to your digestive system.

2. If you have serious pain or recurring pain that you cannot identify, go to see a doctor.

3. Maintain your good habits. Eat good foods in sensible quantities every day, and do Power Exercises and Power Breathing every day. If you have a good stomach, you will keep it. If you had a bad stomach, it will come back as soon as you return to your bad habits.

Prevention is always better than cure.

Remember: Garbage in, garbage out. Good digestion has a greater effect than just solving stomach aches and pains. It will change your emotional disposition and personality. Good digestion will give you a better self-image.

Healing of specific diseases:

Arthritis

The best way to prevent arthritis, or any sickness, is to balance the four corners of the foundation of your health. If you set up positive habits by following the nine steps to health, you should prevent the arthritis before it happens.

Arthritis is basically a circulation problem. If you can keep the blood circulating freely through the joints, they should never develop arthritis. Any time you can increase the flow of blood through the joints with exercise or heat, the discomfort usually disappears. It only follows logically, then, that exercises that increase the blood circulation, like Power Exercises and Power Breathing, will help prevent arthritis, and help reduce the pain and/or heal existing cases. One of my black belt students completely cured his arthritis after he began doing Power Exercises and Power Breathing regularly.

There also seems to be some relationship between bad diet and arthritis. A good, clean diet of natural foods will go a long way to prevent arthritis, and aid in the recovery of existing cases. There is also strong evidence that the swelling of the joints is a long term symptom of food allergies or intolerance. There are documented cases of people who have cured their arthritis after removing one allergen (for example, milk) from their diet. When they re-introduce the food to their diet, the arthritis returns; when they remove the food again, the arthritis disappears. I strongly recommend you consult an allergist and begin an elimination rotation diet to discover if you are, in fact, allergic to a food you are regularly eating.

Controlling Blood Pressure

High blood pressure is almost always stress related. Just look at anyone who is very angry, and you can practically see the blood vessels popping out of his neck and face. Diet can also contribute to high blood pressure: high sodium (salt) content seems to increase blood pressure, and high cholesterol and other fatty foods close up the veins. High blood pressure can cause a cerebral hemorrhage, and low blood pressure can cause cerebral anemia.

The best way to deal with high or low blood pressure is never to get it. The best way to prevent getting abnormal blood pressure is to balance the four corners of the foundation of your health and create lifelong positive habits through the nine steps to health.

To reduce high blood pressure that you already have, reduce the stress, change the diet, and increase the exercise. To reduce the stress you must change your attitude to a more positive one. You must not get so angry at people and situations. Control your temper and turn the negative into positive. Power Exercises with Power Breathing are a great way to reduce stress and calm the mind. They will regulate the autonomic nervous system so that your body is not constantly responding to stress. It is also a good way to strengthen the walls of the blood vessels so that they are not likely to hemorrhage. Advanced Breathing # 3 is especially helpful in reducing high blood pressure (see p. 96). A natural, nutritional diet will help reduce the "clog" problems in the circulatory system, and begin the repairs.

One of my Instructors used to suffer from high blood pressure. He was in excellent condition for a man of fifty, because he trained hard to become an Tae Kwon Do Instructor. Yet, he still had high blood pressure. When I convinced him to change his attitude to a more positive, more tolerant, and more understanding one, his blood pressure began to drop. He then changed his diet to eliminate red meat and unnecessary salt, and eat only natural, nutritional foods; he soon lost about twenty pounds. He also began practicing Power Breathing, and now his blood pressure is completely normal and under control. He is a new man, now that his foundation of health is balanced in all four corners.

Asthma

Asthma is a problem of the lungs. Through Power Breathing and Power Exercises, the lungs can be gradually opened up and made more efficient. The asthma will not completely disappear, but the intense problems, the asthma attacks, can be reduced or eliminated by slowly improving the body's ability to use oxygen.

Good nutrition will also help to reduce fluids and congestion in the lungs, just as bad nutrition will increase congestion. Thus, the four corners of the foundation of health must be kept in good balance. The positive habits in the nine steps to health should help prevent asthma from getting worse, and reduce the number and intensity of asthma attacks. Many of my Tae Kwon Do students who suffer from asthma, even whole families, have reported great decreases in their asthmatic problems since they have begun training.

There has also been a lot of successful research concerning asthma and allergies. Asthma, and asthma-like reactions, are one symptom of food allergy or intolerance. The fact that whole families will sometimes have asthma shows that there is a genetic relationship, very possibly a genetic allergy to the same food that they all eat at the same table. If you suffer from asthma, I strongly recommend you consult an allergist, and begin an elimination rotation diet to discover if you are, in fact, allergic to a food you are regularly eating. Whether you are or are not allergic to a specific food, a positive mental attitude, deep breathing, a natural, nutritional diet, and a powerful exercise program will reduce your asthmatic symptoms greatly.

Diabetes

Diabetes is a disease of the autonomic nervous system, in which the pancreas is not able to produce enough insulin to handle the sugar intake. There is no established proof of the cause of diabetes, but there is a suspicious coincidence between diabetes and a daily diet high in refined sugar and refined carbohydrates. Obviously, a natural, nutritional diet that does not include these unnatural foods would go a long way to prevent this disease from ever beginning. Balancing the other three corners of the foundation of health and following the nine steps to health should prevent you from spending the rest of your life testing your urine and sticking yourself with needles.

One of the things that people who have diabetes already know is that they must eliminate all refined sugar and other unnatural foods from their diet. The difference between whole grain rice and polished white rice can be catastrophic. The amount of insulin necessary for a diabetic can be greatly reduced by proper diet and exercise.

Power Exercises, used in conjunction with Power Breathing, will help balance the autonomic nervous system. Power Breathing will massage the dysfunctional organs and help restore the entire system to balance. Once again, the best exercise for body and mind is Tae Kwon Do. One of my Instructors is a diabetic. He has confounded his doctors by cutting his insulin injections in half since he began Tae Kwon Do training, and he no longer needs some of the other drugs they told him he would have to take for the rest of his life.

If you do not have diabetes, do not put yourself in a high risk group by eating refined sugars and otherwise letting your foundation get out of balance. If you already have diabetes, balance the four corners of your foundation and follow the nine steps to health. You can reduce your insulin dependency, increase your life expectancy, and enjoy every day more.

Cancer

I read one health magazine that reported that one out of every five Americans has cancer. Another article I read stated that one out of every two Americans has the potential to develop cancer. This is not good news for all of us. I know you all want to believe you are the one who does not have it, but some of you have to be the one out of every five. I strongly believe you can improve your chances to prevent and even heal cancer by balancing the four corners of the foundation of your health and by following the nine steps to health.

Medical science has yet to come up with the exact causes of cancer, and any kind of desirable cure. They can surgically remove the cancerous part and the surrounding area, or bombard your body with radiation and/or chemicals in sufficient quantities to poison and kill the cancerous cells without completely killing you. These are not very attractive choices to me.

Medical research has discovered many things that contribute to cancer, like smoking, but it cannot pinpoint a virus or germ, so the researchers are still looking. In my opinion, cancer is a modern disease. The great doctors of 200 years ago would have at least recorded cancer if it were causing deaths. It is one of the most common causes of death today, yet it was virtually unknown a few hundred years ago. What does that tell you? Cancer is also dramatically more prevalent in civilized, technological cultures today, than in the more primitive cultures that still exist. What does that tell you?

So what's happening in our culture that is killing us? I go back to stress and diet. Stress weakens the entire body, including the immune system. Bad diet containing red meats, refined sugars and grains, and chemical additives (not to mention consumption of alcohol, tobacco, or drugs) also weakens the entire body, and prevents it from regenerating (healing) itself properly. When new cells cannot grow naturally, they grow unnaturally -- cancerous.

The best cure for anything, including cancer, is not to get it in the first place. Prevention is much better than cure. What can you do to prevent cancer?

1. Meditation will give you peace of mind and discipline will help you maintain positive thinking. Meditation will help you reduce stress and better deal with it. It will give you a healthy mental attitude.

2. Power Breathing will build up good circulation throughout your entire body, but especially through the internal organs. It will improve your digestion and build up a strong immune system.

3. Choosing only natural, nutritional foods will give your body healthy building blocks with which to repair and rebuild. Eliminating poisons and anti-nutrients will not only eliminate faulty building blocks, it will also not waste useful nutrients on digesting and eliminating useless "foods."

4. Power Exercises will give you the proper exercise your body needs to stay healthy, it will help you release stress and tension, improve your circulation, strengthen your body, and give you energy.

I strongly believe you can prevent any type of cancer. A strong and healthy immune system will keep you healthy. A weak and over-taxed immune system is an army waiting to be conquered. The best way to build up your body's armed forces is to balance the four corners of the foundation of your health, and create the positive habits of the nine steps to health. That way your immune system will kick, punch, and sweep all of the bad cells out of your system and you can be cancer-free.

Especially in the case of cancer, prevention is better than cure.

Other Diseases

There are so many other health problems causing millions of people to suffer that could be reduced or completely eliminated by balancing the four corners of the foundation of health and developing the positive habits of the nine steps to health. Why do people suffer unnecessarily? Many do not know the causes of their problems, and others do not have the self-control or the desire to change.

Finding the cause is not always easy. There is usually one main cause of a health problem, but many contributing factors. For example, acne is related to diet. However, it is also related to hormone balance, personal hygiene, and stress. One person can eliminate sugar and fatty foods to cure his acne, while another, eating the same diet, might have to also reduce his stress and improve his self-image before his skin clears up.

You can reduce or eliminate the likelihood of getting any of the following health problems, including the common cold:

Acne, anemia, bad breath, bladder problems, bronchitis, colds, constipation, diarrhea, hemorrhoids, insomnia, rashes and other skin disorders, sexual disfunction, sinus problems, and ulcers.

If you already have any of these problems, the effects can be greatly reduced or cured also. Just balance the four corners of the foundation of your health, and develop the positive habits outlined in the nine steps to health, and you will be healthier, happier, and able to enjoy life to its fullest.

I believe it is time we took the bull by the horns and faced the situation. The U.S. is the military, economic, and political super-power in the world today. Instead of having one out of five people suffering from cancer, I would like to see us become the health super-power of the world, as well.

HEALTHY LIVING

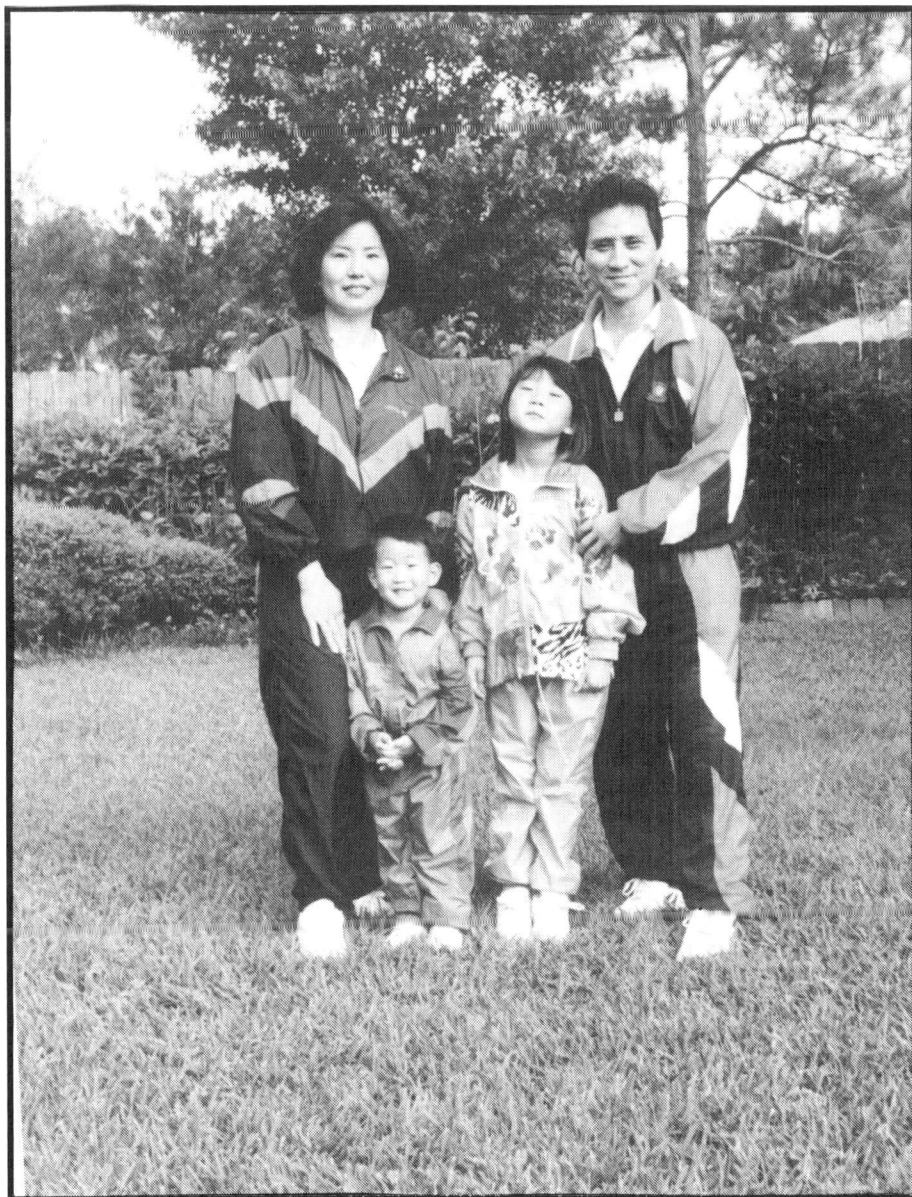

Health is the foundation of a happy life.
A healthy family is a happy family.

We live in an exciting time. Modern technology has given us incredible advantages over our ancestors:

> We can communicate to people on the other side of the world instantaneously through television, telephone, radio, and FAX.

> We can travel at 70 miles an hour in our own town, or fly to any country in the world within one day.

> We can buy fresh fruit and vegetables in summer or winter, frozen and canned vegetables the year 'round, ready made breads, pastas, and pastries, and fresh cut meat, fish, and poultry, all in a single store in our own neighborhood.

> We have machines that wash our dishes, wash our clothes, mow our lawns, clean our carpets, and do virtually any other mindless job that takes away our time.

> We have reduced infant mortality and increased life-expectancy.

No other group of people in history has had the advantages that we have. We have a lot to be thankful for.

Yet, with all of these advantages, too many of us are suffering needless pain. Modern sicknesses that seem incurable have reduced or eliminated our happiness. Even our doctors and psychologists are suffering because they do not know how to release their stress.

The problem is that too many of us have gotten too far away from our nature. We have cut ourselves off from the natural sources of energy, and tried to substitute unnatural sources. We have put our bodies out of chemical balance through incorrect thinking, unnatural breathing, poor diet, and lack of exercise. We have put too much needless stress upon ourselves.

As we move into the 21st century, it will not get any better. The amount of stress is bound to increase. We will not be able to completely avoid stress, but we can get rid of unnecessary stress, so that we can deal with necessary stress much more effectively.

The main thing is to stop worrying so much about everything. Even though you may have read this entire book, you may be worrying about whether you are breathing exactly correctly, or eating just the right foods. That kind of attitude creates more of the stress you are trying to release. You do not need to worry about any of these things. Your body has an amazing system of self-healing. If you can get in touch with your true self and follow your natural instincts, your body will naturally keep the good and get rid of the bad. This is what I mean when I say you must be in harmony with nature.

Health and happiness are waiting for you, as soon as you can stop your bad habits and replace them with good habits. You can release all of your stress, repair damaged tissue, and get rid of all toxins that pollute your body and mind. All you need to do is cooperate with your nature. How?

1. Balance the four corners of the foundation of your health.

2. Develop the positive habits of the nine steps to good health.

The four corners of the foundation of health and the positive habits of the nine steps to good health do not cost you extra money or time to follow. In fact, they do away with a lot of bad habits that are pretty expensive to maintain. This is the most inexpensive and greatest health program ever on earth.

I was the prime example of what stress can do to the human body. Fortunately, I am also a good example of what can be done to recover from stress.

If you suffer from headaches, neck and back aches, stomach aches, and other stress-related problems, I hope you can learn to change before it's too late. Stop the pains before they get a chance to cripple you, like they did to me. Please learn from my experience and my mistakes.

461

I researched meditation, breathing, and nutrition, and organized them into what I believe is a simple and understandable system. I developed Power Exercises and the Aerobic Self-Defense workout so that everyone could have an interesting and beneficial exercise program to fulfill his needs.

Your body was designed to move, and your mind was designed to think. If you do not move your body through work or exercise, it will wither up and become useless. If you do not use your mind to think and imagine, it will also wither up and become useless.

What we consider the traits of "old age" are not really related to time. They are related to lack of use. As we grow older, we stop exercising our bodies and minds. We retire from our jobs, and we retire from life. That's when we become old.

No matter what age you are, if you exercise your body, it will be stronger, healthier, and younger. If you exercise your mind, it will be sharper, clearer, and more creative. By balancing the four corners of the foundation of your health, and developing the good habits in the nine steps to health, you can double your productive life-span. You will be able to achieve your goals, and become successful in your life.

Even if you change all your bad habits and become healthy, you are not finished yet. Health is not something you acquire and then keep forever. In order to maintain health, you must maintain a healthy lifestyle. That doesn't mean you can never eat a fabulous dessert or drink some wine once in a while without hurting yourself. It does mean that you can not eat junk food or drink a lot every day, though. In order to maintain health, you have to maintain healthy living -- you must change your habits (the things you do every day). If your daily habits are good, you can "indulge" once in a while. If you "indulge" every day, your daily habits are not good.

You also must continue to keep the four corners of the foundation of your health in balance, and continue to follow the nine steps to health. If you return to your old bad habits, your old bad health will soon return, as well.

Prevention is better than cure.

462

In life, whatever we set out to do, we can identify 3 stages of development:

1. We have an idea. We have a vision of how we would like to see the world. We set a goal to change it. Ideas can change the world, but not when they remain in someone's brain.

2. We put the idea into action. An idea without action is just a pipe dream. During the action phase is when ideas can begin to change the world. But "the best laid plans of mice and men often go awry."

3. We persist until we achieve our goal. Lots of people have good ideas and try to put them into action. Successful people continue in the face of adversity, until they overcome their problems and achieve their goal.

I have presented you with a good idea: Healthy Living for the rest of your life. I have given you the theory and the step-by-step details to achieve it. It is now up to you to put it into action, and persist until you can achieve your goal. I believe you can change your bad habits to good habits by following the nine steps to good health. I believe you can balance the four corners of the foundation of your health. I also believe you will feel so good that you will continue to maintain these good habits and enjoy healthy living.

Whatever seeds you plant will grow. If you plant healthy seeds, you will have a healthy life. If you plant the seeds of an unhealthy life, what can you expect? Take the first step today. Change your bad habits into good habits, and live happily ever after.

I urge you to share your knowledge with other people. When you teach others, you teach yourself, as well. The act of sharing will build your self-confidence, and motivate you to think positively and remain healthy.

If you can share this knowledge with two other people, and they each share with two more, an so on, we will have a great impact on the world. Through positive thinking, we can build healthier families, healthier communities, a healthier and stronger America, and, ultimately, a healthier and more peaceful world.

Health is the foundation of loving relationships in life.

Health is the foundation of outstanding leadership.

Health is the foundation of becoming a winner in life.

Health is the foundation of world peace.

Health is the Foundation of Success.

INDEX

Notes

[1] Robert Buist, *Food Intolerance: What it is & how to cope with it* (San Leandro: Prism Press, 1984), p. 39.

[2] Buist, p. 22.

[3] Martin Katahn, Ph. D., *The T-Factor Diet* (New York: Bantam Books, 1990), p. 216.

[4] Katahn, pp. 277-311. All subsequent fat gram contents come from this source.